One hundred years of wartime nursing practices, 1854–1953

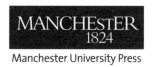

Manchester University Press

Nursing History and Humanities

This series provides an outlet for the publication of rigorous academic texts in the two closely related disciplines of Nursing History and Nursing Humanities, drawing upon both the intellectual rigour of the humanities and the practice-based, real-world emphasis of clinical and professional nursing.

At the intersection of Medical History, Women's History and Social History, Nursing History remains a thriving and dynamic area of study with its own claims to disciplinary distinction. The broader discipline of Medical Humanities is of rapidly growing significance within academia globally, and this series aims to encourage strong scholarship in the burgeoning area of Nursing Humanities more generally.

Such developments are timely, as the nursing profession expands and generates a stronger disciplinary axis. The MUP Nursing History and Humanities series provides a forum within which practitioners and humanists may offer new findings and insights. The international scope of the series is broad, embracing all historical periods and including both detailed empirical studies and wider perspectives on the cultures of nursing.

Previous titles in this series:

'Curing queers': Mental nurses and their patients, 1935–74
Tommy Dickinson

Who cared for the carers? A history of the occupational health of nurses, 1880–1948
Debbie Palmer

ONE HUNDRED YEARS OF WARTIME NURSING PRACTICES, 1854–1953

EDITED BY JANE BROOKS AND CHRISTINE E. HALLETT

Manchester University Press

Published by Manchester University Press
Altrincham Street, Manchester M1 7JA
www.manchesteruniversitypress.co.uk

British Library Cataloguing-in-Publication Data
A catalogue record for this book is available from the British Library

Library of Congress Cataloging-in-Publication Data applied for

ISBN   978 0 7190 9141 4   hardback

ISBN   978 0 7190 9142 1   paperback

First published 2015

Typeset by Servis Filmsetting Ltd, Stockport, Cheshire
Printed in Great Britain by Bell & Bain Ltd, Glasgow

To
James Campbell
and
Keith Brindle

Contents

Contents

Figures

Contributors

Jane Brooks is a lecturer in the School of Nursing, Midwifery and Social Work at the University of Manchester, Deputy Director for the UK Centre for the History of Nursing and Midwifery and editor of the UK Association for the History of Nursing Bulletin. Her most recent publications include articles on the feeding work of nurses after the liberation of Bergen-Belsen and nursing during the 1943/4 typhus epidemic in Naples. She has previously published on the history of nursing work with older adults in the UK.

Christine Hallett is Professor of Nursing History in the School of Nursing, Midwifery and Social Work at the University of Manchester and the Chair of the UK Association for the History of Nursing. Her most recent publications include *Containing Trauma: Nursing Work in the First World War* (2009), *Veiled Warriors* (2014) and the popular work, *Celebrating Nurses* (2010), which has been published in the UK, USA and Australia.

Maxine Dahl trained as a registered nurse in Brisbane, Australia before joining the Royal Australian Air Force (RAAF) in late 1979. During her time in the RAAF, Maxine worked in Defence health facilities, nursing education and health management and policy. She transferred to the RAAF Reserve force in 2004. Her interest in flight nursing began during her RAAF service and became the focus for her doctoral studies, which were completed in 2010.

Charlotte Dale recently completed her PhD, in the UK Centre for the History of Nursing and Midwifery at the School of Nursing,

Midwifery and Social Work, University of Manchester. Her thesis, upon which her chapter in this volume is based, is entitled: 'Raising professional confidence: The influence of the Anglo-Boer War (1899–1902) on the development and recognition of nursing as a profession'. She is a holder of the Monica Baly Bursary and Mona Grey Prize and received research expenses' funding from the Wellcome Trust to support her research into this area of nursing history.

Kirsty Harris completed her award-winning history PhD on the labour history of Australian Army nurses in the First World War in 2007. She is currently an honorary fellow at the University of Melbourne and has published a number of academic articles on military nursing work during the First World War. Her first book, *More than Bombs and Bandages: Australian Army Nurses at Work in World War I*, was published in 2011. Her current research interests include examining the nursing of Spanish influenza victims in 1918–19 and the frontline experiences of Empire women at Gallipoli in 1915.

Carol Helmstadter has published widely on the history of nursing reform in nineteenth-century England in both nursing and history journals. *Nursing Before Nightingale 1815–1899* (2011) co-authored with Judith Godden, was published by Ashgate. This work studies social and religious discipline and professional expertise in nursing reform in England 1800–90. In 2008 the Canadian Nurses Association made her a centenary nurse for her contributions to nursing history.

Angela Jackson is a doctor of History who specialises in the subject of the Spanish Civil War 1936–39, particularly relating to the roles played by women in the conflict and the interactions between soldiers and civilians. Her books have all been translated into Catalan or Spanish, the latest being the biography of an English nurse who worked close to the front lines in that war, *'For us it was Heaven': The Passion, Grief and Fortitude of Patience Darton from the Spanish Civil War to Mao's China* (Sussex Academic Press, 2012).

David Justham initially studied chemistry before becoming a nurse. He has recently retired from his post as lecturer with the University of Nottingham's School of Nursing, Midwifery and Physiotherapy.

Justham previously held posts within occupational health, and the NHS administration. He has recently completed his PhD, which considered nursing practices in the management of infections in hospitals between 1929 and 1948 at the UK Centre for the History of Nursing and Midwifery at the School of Nursing, Midwifery and Social Work, University of Manchester.

Jan-Thore Lockertsen is a theatre nurse and a PhD student at the University of Tromso, where he also teaches theatre nursing. Lockertsen belongs to the research group 'Patient-related nursing research'. His research interests are wartime nursing and history of theatre nursing in Norway.

Barbara Maling is an assistant professor in the School of Nursing at the University of Virginia and an acute care nurse practitioner in Charlottesville, Virginia. Her historical research addresses the diversity of Southern nursing care providers during the American Civil War with a focus on black nurses (enslaved and free) in Virginia.

Debbie Palmer is an associate research fellow in the Centre for Medical History, University of Exeter, working on the 'History of stress', funded by the Wellcome Trust. Her particular interest is occupational stress in the 1960s and 1970s. She is a registered general nurse and her PhD examined the history of nurses' occupational health, 1890–1948.

Cynthia Toman retired from the University of Ottawa where she was the Director of the AMS Nursing History Research Unit and Associate Professor. She is now an Adjunct Professor at the University of Ottawa. Toman's publications include *An Officer and a Lady: Canadian Military Nursing and the Second World War* (2007) and and she is co-editor of *Place and Practice in Canadian Nursing History* (2008). She is currently working on First World War Canadian military nurses, upon which her chapter in this book is based.

Acknowledgements

This edited book began in June 2011 when the editors held a day workshop in Manchester. The workshop was generously funded by the Wellcome Trust and we were able to invite internationally renowned colleagues in the history of nursing and war. The day was a great success and everyone expressed interest in developing it as a book. We are most grateful to everyone who participated.

The image of a Koulali Hospital ward is copyrighted to the Wellcome Library, London, and is here published by kind permission.

We would like to thank the National Library of Australia's Pictures Collection, NLA MS 3962, for the image of Staff Nurse Edith Rush, nursing on Lemnos Island during the Gallipoli campaign, 1915. The image is part of the collection of letters and photos of Staff Nurse (later Sister) Anne Donnell, AANS.

We are grateful for the kind permission from Library and Archives Canada, to publish the following images; The Dowager Empress Maria Fedorovna, accompanied by Princesses Olga and Tatiana and Grand Duchesses Cyril and Maria Pavlowa at the opening of the Anglo-Russian Hospital at the Dmitri Palace, 1 February 1916, Petrograd (PA-157337). The image probably depicts the nursing personnel of the Anglo-Russian Field Hospital, June 1916 (PA-157333), two nursing sisters with wounded soldier at the Anglo-Russian Hospital in the Dmitri Palace, Petrograd, 1916 (PA-157356) and the image of a group of armed Russian soldiers with automobile, Petrograd, 1917 (PA-157327).

We would like to thank the Royal Australian Air Force Museum, Point Cook, for permission to use the five images related to Australian Air Force nursing in the Korean War; including the photograph of the flight pannier, Sister Cathie Daniel with patient flying from Korea to Iwakuni, a recently arrived load of unidentified patients being cared for by RAAF nurses on transfer from Korea to Iwakuni, with unidentified nursing sisters, Sister M. Larsen reviewing an unidentified patient, and finally Casualty Air Evacuation Flight – BCCZMU.

We would like to thank Gerd Semb and Kari Roll Klepstad for their permission to reproduce the images in Chapter 11. Images of the Norwegian Mobile Army Surgical Hospital are reproduced by kind permission of Ragnhild Strand. Images of Patience Darton; Penny Phelps; Dr Reggie Saxton; the cave hospital at La Bisbal de Falset and interior of a cave hospital, in Chapter 8, are from the collection of Angela Jackson. She would like to express her thanks to the veterans and families who supplied these. Every attempt has been made to locate the original copyright holders. The author and editors would be grateful for any information related to these copyright holders.

We are most grateful for the support of their Head of Department, Karen Luker and the School of Nursing, Midwifery and Social Work for supporting this project. We should also like to thank Professor Michael Worboys of the Centre for the History of Science, Technology and Medicine, at the University of Manchester and Professors Peter Gatrell and Bertrand Taithe from the Humanitarian and Conflict Response Institute, also at the University of Manchester, for encouraging the history of nursing and war. Thank you also to Joanne Smedley for her secretarial assistance.

An especial thank you goes to Emma Brennan of Manchester University Press for her unfailing patience and continued interest in the project. We are also most grateful to the anonymous reviewers who spent so much of their valuable time helping us improve this volume.

Our greatest thanks go to our husbands, families and friends.

Abbreviations

AANS	Australian Army Nursing Service
AGH	Australian General Hospital
AIF	Australian Imperial Force
AMS	Army Medical Museum
AWM	Australian War Memorial
BAOR	British Army of the Rhine
BCCZMU	British Commonwealth Communications Zone Medical Unit
BCFK	British Commonwealth Forces Korea
BCOF	British Commonwealth Occupation Force
BL	British Library
BNA	British Nursing Association
CAEF	Casualty Air Evacuation Flight
CAMC	Canadian Army Medical Corps
CCS	Casualty Clearing Station
CLA	Cornwall Lunatic Asylum
CLAVC	Cornwall Lunatic Asylum Visiting Committee
CNMC	Children's National Medical Centre
CRO	Cornwall Record Office
FNM	Florence Nightingale Museum
IODE	Imperial Order Daughters of the Empire
LAA	Light Anti-Aircraft
LAC	Library and Archives, Canada
LCC	London County Council
MML	Marx Memorial Library, London
MO	Medical Officer
MPA	Medico-Psychological Association

NAWU	National Asylum Worker's Union
NORMASH	Norwegian Mobile Army Surgical Hospital
ORT	operating room technicians
QAIMNS	Queen Alexandra's Imperial Military Nursing Service (QAs)
QARANC	Queen Alexandra's Royal Army Nursing Corps
RAAF	Royal Australian Air Force
RAF	Royal Air Force
RAMC	Royal Army Medical Corps
RN	registered nurse
SDEC	South Devon and East Cornwall Hospital
SJAB	St John's Ambulance Brigade
SLV	State Library of Victoria
TFSH	Tungt feltsykehus (Norwegian field hospital)
UCH	University College Hospital, London
UKCHNM	United Kingdom Centre for the History of Nursing and Midwifery
UN	United Nations
UNRRA	United Nations Relief and Rehabilitation Administration
US MASH	United States Mobile Army Surgical Hospital
VAD	Voluntary Aid Detachments
WSQs	Wing Sick Quarters

Introduction: The practice of nursing and the exigencies of war

Jane Brooks and Christine E. Hallett

The nature of nursing work has always been contested. Encompassing both fundamental skills and the application of medical technologies, nursing inhabits the borderlands between the delivery of scientific solutions and the creation of conditions, in patients and their environments that will permit healing. This can create tension and conflict in the minds of care-givers, who can feel uncertain about the boundaries of their practice. In wartime, these apparent contradictions hold an even greater tension, especially when trained and untrained nurses work together, often with very different ideas about the purpose of their wartime work.[1] At times, the crisis created by large numbers of traumatic injuries and destructive environments leads to emergency situations in which the boundaries of healthcare practice may actually dissolve. *One hundred years of wartime nursing practices, 1854–1953* examines these issues in a number of scenarios, taking the emergence of professional military nursing during the Crimean War (1854–56) as its starting point, and ending with the highly technical work of trauma nurses and 'flight nurses' during the Korean War (1950–53).

Previous histories of nursing and war have tended to fall between a number of paradigms, including women's history, medical history and nursing history. The early historiography of women and war focused on the advantages gained by women during a war.[2] More recently, women's historians have identified that, although women may gain advantages during war, through employment and an expansion of their societal roles, these advantages are lost at the war's end, when women are returned to the home.[3] Gail Braybon and Penny Summerfield's text, *Out of the Cage* (1987) was particularly influential in the development of this thesis.[4] Traditional histories of wartime medicine, such as Roger Cooter, Steve Sturdy and Mark Harrison's *War, Medicine and Modernity*, have problematised the notion that 'war is good for medicine'. They acknowledge that war does bring scientific innovation and medical reform, though the human costs may be excessive.[5]

Existing works on the history of nursing in wartime have focused predominantly on the development of 'official' nursing services. Jan Bassett's work on the Australian Army Nursing Service, Anna Rogers's book on the development of the New Zealand Army Nursing Service and Mary Sarnecky's monograph on the US Army nurses provide useful insights into their respective countries' military nurses.[6]

Most histories of British military nursing services have lacked critical analysis, and have taken almost entirely celebratory approaches to their subjects. Ian Hay's *One Hundred Years of Army Nursing* (1953) and Juliet Piggott's *Queen Alexandra's Royal Army Nursing Corps* (1975) are among the earliest examples of this genre.[7] Eric Taylor's, *Wartime Nurse: One Hundred Years from the Crimea to Korea, 1854–1954*, also lacks analysis.[8] It is the most recent text to consider a century of war, but its approach is intentionally populist and narrative rather than critical.

This volume represents a radical departure from earlier approaches. Where twentieth-century texts focused on either traditional celebratory narrative or feminist revision, the studies reported here tackle the multiple roles of nurses in wartime and the ways in which military nurses negotiated their clinical space. We explore their engagement with fundamental nursing care and traditional nursing practices, but also consider how nursing work was subverted by the need to engage in the emergencies created by warfare.

We argue that the shifting boundaries of clinical practice challenged the role boundaries of nurses and impacted on their identities as nurses. A number of recent texts have concerned themselves with the duality of the nurses' wartime experiences in which their worth as women appears to have taken precedence over their clinical worth. Cynthia Toman's *An Officer and a Lady* has considered the work of Canadian nursing sisters during the Second World War. Christine Hallett's *Containing Trauma* has considered British nurses' work during the First World War, whilst Kirsty Harris's *More than Bombs and Bandages* has explored the work of Australian nurses during the First World War.[9] Collectively, these twenty-first-century texts began a shift towards the study of nursing practices which forms the focus of the present volume. *One hundred years of wartime nursing practices, 1854–1953* explores the practices of nursing from the mid-nineteenth to the mid-twentieth centuries. It is appreciated that not all wars in this period have been covered in the text. Both the Franco-Prussian (1870–71) and Russo-Japanese (1904–5) wars are, for example, absent. However, the contributions in this volume do demonstrate both the continuities and the changes in wartime nursing during the one hundred years, from 1854 to 1953.

The gendered nature of wartime nursing

One of the fundamental questions asked by this volume is: 'What is military nursing work and how does it differ from the work of other carers and clinicians?' Enmeshed within this question are issues about the gendered nature of both nursing and soldiering. The book examines cultural expectations about what constituted 'women's work' in several eras and addresses the thorny issue of what makes female nurses different from male orderlies in military settings. Was it simply the refusal of military medical authorities to permit women within more than a few miles of the 'front lines' of battle that dictated the need for orderlies in army medical services, or were there more complex reasons, embedded in notions of female sensibility, or taboos about the female nurse's handling of the injured male combatant's body, behind the complex interplay of different clinical roles in military scenarios?[10]

Engagement in war is essentially problematic for nursing and nurses. The presence of women, especially middle-class women, who were not part of the army's entourage, was anathema for most of the nineteenth century. By the end of the Crimean War, a place for female nurses in war zones may have been established, but their involvement in warfare remained highly contested until the late twentieth century. Lucy Noakes has shown that women's involvement in paramilitary organisations such as the First Aid Nursing Yeomanry, the Women's Auxiliary Force and the Women's Volunteer Reserve were among the most problematic of their choices during the first part of the twentieth century. The wearing of khaki uniforms and the engagement in parade and drill sent a clear message to the military authorities that their members aligned themselves with the male military 'war effort'.[11] The responses of military authorities were to view these efforts as a trespass on their own exclusively male domain. Noakes argues that states were determined to make use of women's labour, while resisting any pressure to offer them legitimacy, and to protect their rights in either the army or the civilian workforce.[12] Nurses were able to overcome these restraints. By presenting themselves as engaged in a purely female pursuit, and by wearing highly feminine uniforms, grey or blue and white, rather than khaki, they won for themselves the right to practise close to the battlefield and to be recognised as legitimate participants in the war effort.

Yet their roles remained replete with contradictions. Patricia D'Antonio has observed that the image of the wartime nurse is one in which compassionate, heroic carers demonstrate both competence and organisational skill. Yet, the realities of their day-to-day work 'provided little heroic glamour'. In fact, the realities of nursing work often involved 'the care of patients with ugly fragmentation wounds, or with soft body tissues reduced to devitalised pulp, or with faces shot away, or stomachs blown wide open'.[13] Thus, the motivations for nurses to engage in 'war work' were varied. For some, nursing was a humanitarian service and therefore arguably antithetical to the ethos and actions of war. For these nurses, the engagement in 'war work' may have proved highly paradoxical. For others wartime nursing was an opportunity to demonstrate nursing expertise. Still others viewed war nursing as an openly patriotic endeavour. For most, their motives were probably a combination of all three.[14] This book demonstrates that war became an arena in which the value of female nurses and nursing work came to be recognised; within war, nurses could foster new roles and opportunities.

Nursing, power and humanity

In her exploration of the US Army Nurse Corps' involvement in the Vietnam War, Kara Dixon Vuic, exposed the tensions and contradictions inherent in the position of the wartime nurse: the only female actor permitted to play a role close to the front lines, yet absorbed in

humanitarian work.[15] Dixon Vuic argued that 'wartime service ...
became a source of power for women who sought unparalleled opportunities and national recognition'.[16] In this way, nurses were implicated
in the highly destructive process of warfare, even as they presented
themselves as the humanitarian carers of those it damaged. These contradictions were most elegantly – and most shockingly – exposed in the
writings of philanthropist and First World War hospital 'directrice',
Mary Borden, whose book, *The Forbidden Zone*, offered a swingeing
exposé of the complicity of army medical and nursing services in perpetuating the trauma of war. Her oblique and subtle dissection of the
field hospital's work and routines revealed the truth of the matter: that
such institutions were merely 'patching up' men to be returned to the
horrors of the front lines, further damaged, and possibly killed.[17]

Complementing Borden's work, preceding it, yet taking further its
message was the writing of her colleague, trained American nurse,
Ellen La Motte, whose *The Backwash of War* laid bare the realities
of war-wounds and questioned the role of the nurse in perpetuating
the torture of those sent to the battlefield. Her writing, which carried
strangely contradictory qualities, both incisive and surreal, suggested
that military nursing might, in fact, be, quite literally, a 'dead end'
occupation.[18]

Nursing work and nursing knowledge

A recent study of twenty-first century American military nurses
focuses on the highly technical nature of modern military nursing in
Iraq and Afghanistan. Exploring the work of 37 US military nurses,
Elizabeth Scannell-Desch and Mary Ellen Doherty choose to emphasise nursing work in mobile surgical field hospitals, fast-forward
teams and medevac aircraft, as well as in base and city hospitals.[19]
The focus on the drama and technology of emergency treatment is
perhaps typical of society's current fascination with all things technical and may, as such, be fuelled by a drive from within the nursing
profession to demonstrate its own legitimacy. Military nurses' need
for a high level of scientific knowledge and technical skill is emphasised, and can be seen as part of a century-long drive to develop a
legitimate knowledge base for nursing practice.

Nurses have often found it easier to argue for a scientific basis to their practice than for the artistry inherent in their skills, arguably because of the intimate nature of nursing care, and its association with body work and dirt. Linda Nochlin's exposition on the historical barriers to women in the art world, offer some interesting comparisons. Nochlin maintains that women were objects of the artists, rather than creators of art and that art takes time to practice, time that was not available to women.[20] Because of its association with menial tasks, nursing work was never elevated to the level of 'artistry'. Furthermore, the increasing scientific emphasis of medicine and the desire of professional nursing from the mid-nineteenth century to associate itself with this movement, discouraged nurses from identifying their work as artistic.[21]

As Jocalyn Lawler argues, nursing takes place 'behind the screens'. Thus the nurse's work with her patient fuels the fear of outsiders of a loss of privacy, of integrity – of identity itself.[22] Alison Bashford maintains that, 'the powerful cultural link drawn between middle-class femininity, female bodies and moral/physical purity, is particularly significant for any nurse'.[23] Such anxieties are exacerbated when the nurse is young, female and single and her patient is young and male. It is arguable that on active service overseas such concerns about morality were combined with nurses being women, 'out of place', a concept that is central to Mary Douglas's thesis on the fear of dirt.[24] Dirt is acceptable in certain defined spaces, but once it moves into the areas that should be clean, it becomes highly problematic. In the same way, nurses as women can function within the acceptable sphere of the civilian hospital, but once removed to the masculine world of war, their place is contentious. But the ambivalence of the hidden work of the nurse goes further than this. Nurses perform their work away from the public gaze, in direct contrast to other professional groups: the surgeon in the operating theatre, the teacher in the classroom and the lawyer in court.[25] This 'hiddenness' has a number of consequences. It fuels the fear of what is occurring, but it preserves the dignity of the patient who is nursed. Nevertheless, when the patient emerges into the public world once more, the memories of the intimate body care are quickly and deliberately forgotten. Thus the nurse's work becomes even more invisible.[26] The work of the young female nurse with male soldier patients magnifies these difficulties and so the work of the wartime nurse is subsumed in the public discourse under her heroism and bravery. This hijacking of nurses' achievements to fuel pro-war propaganda was at times adopted as part of a deliberate government project.[27]

In her paper, 'Intelligent interest in their own affairs', Christine Hallett focused on how nurses constructed a knowledge base for themselves, out of their wartime nursing experiences.[28] As new challenges, from gas gangrene to shell shock, confronted them, nurses developed new treatments and approaches that enabled them to expand the scope of their practice. The ways in which they incorporated this new knowledge into a nascent corpus of 'nursing' knowledge included the reproduction of excerpts from scientific papers, and the incorporation of both invited articles by doctors and essays by nurses into the pages of professional journals, most notably the *British Journal of Nursing*. The work of nurses was sometimes crucial in enabling medical officers to implement new 'scientific' treatments, many of which were highly speculative. The efforts of the nurses in caring for patients undergoing experimental regimes were essential in sustaining life, while their professional observations enabled the modification of doses or frequencies of interventions in order to maximise the efficacy of treatments and chances of success.

This volume goes beyond such analysis of nursing knowledge to examine how nurses practising in wartime gave meaning and significance to their actions *as* actors, regardless of scientific rationales. Carol Helmstadter, Barbara Maling and Cynthia Toman identify the importance of the nurse as a woman and as a political actor in war.[29] While the nineteenth-century reformed nurse had been viewed as inhabiting a purely domestic sphere (the hospital ward), female nurses' involvement in war brought them out of this domestic realm and placed them on a 'world stage' in the 'masculine sphere' of war. This meant that their work was highly visible and likely to be widely publicised. Hence, their nursing work could therefore be re-cast as patriotic service and could be interpreted as a highly political act. Key to the success of the female nurses' presence in the early days of wartime nursing was the image of Florence Nightingale as 'saintly warrior', genteel and self-sacrificing, and this trope continued to be used to protect the image of the military nurse well into the twentieth century.[30]

The focus of this book is on the nature of nursing work and its impact on role boundaries. Charlotte Dale and Kirsty Harris argue for the significance of patient-feeding as a core nursing practice that was underpinned by nutritional knowledge, but which required skills of improvisation in scenarios where food supplies were not readily available.[31] David Justham similarly argues that at a time when antibiotics were not yet available, good nursing care, coupled with an ability to implement complex technologies such as blood transfusion and antiseptic wound treatment meant the difference between life and death.[32] Jane Brooks, Jan-Thore Lockertsen and Maxine Dahl explore the ways in which trained, skilled nurses were able to take on increasingly complex care in hostile environments.[33] Debbie Palmer reminds the readers that the draw of wartime nursing and the adventure and 'glory' that it can bring, comes with a price that needs to be paid by the civilian patients at home. As trained nurses clamoured to engage in overseas service, the hospital wards were left with ever-decreasing staffing numbers and more inadequately trained nurses.[34]

Structure of the book

The book is divided into three sections. Part I: 'Gentlemen's wars' considers the significant wars of the nineteenth century. The section commences with Carol Helmstadter's chapter on the Crimean War. Helmstadter argues that previous histories of female nursing during this war have identified nursing as an essentially domestic task, arising as it did from the work of charwomen.[35] Nevertheless, she demonstrates that the nature of the diseases and injuries sustained by the soldiers in the Crimea, would have required far greater skill than mere 'household domestic' work. Anne Summers has argued that the 'reformed nurse became visible' during the nineteenth century, through a variety of local, national and international institutions. This process took place locally through the hospital systems, nationally through the development of the female army nursing service, and internationally through 'service in wars and under the aegis of the Red Cross and other relief agencies'. Accordingly, Summers continues: 'Domestic service and pastoral mission were the twin pillars of this apparently modern edifice.'[36] As Helmstadter demonstrates in her chapter, while some of the most accomplished clinical nurses in the Crimea were the working-class hospital nurses and the Anglican and Catholic Sisters, their work was neither exclusively missionary not solely domestic, but involved complex dressings and the labour-intensive care of typhoid victims.

Historian Jane Schultz has demonstrated that Florence Nightingale's image was of some importance in promoting the legitimacy of female war service in the American Civil War, arguing that Nightingale's 'saintly warrior image – a curious emulsion of masculinised feminine traits' provided a vital exemplar that American women could use to argue for a more active, progressive role in wartime.[37] Barbara Maling takes up this theme in Chapter 2 on nursing in the South during the American Civil War, in which she argues for Nightingale's influence in legitimating nursing work outside the home for prosperous women, a development that had important implications for the nursing of troops during the war and the place of female nursing in a hitherto almost entirely masculine space.[38]

Charlotte Dale's chapter on the work of the nurses caring for soldiers suffering from typhoid during the Boer War demonstrates the significance that a skilled nursing service could have on dangerously ill men in a war zone.[39] In her critical discussion of the care that the men received, Dale argues that, at the beginning of the Second Anglo-Boer War in 1899, there were three distinct groups of female nurses: the Army Nursing Reserve; civilian nurses who were not formally a part of the army; and volunteers, many of whom came under the auspices of the Red Cross. The success of the care was partly dependent on which type of nurse cared for the soldier. Dale is particularly critical of the regular army nurses for whom hands-on care was anathema. It was, Dale demonstrates, those members of the Reserve who had been civilian hospital nurses prior to their venture to South Africa and were convinced of the importance of bedside care, who provided the intensive nursing required and who clearly established 'the need for trained nursing care to ensure successful outcomes'.[40] Helmstadter argues that one of the reasons for sending female nurses to the Crimea was that there were simply no trained men in nursing, the work of the hospital nurse having arisen from female domestic service.[41] Nevertheless, by 1902, Dale argues, the importance of a female military nursing service in Britain was firmly established, with the creation of the Queen Alexandra's Imperial Military Nursing

Service. The military medical services in the USA clearly also felt that a female military nursing service was vital in order to care for its soldiers, and the US Army Nurse Corps was founded in 1901.[42] Similarly, the Canadian Army Medical Corps established a permanent nursing service in 1904.[43] The wars of the mid- to late-nineteenth century had therefore firmly established the importance of a female military nursing service and had given women a place in the masculine theatre of war, but their place as women in a war zone would continue to be contested.

Part II: 'Industrial war', focuses on the First World War. Following the establishment of military nursing services in a number of countries at the beginning of the twentieth century, the position of women nurses in the military was, if not welcomed, then tolerated as a necessity. Key scientific discoveries from the latter half of the nineteenth century, such as an understanding of the transmission of plague, a vaccine for typhoid, radiography, the widespread use of anaesthesia in surgery and the use of the thermometer also necessitated skilled assistants to administer innovative treatments and medications.[44] Trained female personnel were ideally placed to act as these assistants. This part opens with Christine Hallett's chapter on the 'total nursing care' required for the helpless victims of poison gas. Hallett asserts that while the nurses did sometimes act as 'observers when reporting on major scientific decisions', they also took full responsibility for their own skilled and technical work, keeping patients from asphyxiating, bathing their damaged eyes and treating burns. Nurses were working with the latest science, even if some of that science was erroneous. Steve Sturdy has argued that the 'case of chemical warfare' was in fact part of the development of 'war as experiment'[45] and, as Hallett argues in her chapter, nurses engaged fully in the innovative scientific treatments used to combat the unforeseen catastrophes created by gas poisoning. But few medics or medical journals acknowledged their work.

This lack of acknowledgement of the work of the nurse finds corroboration in Kirsty Harris's exploration of the often overlooked feeding work of nurses on hospital ships and in the Middle Eastern theatres of the First World War. Invalid nutrition was a central aspect of nursing work in the late nineteenth to early twentieth centuries (as already shown in Chapter 1 on the Crimean War).[46] Harris's chapter demonstrates that despite a number of scientific advances, frequently, there was little the medical profession could do and that nutrition and what Therese Meehan has described as 'careful nursing' were the common arsenal of treatment options.[47] Harris demonstrates that the feeding of the soldier in the First World War was skilled and technical work. Ensuring that the malnourished soldiers received adequate nutrition required improvisation and innovation on the part of the nurses, as well as patience and tenacity in grappling with the red tape of the military machine. Nevertheless, the work was largely ignored by the medical profession, medical scientists and the military authorities. Brooks reported similar findings with reference to the liberated persons of Bergen-Belsen at the end of the Second World War.[48]

If the clinical work of nurses in the First World War was largely ignored by the authorities, the potential of female nurses as political instruments was not, as Cynthia Toman illustrates in her exploration of the political work of nurse Dorothy Cotton as an 'ambassador' in Petrograd.[49] In Chapter 6, Toman argues that the clinical work undertaken at the Anglo-Russian Hospital was not particularly remarkable, and it is clear from this chapter that little clinical nursing was performed during the latter stages of the hospital's existence, once the Bolsheviks were in power. However, Toman suggests that the hospital functioned as a 'realm of diplomacy', especially during the early months of the war when the Allies were keen to offer Russia all the support they could. Nurses serving overseas could be used as instruments of the state.

Debbie Palmer's work focuses on the nurses left behind during this conflict and examines their health and work in a wide variety of settings and workplaces. She focuses, in Chapter 7, on two very different hospitals in the South-West of England, a provincial voluntary general hospital (the type that was paid for by local benefactors and could recruit middle-class women into its nursing establishment) and the local asylum for the mentally ill and those with epilepsy, largely nursed by working-class recruits. The First World War confirmed the value of nurses and their vital role as clinicians, political instruments and morale raisers for the troops. Nevertheless, as Palmer's chapter demonstrates, the war also identified the weaknesses in the nascent profession: there were too few trained nurses and too many who wished to escape the drudgery of hospital work.[50] The neophyte profession struggled to claim a particular ground for itself. Moreover, Palmer's work suggests that the social class of both patients and nurses in an institution impacted on their perceived value and, hence, on their working and living conditions. The asylum suffered from worsening recruitment and retention and increasingly poor diet and accommodation for the nursing staff. By contrast, the adverse effects of the war on the voluntary hospital were far fewer.

Part III considers the 'Technological warfare' of the mid-twentieth century. Angela Jackson's chapter on the work of the nurses of the International Brigades, and the transmission of their knowledge to young untrained Spanish girls, demonstrates the clinical talent that was developing among nurses from around the world and the determination of these women to work against fascism.[51] Jackson's descriptions of the 'theatre nurse [who] might work for thirty-six hours at a stretch or face a constant stream of almost impossible choices in triage', or the nurse who delivered babies 'by the roadside or in the soot and grime of a disused railway tunnel', provide a stark portrayal of the conditions under which International Brigade nurses worked, and also demonstrate of their ability to improvise and innovate. Set against their clinical abilities are the short-lived changes in Spanish attitudes towards women workers and the crucial role of the untrained Spanish girls who assisted the International Brigade nurses at a time when bedside nursing in Spain was more usually undertaken by nuns, and technical nursing work by male 'practicantes'.[52]

David Justham's work on wound care, prior to the discovery of penicillin demonstrates the considerable skill required by nurses to maintain wound healing and prevent infection (see Chapter 9). The prevailing attitudes of nurses and their procedural training did not necessarily follow the modern principles of wound healing.[53] Justham's argument suggests that this narrowness of vision was partly to blame for the lack of value placed on the growing realisation that maggots could and did assist in wound healing in an era when antibacterial and antibiotic treatments were not available. Moreover, he suggests this antipathy may also have been grounded in the belief that sanitarianism and cleanliness were paramount and that maggots were 'dirt out of place'.

Jane Brooks's chapter focuses on the last months of the Second

12

World War and explores the humanitarian work of trained and volunteer nurses after the liberation of Bergen-Belsen in 1945.[54] The lack of trained nurses from the Allied nations necessitated the use of German army nurses as well as male medical students and Red Cross volunteers. Brooks argues that the choice of German army nurses to care for mainly Jewish victims of the Holocaust appears at first an odd and perhaps cruel choice. Nevertheless, she maintains, these nurses were trained and the decision to use them demonstrates an acknowledgement of the particular skills that trained nurses had over their untrained colleagues. Ultimately, Brooks argues, it was the clinical wisdom of the trained nurses of all nationalities that enabled many of the victims to rehabilitate.

Jan-Thore Lockertsen's chapter focuses on the Korean War, described by North American historian Mary Sarnecky as the 'forgotten war'.[55] In Chapter 11, Lockertsen examines the work of the nurses of the Norwegian Mobile Army Surgical Hospital (NORMASH). Lockertsen explores the challenging work undertaken in the operating theatres and hospital wards by nurses without any previous military training. Moreover, as with previous wars, the paucity of trained nursing staff led to the requirement to use local untrained staff and the need for trained nurses to supervise those staff.[56] In the Korean War this included orphaned and refugee boys, who undertook their work with eagerness. As one of his oral history participants maintained, 'It was amazing to see what the boys could do.'

Finally, Maxine Dahl's chapter details the work of the flight nurses during the Korean War. She discusses the involvement of nurses in this developing area of wartime emergency care.[57] Dahl argues that the air evacuation system which had originated during the Second World War was an exciting nursing innovation for the service of the Royal Australian Air Force (RAAF) permitting them, for the first time, to act autonomously, rather than under the direction of a medical officer. During the Korean War, the RAAF nurses evacuated the wounded from Korea to Japan. By the end of 1953, they had evacuated over 12,762 patients, with a variety of injuries and conditions. Dahl maintains that the oral history participants for the study understated the seriousness of their work, but they admitted caring for patients who were badly burnt, with chest wounds or with amputations. Of crucial importance to this chapter is the exploration of the range of work-roles in which the nurses engaged, including, pre-flight assessment of the injured, briefing the pilots on the health status of their patients and potential problems that may have been caused by particular altitude or speed and providing in-flight nursing care.

Conclusion

This book brings together a number of highly original contributions, some by established scholars exploring new aspects of nursing history; others by exciting new thinkers in the discipline. The three themes chosen to structure the book, while standing in a chronological sequence, also reflect some of the current trends in scholarship. In exploring women's nursing contributions to the wars of the nineteenth century, the book focuses on the ways in which gendered notions of women's work – and of 'womanhood' itself – both drove and constrained the emergence of wartime nursing as a recognised discipline. In considering the work of First World War military nurses, we explore the dangerous military and political worlds in which nurses negotiated their practice. Not only did they face the challenges posed by highly destructive innovative weapons such as toxic gases, and survive in what had hitherto been an almost exclusively male domain; they also negotiated the shifting terrain of a highly unstable political world.

In its exploration of multiple nursing roles during the wars of the mid-twentieth century, the book focuses attention on the consequences of 'total warfare' – a shift in strategy characterised by highly destructive technologies. In doing so, it considers the responsiveness (and yet also the instability) of nursing work, as crisis scenarios gave rise to improvisation and the – sometimes quite dramatic – breaking of practice boundaries. We examine how those boundaries, once broken, could again coalesce around practice whose scope was, both broader and more stable than previously.

In *One hundred years of wartime nursing practices* we explore the ways in which the exigencies of wartime practice – the ways in which nurses faced the crises created by the deliberate unleashing of forces designed to damage human beings – led to an expansion of the scope of nursing work that, in turn, impacted on the professional identity of nursing itself. By rising to the challenges posed by a need

14

to blend both the apparently mundane and highly gendered work of caring for patients' physical and emotional needs with the clearly scientific and intricate work of implementing the latest technologies, nurses influenced not only the expectations of the societies in which they operated but their own thinking about the significance of their practice.

Notes

1 Janet S. K. Watson, 'Wars in the wards: The social construction of medical work in First World War Britain', *Journal of British Studies* 41, 4 (October 2002), 484–510. For further work by Watson, on women's nursing engagement in war, see Janet S. K. Watson, 'Khaki girls, VADs and Tommy's sisters: Gender and class in First World War Britain', *The International History Review* 19, 1 (February 1997), 32–51; Janet S. K. Watson, *Fighting Different Wars: Experience, Memory, and the First World War in Britain* (Cambridge, Cambridge University Press, 2007).

2 Arthur Marwick, *Total War and Social Change* (Basingstoke, Palgrave Macmillan, 1988).

3 Penny Summerfield, *Reconstructing Women's Wartime Lives: Discourse and Subjectivity in Oral Histories of the Second World War* (Manchester, Manchester University Press, 1998); Jeremy A. Crang, 'Come into the army Maud': Women, military conscription, and the Markham Inquiry', *Defence Studies* 8, 3 (2008), 381–95; Deborah Montgomerie, 'Assessing Rosie: World War II, New Zealand women and the iconography of femininity', *Gender and History* 8, 1 (1996), 108–32; Phil Goodman, '"Patriotic femininity": Women's morals and men's morale during the Second World War', *Gender and History*, 10, 2 (1998), 278–93; Sonya O. Rose, *Which People's War? National Identity and Citizenship in Britain, 1939–1945* (Oxford, Oxford University Press, 2003); Lucy Noakes, *War and the British: Gender, Memory and National Identity* (London, I. B. Tauris, 1998); Lucy Noakes, *Women in the British Army: War and the Gentle Sex, 1907–1948* (London, Routledge, 2006); Judith Gardam and Hilary Charlesworth, 'Protection of women in armed conflict', *Human Rights Quarterly* 22 (2000), 148–66.

4 Gail Braybon and Penny Summerfield, *Out of the Cage: Women's Experiences in Two World Wars* (London, Pandora, 1987).

5 Roger Cooter, Steve Sturdy and Mark Harrison, *War, Medicine and Modernity* (Stroud, Sutton Publishing, 1998).

6 Jan Bassett, *Guns and Brooches: Australian Army Nursing from the Boer War to the Gulf War* (Melbourne, Oxford University Press Australia, 1992); Anna Rogers, *While You're Away: New Zealand Nurses at War, 1899–1948* (Auckland, Auckland University Press, 2003); Mary Sarnecky, *A History of*

the US Army Nurse Corps (Philadelphia, University of Pennsylvania Press, 2000).

7   Ian Hay, *One Hundred Years of Army Nursing* (London, Cassell & Co., 1953); Juliet Piggott, *Queen Alexandra's Royal Army Nursing Corps* (London, Lee Cooper, 1975).

8   Eric Taylor, *Wartime Nurse: One Hundred Years from the Crimea to Korea, 1854-1954* (London, Robert Hale, 2001).

9   Christine Hallett, *Containing Trauma* (Manchester, Manchester University Press, 2009) and Kirsty Harris, *More than Bombs and Bandages* (NSW, Big Sky Publishing, 2011).

10 For further discussion of the shattered male body and the reaction to it by nurses and other women, see, Joanna Bourke, *Dismembering the Male: Men's Bodies, Britain and the Great War* (London, Reaktion Books Ltd, 1999).

11 Lucy Noakes, 'Eve in khaki: Women working with the British military 1915-1918', in K. Cowman and L. Jackson (eds), *Women and Work Culture* (Farnham, Ashgate, 2004).

12 Noakes, *Women in the British Army*. See also: Cynthia Enloe, *Does Khaki Become You? The Militarization of Women's Lives* (London, Pluto Press, 1983).

13 Patricia D'Antonio, 'Nurses in war', *The Lancet* 360 (December 2002), 7–8.

14 Watson, 'Wars in the wards'; Watson, 'Khaki girls, VADs and Tommy's sisters', and Watson, *Fighting Different Wars*.

15 Kara Dixon Vuic, *Officer, Nurse, Woman: The Army Nurse Corps in the Vietnam War* (Baltimore, Johns Hopkins University Press, 2010); Kara Dixon Vuic, 'Wartime nursing and power', in Patricia D'Antonio, Julie A Fairman and Jean Whelan, *The Routledge Handbook on the Global History of Nursing* (Abingdon, New York, Routledge, 2013), 22–34.

16 Dixon Vuic, 'Wartime nursing and power', 25.

17 Mary Borden, *The Forbidden Zone* (London, William Heinemann Ltd, 1929). See also: Laurie Kaplan, 'Deformities of the Great War: The narratives of Mary Borden and Helen Zenna Smith', *Women and Language* 27, 2 (2004), 35–43.

18 Ellen La Motte, *The Backwash of War: The Human Wreckage of the Battlefied as Witnessed by an American Hospital Nurse* (New York, G. P. Putnam's Sons, 1916), 11.

19 Elizabeth Scannell-Desch and Mary Ellen Doherty, *Nurses in War: Voices from Iraq and Afghanistan* (New York, Springer, 2012).

20 Linda Nochlin, *Women, Art, and Power and Other Essays* (London, Thames & Hudson, 1989).

21 For further discussion on the developments of a more scientific training and knowledge base for nurses, see for example, Anne Marie Rafferty, *The Politics of Nursing Knowledge* (London, Routledge, 1996); Monica Baly, *Florence Nightingale and the Nursing Legacy* (London, Whurr Publishers,

1997); Sue Hawkins, *Nursing and Women's Labour in the Nineteenth Century* (Abingdon, Oxon, 2010).

22 Jocalyn Lawler, *Behind the Screens: Nursing, Somology, and the Problem of the Body* (Melbourne, Churchill Livingstone, 1991).

23 Alison Bashford, *Purity and Pollution: Gender, Embodiment and Victorian Medicine* (Basingstoke, Macmillan, 2000), 22.

24 Mary Douglas, *Purity and Danger: An Analysis of the Concepts of Pollution and Taboo* (London, Routledge, 1966).

25 Hallett, *Containing Trauma*, 6.

26 Lawler, *Behind the Screens*, Jocalyn Lawler (ed.), *The Body in Nursing: A Collection of Views* (Melbourne, Churchill Livingstone, 1997).

27 Trudi Tate, *Modernism, History and the First World War* (Manchester, Manchester University Press, 1998).

28 Christine Hallett, "'Intelligent interest in their own affairs": The First World War, The British Journal of Nursing and the construction of nursing knowledge', in D'Antonio, Fairman and Whelan, *The Routledge Handbook on the Global History of Nursing*.

29 See Carol Helmstadter, 'British military nursing in the Crimean War'; Barbara Maling, 'American "Nightingales": The influence of Florence Nightingale on Southern nurses during the American Civil War'; and Cynthia Toman, 'Eyewitness to revolution: Canadian military nurses at Petrograd, 1915–17', in this volume.

30 Jane Schultz, 'Nurse as icon: Florence Nightingale's impact on women in the American Civil War', in Simon Lewis and David T. Gleeson, *Civil War – Global Conflict* (Columbia, University of South Carolina Press, 2014).

31 See Charlotte Dale, 'Traversing the veldt with "Tommy Atkins": the clinical challenges of nursing typhoid patients during the Second Anglo-Boer War, 1899–1902', and Kirsty Harris, 'Health, healing and harmony: invalid cookery and feeding by Australian nurses in the Middle East in the First World War', in this volume.

32 See Christine Hallett, "'This fiendish mode of warfare": Nursing the victims of gas poisoning in the First World War', and David Justham, "'Those maggots – they did a wonderful job": The nurses' role in wound management in civilian hospitals during the Second World War', in this volume.

33 See Jane Brooks, "'The nurse stoops down ... for me": Nursing the liberated persons at Bergen-Belsen'; Jan-Thore Lockertsen, 'The Norwegian Mobile Army Surgical Hospital: Nursing at the front', and Maxine Dahl, 'Moving forward: Australian flight nurses in the Korean war', in this volume.

34 See Debbie Palmer, 'The impact of the First World War on asylum and voluntary hospital nurses' work and health', in this volume.

35 F. B. Smith, *Florence Nightingale: Reputation and Power* (Beckenham, Kent, Croom Helm, 1982), 43–4; Mark Bostridge, *Florence Nightingale: The*

Making of an Icon (New York, Farrar, Straus and Giroux, 2008), 232; Anne Summers, *Angels and Citizens: British Women as Military Nurses 1854–1914* (New York, Routledge & Kegan Paul, 1988), 51–2.

36 Anne Summers, *Female Lives, Moral States: Women, Religion and Public Life in Britain, 1800–1930* (Newbury, Threshold Press, 2000), 81.

37 Schultz, 'Nurse as icon'.

38 See Maling, 'American "Nightingales"'.

39 See Dale, 'Traversing the veldt'.

40 See Dale, 'Traversing the veldt'.

41 Personal communication from Carol Helmstadter (14.3.2013) LMA/H01/ ST/NC15/37/2, Florence Lees' report on her nursing experience in the Franco-Prussian War 1870–71, p. 57: There does not exist in England any training school for men. Florence Nightingale's annotation: 'Yes, there is at Netley [but of course this was for army men].'

42 Sarnecky, *A History of the US Army Nurse Corps*, 1.

43 Cynthia Toman, *An Officer and a Lady: Canadian Military Nursing and the Second World War* (Vancouver, University of British Columbia Press, 2007), 4.

44 Molly Sutphen, 'Striving to be separate? Civilian and military doctors in Cape Town during the Anglo-Boer War', in Cooter, Harrison and Sturdy, *War, Medicine and Modernity*, 50; Roy Porter, *The Greatest Benefit to Mankind: A Medical History of Humanity from Antiquity to the Present* (London, Fontana Press, 1999), 344–6.

45 Steve Sturdy, 'War as experiment. Physiology, innovation and administration in Britain, 1914–1918: the case of chemical warfare', in Cooter, Harrison and Sturdy (eds), *War, Medicine and Modernity*, 65–84.

46 See Helmstadter, 'British military nursing in the Crimean War'.

47 Therese Connell Meehan, 'Careful nursing: a model for contemporary nursing practice', *Journal of Advanced Nursing* 44, 1 (2003), 99–107.

48 Jane Brooks, '"Uninterested in anything except food": Nurse feeding work with the liberated inmates of Bergen-Belsen', *Journal of Clinical Nursing* 21, 19 (2012), 2958–65.

49 See Toman, 'Eyewitness to revolution'.

50 See Palmer, 'The impact of the First World War on asylum and voluntary hospital nurses'.

51 See Angela Jackson, 'Blood and guts: Nursing with the International Brigades in the Spanish civil war, 1936–39', in this volume.

52 Josep Trueta, *Trueta: Surgeon in War and Peace. The Memoirs of Josep Trueta* (translated by Meli and Michael Strubell) (London, Victor Gollancz, 1980), 91; Isabel Anton-Solanas, 'Nurses, practitioners and volunteers: the dissolution of professional and practice boundaries during the Spanish Civil War (1936–39)' (unpublished PhD thesis, Manchester University, 2010).

53 See Justham, '"Those maggots – they did a wonderful job"'.

54 See Brooks, '"The nurse stoops down … for me"'.
55 Mary Sarnecky, 'Army nurses in "the forgotten war"', *American Journal of Nursing* 101, 11 (2001), 45–9.
56 See Lockertsen, 'The Norwegian Mobile Army Surgical Hospital'.
57 See Dahl, 'Moving forward'.

Part I
Gentlemen's wars

1

Class, gender and professional expertise: British military nursing in the Crimean War

Carol Helmstadter

Modern historians have suggested that nursing in the Crimean War was largely a form of housekeeping and that the only major contributions made by the female nurses whom the government sent to the East were the introduction of night nursing and small personal attentions to the soldiers.[1] Certainly, the roots of hospital nursing did lie in domestic service but did military nursing in the 1850s really largely consist of household duties? War and other emergencies test the mettle of nurses, often increasing their competencies, expanding their scope of practice and demonstrating more publicly the abilities of a historically undervalued profession. The Crimean War 1853–56 provides an especially interesting example because nursing itself was undergoing a profound transformation at the time.

At the beginning of the nineteenth century nurses were fundamentally charwomen who primarily did the laundry, cleaning, sewing and cooking. These were indeed their principal duties but they did help with the less important parts of patient care – ambulation and cleaning up after all the bleedings, vomitings, purgings, and washing incontinent patients.[2] These nurses needed absolutely no qualifications or hospital experience to be hired at full salary and they reported to a matron who was not a nurse but rather a housekeeper who had no responsibility for nursing care.[3]

By 1854, however, the new scientific medicine had become established in the London teaching hospitals, transforming British medicine and shifting the centre for medical research and education from Edinburgh to London. Because it treated more acutely ill

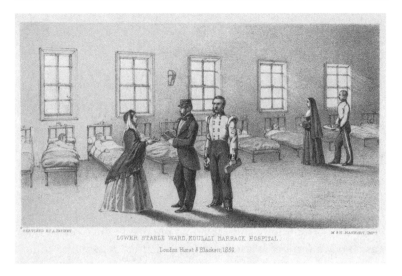

1.1 Koulali Hospital Ward 1856

patients and used supportive, as opposed to depleting, therapies the new hospital practice made the old nurses obsolete.[4] The new medicine required reliable, clinically experienced nurses who could take responsibility for critically ill patients and carry out medical orders intelligently and with good judgement. By the 1850s some hospital nurses and some religious Sisters met these criteria but they formed a tiny minority of the nursing workforce. As a result, the hospital nurses whom the British government sent to nurse the soldiers during the Crimean War were a very disparate group. Some were very much like the nurses at the beginning of the century while others were highly competent practitioners; most fell between the two extremes.[5] Unlike contemporary American hospitals, which often employed male nurses in the men's wards, in the British hospitals nurses were all women because they evolved from charwomen.[6]

This chapter explores the importance of nursing knowledge in the mid-nineteenth century context of a different understanding of disease and a different construction of women's role in a society that was becoming increasingly defined by social class. I look first at the way disease was understood and treated and what that meant for what nurses had to know. I then consider two barriers that prevented the public from grasping that efficient nursing required the kind of knowledge base which, at that time, could only be gained through clinical experience. The first barrier was the persistence of the image of nurses as working-class women who really were essentially domestic servants at the beginning of the nineteenth century. At mid-century they retained their housekeeping duties: cleaning, laundry, mending and, in addition, cooking. Although by 1854 in order to deemed competent nurses had to have a very considerable base of specific nursing knowledge, the nurses' multiple roles were confusing to the public. Second, the Victorian construction of gender and the concept of women as naturally and innately accomplished nurses was in direct opposition to an understanding of nursing as based on clinical knowledge.

A different understanding of disease and hence of nursing care

In the Crimean War four different combatants, Britain, France, Sardinia and the Ottoman Empire fought Russia on two continents in many locations but, because it is so well documented, this chapter deals only with British nursing on the Black Sea littoral. When Britain and France declared war on Russia at the end of March 1854 the Turks were already fighting the Russians. A Russian army had invaded Ottoman territory in Bulgaria and was besieging the fortress of Silistria on the Danube. Hoping to prevent the Russians from advancing further into Bulgaria, British and French troops began landing in Varna in June 1854. However, in that same month diplomatic pressure forced the Russians to withdraw their troops, leaving the allied armies in Bulgaria with no enemy to fight. The allies then decided to invade the Crimea and destroy the powerful Russian naval base of Sevastopol.[7] The siege of Sevastopol would become the most publicised part of the war.

The British army was a very sick army when it left Bulgaria for the Crimea. Bowel disease had always been the primary medical problem of field armies but it was even worse in 1854 because the Crimean campaign coincided with one of the four worst nineteenth-century cholera pandemics.[8] So many soldiers died of cholera in Varna that there was no time for funerals. The bodies were simply carted out of the hospital at night and thrown into pits.[9] At that time doctors identified three kinds of bowel disease: diarrhoea, dysentery and cholera. They classified diarrhoea into five categories, each requiring a different treatment. Choleraic diarrhoea was treated with drugs including castor oil; summer diarrhoea was treated with laxatives, mercury and ipecac in mild cases, and in more severe cases with leeches, blisters and poultices; congestive diarrhoea was treated with warmth, rest, fomentations, analgesics, diaphoretics and mercurials; atonic diarrhoea was treated with drugs; scorbutic diarrhoea received the same treatment as dysentery. Dysentery, which was characterized by blood and mucus in the stool, and cholera, diagnosed by rice water stools, were treated with rest, warmth, nutritious diet, drugs, fomentations, poulticing and massage.[10]

What did nursing care consist of in the 1850s, what did nurses need to know and what were fomentations, mercurials and blisters? Patient care was based on a different understanding of disease and its causation. Doctors believed morbid materials, derived from miasmas or from a poor or immoral life style, invaded the body and were the cause of the various illnesses. Symptoms such as vomiting, diarrhoea, rashes and open sores were the body's way of ejecting the disease-producing matter and were actually wholesome efforts of the body to heal itself. Therefore doctors tried to encourage these processes with emetics, cathartics, or by creating open sores with chemicals.[11] Hence many treatments nurses administered were very different from modern therapies.

Mercury compounds were a mainstay of treatment in the earlier part of the century. Doctors prescribed huge doses because mercury was considered efficacious for almost all ailments.[12] An extreme example is the salivating treatment, considered a cure for syphillis. Nurses gave increasing amounts of mercury until the patients suffered severe mercury poisoning, spitting out 2½–3 pints of saliva a day.[13] Alcohol was considered a stimulant, and since it was believed that most people died of exhaustion rather than of cardiac or respiratory arrest, doctors prescribed enormous amounts of wine and brandy.[14]

A blister was essentially an open sore, usually produced by a poultice made with mustard or Spanish fly, or sometimes doctors just poured nitrous acid directly onto the skin. Open sores were believed to attract the morbid materials causing the disease and allow them to escape from the body. A blister at the nape of the neck, for example, was thought to relieve cerebral inflammation.[15] George Lawson, a young army surgeon, was smitten with Crimean fever in May 1855. 'I have ... had a very severe attack of fever,' he wrote his parents', and am now suffering from the results, and the treatment. I am ... very weak, but what troubles me most is a terrible sore state of the back of the neck from continued blistering ...'[16] In the same month Florence Nightingale also suffered a near-fatal attack of Crimean fever. When her friend Selena Bracebridge came to Balaclava to take her back to Scutari, Nightingale wrote her family: 'I think seeing her did me more good than all their [the doctors'] blisters.'[17]

Blisters were left on as long as 12 or even 24 hours and caused excruciating pain. If left on too long, they could create third-degree burns. They had to be dressed in the same way as wounds – with poultices, usually made of bread or linseed. Blisters were standard treatments for fevers and were also used as stimulants to promote the energies of the nervous and circulatory systems or of particular organs.[18] Poultices were a major method of dressing blisters and surgical and other wounds. Hospital nurses were still making 14 or 15 poultices a day in the 1870s because nearly all wounds became infected and required dressing.[19]

Fomentations consisted of flannels soaked in hot water that was usually medicated, and then applied to the affected part or wound. If not properly applied they could do more harm than good. For example, the Crimean War surgeons trusted only Rev. Mother Francis Bridgeman and her team of experienced nuns to apply chloroform fomentations. The sisters soaked blankets cut into small pieces in boiling water, had the orderlies wring them almost dry, then applied them to the soldier's abdomen, and finally, sprinkled chloroform on them. Then they gave the soldier a bit of ice and some brandy to settle his stomach.[20]

We now know that symptoms such as open sores, diarrhoea, or vomiting do not cure disease and we would never deliberately create wounds or treat diarrhoea with castor oil, emetics, or mercurials, but it is important to remember that in the 1850s these therapies were based on the latest scientific knowledge and on a completely different interpretation of disease processes. From a nursing point of view, nurses needed significant knowledge and experience when applying and tending blisters, fomentations or mercurials for there was a very narrow margin between achieving the desired result and killing the patient. After bowel disease, fevers were the commonest class of malady suffered during the war. Most fever patients needed spoon-feeding, sometimes a spoonful of ice, beef tea, or wine every five minutes throughout the day and night, although every half hour was more standard. The third most prevalent disease was scurvy for which the treatment was purely dietetic.[21] Until April 1855 the men's diet consisted entirely of hard tack, salt meat, and rum so scurvy developed rapidly. Many men could not eat the hard biscuits because of the state of their gums. Furthermore, underlying scurvy complicated other diseases and slowed the healing of wounds. Surgeon-General Thomas Longmore wrote that in the winter of 1854–55 scurvy affected almost every officer and man to a greater or lesser extent.[22]

The fourth most common condition was frostbite which the nurses considered the worst affliction. The army had expected the war to be over quickly, before winter set in, and had not supplied the men with winter clothes. In the bitter Crimean winter the under-dressed soldiers' flesh and clothes often froze together in one piece. When the nurses cut off their clothes the flesh came off with them, exposing the fascia and muscles, and this was far more painful than wounds.[23] Because it did not attack exposed parts such as the face, ears and nose, but usually started in the toes and feet, Longmore thought what was commonly called frostbite in the Crimea was not true frostbite but rather gangrene. He pointed out that many cases diagnosed as frostbite occurred when the temperature was above the freezing point.[24]

Then a severe epidemic of typhus occurred, reaching its peak in the first part of April 1855, and typhus often led to extensive bedsores and gangrene. Nursing care consisted of opium for pain and trying to increase the patient's strength with food, stimulants, and tonics given frequently in small amounts. There was also hospital gangrene that attacked many men on the transports from Balaclava to Scutari. If the gangrene started in a limb, it had to be wrapped in cotton wool and kept warm. If it spread up the limb, the surgeons amputated. There were also a few cases of gas gangrene.[25] Finally, because there was no nursing care whatsoever on the transports on what could be a ten-day trip from Balaclava to Scutari, many men had enormous bedsores covering their neck, back and hips, sores that were so extensive they eventually killed them.[26]

Curiously, venereal disease is almost never mentioned in the official reports although it was a common problem among the soldiers. One of the few references to it occurred when the Scutari General Hospital opened in June 1854. Within sixteen days it held 565 patients, largely venereal and diarrhoea cases.[27]

As opposed to men in the field hospitals, wounds accounted for only a small number of the soldiers in the base hospitals.[28] Unlike the Southern nurses who worked on the battlefield in the American Civil War a few years later, the British nurses worked only in base hospitals.[29] Gunshot wounds were, of course, first treated in the field hospitals but many complications could occur after the men had been transferred to the base hospitals. Secondary haemorrhage, which could strike within a few days to three weeks or more, was frequent and usually fatal. Pyaemia, or abscesses in the viscera, was common, especially in gunshot wounds of bones, and it also was usually fatal. As well, gunshot wounds were especially liable to erysipelas, a diffused, spreading inflammation of the skin involving the subcutaneous tissue and usually accompanied by fever. Surgeons dreaded it because it spread so easily and could suppurate and attack deeper structures.[30] Treatment consisted of isolation and maintenance of constitutional strength, again by frequent feedings of beef tea, milk and any light food the patient could eat, plus wine and other alcoholic stimulants. As Longmore pointed out, this treatment required 'judicious and careful nursing'. Local treatment of erysipelas differed from surgeon to surgeon: some used fomentations and linseed poultices, others leeches, cupping and repeated punctures followed by fomentations.[31] Finally, in the warm weather what appeared to be the common housefly abounded in the Crimea, literally swarming on the patients' faces and any exposed parts, and invading the men's wounds with maggots. The staff covered the men's faces and wounds that were exposed to the air with cotton net gauze.[32]

Doctors ordered leeching and cupping which were usually nursing responsibilities, but in contrast to the Peninsular War 1808–14, the surgeons bled sparingly.[33] However, numerous advances in medicine over the first half of the century generated a great deal more skilled work for the nurses than had been the case at the beginning of the century. New surgical procedures plus anaesthesia – and the Crimean War surgeons used chloroform for major surgery in all but one division – meant far more complicated long-term post-operative care as well as post-anaesthetic nursing care.[34] Furthermore, the new emphasis on supportive, rather than depleting, therapies meant that at a time when there was no intravenous therapy, medical nurses had to spend a great deal more time giving their patients fluids and food both by mouth and when they could not eat or drink, by rectum.

Most important of all nursing competencies were assessment skills. John Flint South, senior surgeon at St Thomas' Hospital in London, pointed this out in 1857 when he wrote that without his Sisters' watchfulness and knowledge of symptoms that required immediate attention, many of his patients would have died.[35] This kind of knowledge could only be gained by long experience. In Scutari these skills were especially helpful in the evenings when the doctors did not examine all their patients as they did on their morning rounds. They generally only looked at those patients about whom they were worried and passed by the others in the dark. For example, when one evening one of the Anglican Sisters found a soldier suffering from severe dyspnoea, she sent for a doctor who then ordered treatment.[36] All of this nursing work was obviously labour-intensive and time-consuming and required the kind of specific knowledge and judgement that defined the new professions that were emerging in the nineteenth century.

A different construction of gender and a heterogeneous nursing team in an age when class defined society

At the first pitched battle, the Battle of the Alma on 20 September 1854, the army's medical department was almost completely unprepared to care for the wounded and dying. The terrible mortality and destruction of the army and the inadequate medical care in that first dreadful winter were no worse than conditions in many previous campaigns, most recently the Peninsular War, but in the early nineteenth century there were no soldiers who were adequately literate to write home and no newspaper correspondents to make the public aware of the horrible conditions.[37]

By contrast, in the Crimea there were newspaper reporters. They were impressed by the efficient way in which the Daughters of Charity ran the French army's base hospitals. These correspondents attributed the Sisters' success to their gender. Construing nursing as an innate characteristic of women was an important part of the Victorian ideal of a society divided into a public, or male sphere and a private, or domestic sphere to which women were relegated. This cultural assumption posited that women's natural abilities placed them in a subordinate position where they should cultivate sentiment and domestic skills of which nursing was one prominent example. Because of their greater natural endowments and intellectual superiority, the talents of men lay in intellectual and public endeavours.[38] Because nursing was an inborn feminine talent, women needed no special training or experience to nurse effectively: their tender words and motherly attributes would alleviate the soldiers' sufferings.[39]

Complicating this understanding of woman's nature was the fact that British society was becoming increasingly defined by class. It was assumed that the nursing talents of upper-class ladies were superior to those of working-class women. One of the Anglican Sisters explained about the orderlies: 'Of course men whose hands were hard and horny through labour, hands used once perhaps to the plough and more recently to the firelock, were not fitted to touch, bathe and dress wounded limbs, however gentle and considerate their hearts might be,'[40] This applied to the working-class nurses whose hands were hardened by all the cleaning they had to do.

When the newspaper accounts appeared describing the way the British wounded and dying soldiers were neglected while the French Sisters took such good care of their soldiers following the Alma, a public outcry arose. The British government felt obliged to recruit women with their supposed special inborn nursing abilities for the army. In October 1854 they despatched Nightingale and 38 female nurses to the East. By the end of the war the government had sent over 200 women.[41] The government also immediately began spending immense amounts of money on its military machine and also made major improvements in the army's administrative structure so that by the second year of the war the army was very well supplied and maintained.[42] However, the first winter of the campaign was one of indescribable suffering and presented the nurses with their greatest challenge. Between October 1854 and the end of April 1855 approximately 35 per cent of the soldiers died due to overwork, insufficient shelter, exposure to wet and cold in the trenches and the dreadful diet. Furthermore, because the hospitals were so overcrowded it was impossible to separate the sick from the wounded and many men who entered the hospital with a good prognosis died of diseases contracted there.[43]

Before the government nurses arrived on 4 November 1854 there were a few soldiers' wives who looked after their husbands and some actually nursed in the field hospital tents but we have no systematic records for them.[44] However, we do have records for the nurses whom the government recruited and who worked in the base hospitals. They were a very heterogeneous group: 9 Anglican Sisters, 28 Roman Catholic nuns, 128 working-class, paid hospital nurses and 54 ladies, most of whom, as befitted a lady, were not paid.[45] Both the Anglican and the Roman Catholic Sisters were clinically experienced nurses with one exception of five Catholic nuns who ran an orphanage and had no hospital experience. Because they were not effective nurses Nightingale sent them home in December 1854. Miss Nightingale, the *Lancet* explained in January 1855, had already 'dispensed with the services of five white-veiled nuns, who proved only in the way, and were of no use as nurses in the management of sponges, bandages, wounds, &c.'.[46] Like these five nuns, the 54 secular lady nurses, with a very few exceptions, had no real hospital experience either.[47]

Nearly all the working-class nurses came highly recommended from teaching hospitals and most had real nursing expertise. Here Nightingale had a real advantage over the Confederate matrons, during the American Civil War, who had to rely on ladies and slaves who had no hospital experience.[48] However, the clinically experienced working-class nurses, like many of the lady nurses, lacked the necessary discipline to work as a team in a military hospital. There were canteens attached to all the military hospitals where alcohol was freely sold. For example, at the Scutari Barrack Hospital the canteen was located in the square that the hospital formed, enabling many hospital nurses to be habitually drunk.[49] Drunkenness, Nightingale wrote, was 'tacitly admitted as unavoidable among Nurses in London

Hospitals'. This was not surprising because drink was a severe problem in all levels of British society at the time. Nevertheless, it did not facilitate good nursing. In her first year in the East she dismissed 12 of the 54 hospital nurses then under her supervision for incorrigible drunkenness.[50] Despite her goal of a respectable nursing service, Nightingale kept on a number of women who drank to excess or who were not what the Victorians called 'respectable women', because these women had the necessary knowledge to nurse effectively. Still, she kept a close eye on these nurses and trusted no working-class nurse until she had known her for some time.[51]

From June until 4 November when Nightingale arrived with her first party of 38 nurses nursing care in the base hospitals was entirely in the hands of orderlies and would remain so in many wards for the rest of the war because many doctors would not allow women in their divisions.[52] The orderlies were commandeered from among the convalescent soldiers and were given absolutely no training. The Commander-in-Chief of the army felt he needed every able man for the front and ordered that only men 'who were unfit for field duties owing to sickness' could be used as orderlies. Then these men were sent back to the front as soon as they were well enough so they did not have the opportunity to learn from experience.[53]

The orderly's job was well-nigh impossible. He had to stand in line for hours at the purveyor's office to procure the meat and bread for his patients, then take the meat to the kitchen, wait for it to be cooked, and then carry it up to his wards. Next he himself had to cook the 'extras'. Extras were supplements for the men's diets – chops, eggs, rice puddings, jellies, wine and spirits – which doctors ordered for individual patients. In the London hospitals the nurses had sculleries where they could cook the extras but the orderlies either had to cook the food on the ward stoves – which were designed for heating, not cooking – or in some out-building, using either their own kits or borrowing pots from the patients.[54] The orderlies obviously had little time for nursing care and generally were not interested in it, frequently finding it distasteful. As did many hospital nurses, they often drank the men's stimulants themselves, did not implement doctors' orders if they could get away with it and stole articles and money from dying and dead patients.[55] They also frequented the infamous hospital canteens. The army doctors and the commissioners whom Parliament sent out to investigate the hospitals all agreed that the orderlies were the worst failing in the army's medical department.[56]

Patient care and moral supervision in a highly class defined society

When they first arrived in Scutari the government nurses worked primarily among the wounded, the post-operative men and the acute medical cases.[57] Their other main duties were washing and preparing the surgical cases for the surgeons' visits, dressing wounds and taking orders for the extras from the surgeons. They then got the food and wine from Nightingale's extra kitchen. One of the first things Nightingale did on arrival in Scutari was to establish special 'extra kitchens' to facilitate the extras cooking.[58]

The nurses' work changed considerably at the end of December 1854 when the Army Medical Board sent out dressers to do the wound care. Dressers were advanced medical students, thus called because they were originally the surgeon's apprentices who did his patients' dressings. Apparently the War Office thought the medical students would do a better job than the nurses. Nightingale objected to the government's sensitivity to public opinion. The War Office, she said, 'does not care whether its one remedy neutralises the other, but tries both to humour the country'.[59] The dressers worked only in the surgical wards so in the medical wards the nurses continued to dress bedsores.[60]

Not only did the nurses have less work with the arrival of the dressers but in the same month the government sent a second party of 45 women so that Nightingale had a much larger staff than her original 38. She therefore reorganised the nursing so that the lady nurses, who, by this time, she realised were almost all ineffectual in the clinical situation, were each assigned one or two working-class nurses who gave the basic nursing care while the lady nurse superintended.[61] But as one of the Roman Catholic nuns pointed out, *'How could they superintend without some knowledge of the work?'*[62] However, if the ladies could not understand the nursing work they could superintend what the Victorians called the nurses' 'morals'.

Morals had a somewhat different meaning in the mid-nineteenth century: morals encompassed what we would now call repectability and responsible work habits as well as ethical behaviour. The search for moral order, or what we call social order and better work discipline, was a constant theme in British hospitals at this time. Hospitals were situated on the fringes of orderly society and were grouped together in official records with reformatories and prisons.[63] Moral disorder or 'lack of order and regularity', as the Victorians sometimes put it, was not limited to these peripheral institutions but permeated society as a whole. The earlier nineteenth century was an age of excess, disorder and riots. The upper classes attributed the unrest to a lack of moral restraint on the part of working-class individuals. Hence they tried to 'elevate the character' of working-class people by emphasising the need for the system and regularity which, in the case of many hospital nurses, was sadly lacking.[64]

Spencer Wells, later famous as one of the first successful abdominal surgeons, approved of the hospital nurses but was originally wary of the lady nurses. After only a few days in one of the military hospitals, however, he decided that educated ladies supervising hospital nurses was an excellent system once the inefficient ladies had been weeded out. Superintending the nurses' morals was more practical than it appeared on the surface: lady nurses saw that the working-class nurses carried out medical directives promptly, refrained from drinking and from what Nightingale called flirting with the soldiers and orderlies. Equally important, the ladies could be trusted with wine and spirits.[65]

Placing clinical experience ahead of social class Nightingale made Eliza Roberts, a working-class woman, her chief nurse because of her extraordinary nursing knowledge. Roberts used crude language and had coarse manners but she was respectable in the sense that she did not drink and she was completely dedicated to her work. Nightingale also gradually began creating a division of labour among her nurses. Because of the extra diet system, all the nurses still did a good deal of cooking, but Nightingale started using the clinically expert nurses entirely for patient care and the extras, assigning less able women exclusively to the laundry, cleaning and sewing. The government provided all the army hospitals with lady superintendents and female nurses and they all made major improvements.[66] By February 1855 with the vastly improved government supply system and better nursing, these hospitals were achieving a high standard of nursing care. 'I have seen upward of 200 sick arrive unexpectedly from the Crimea', one of the doctors wrote. The men were:

> landed, distributed to wards according to diseases, thoroughly washed, or bathed by immersion, put into bed, and prescribed for, varied nourishment given, and medicine administered within a couple of hours.[67]

Social class, gender and professional expertise

This very disparate group of nurses demonstrated clearly that clinical experience was absolutely essential if the soldiers were to be properly cared for: nursing in the 1850s was far more than household management or small personal attentions 24 hours a day. But although nursing practice was becoming increasingly professional many contemporaries failed to recognise this: they could not forget nursing's working-class origins in domestic service. Indeed, class and gender would place almost insurmountable hurdles in the nurses' struggle for professional recognition. Given the strictly segregated class structure of Victorian society – Victorian ladies simply could not mix with working-class women – ladies doing what was considered the menial work of nursing side by side with working-class women caused innumerable difficulties. Mother Mary Clare Moore, the Superior of the Convent of Mercy in Bermondsey, was a very open-minded and tolerant lady but she found working together with the working-class nurses very difficult. Her bishop warned her that the working-class nurses would give her and her Sisters 'many opportunities to learn and practise mortification'. Moore later wrote, 'The very fact of being associated with the [hospital] nurses, who, although respectful to the Sisters, were persons of doubtful character and almost daily intoxicated, caused great pain and uneasiness.'[68]

Another illustration of these problems was the 'equality system'. Before the second party of nurses left for the East, Sidney Herbert, Nightingale's friend and mentor in the War Office, told them they 'all went out on the same footing as hospital nurses, and that no one was to consider herself above her companions'. No sooner did they arrive in the East than the ladies decided that a stop had to be put to the equality system. For them the nurses were domestic servants who should wait on them as well as on the patients. Furthermore, they found associating with working-class women highly objectionable. 'We were compelled', one of the ladies wrote, 'to listen to the worst language, and to be treated not unfrequently with coarse insolence. Whispers were heard amongst them that they had come out to nurse the soldiers and not to sweep, wash and cook.' The ladies decided that in order to maintain their authority it was essential to stop wearing the same uniform as the hospital nurses and they decided:

> It was necessary for their own comfort and for the good of their work that in every possible way the distinction should be drawn. None but those who knew it can imagine the wearing anxiety and the bitter humiliation the charge of the hired nurses brought upon us.[69]

Gender played a rather ambiguous role. On the one hand, as we have seen, it was believed that women, and especially upper-class women, had an inborn, innate ability for nursing, an ability that men lacked. This had been the major reason why the government sent female nurses to the East. On the other hand, the Victorian convention was that women did not belong in the public arena of a military hospital. Thus many doctors resented the female nurses and would not allow them in their wards. This was especially true of the older men but there were also young doctors who felt women did not belong in army hospitals.[70] Dr David Greig, who graduated from Edinburgh in 1853 at the age of 21, considered the working-class nurses 'like the better class of nurse at home'. He thought they did their best but they told him they were unhappy in the East. 'So much for females when they find their way where they have no business',[71] he concluded. Yet, regardless of gender, the nursing work of the inexperienced lady nurses was just as inadequate as that of the untrained orderlies and clearly demonstrated that hospital experience was essential.

It has been suggested that female nurses were 'the last thing the Crimean War soldiers needed'.[72] It was true that the soldiers did not necessarily need *female* nurses but they desperately needed clinically experienced nurses. Because there were no male nurses in the British teaching hospitals, which is where nearly all the clinically experienced nurses came from, the only expert nurses on whom the army could draw were female. Their gender, however, produced such strong resistance from the army that in 1855 Sidney Herbert thought it would be impossible to maintain female nursing as a permanent military service.[73] Female nurses did eventually become a reality in the armed forces, but it was not because they were women but because the hospital nurses had the necessary experience and knowledge to work with acutely ill and severely wounded men.

Notes

1 F. B. Smith, *Florence Nightingale: Reputation and Power* (Beckenham, Croom Helm, 1982), 43–4; Mark Bostridge, *Florence Nightingale: The Making of an Icon* (New York, Farrar, Straus and Giroux, 2008), 232; Anne Summers, *Angels and Citizens: British Women as Military Nurses 1854–1914* (New York, Routledge & Kegan Paul, 1988), 51–2.

2 Archives of Charing Cross Hospital, Minutes of Board of Governors, vol. 2, 75–9.

3 Brian Abel-Smith, *A History of the Nursing Profession* (London, Heinemann, 1964), 8–9; Carol Helmstadter and Judith Godden, *Nursing Before Nightingale 1815–1899* (Farnham, Ashgate, 2011), 8–11, 25–6; John Flint South, *Facts Relating to Hospital Nurses* (London, Richardson Brothers, 1857), 10.

4 Cairn Berkowitz, 'The beauty of anatomy: Displays and surgical education in early nineteenth-century London', *Bulletin of the History of Medicine* 85, 2 (2011), 250; United Kingdom House of Commons Sessional Papers (*Parliamentary Papers*) 1864, vol. 28, 484–5.

5 Helmstadter and Godden, *Nursing Before Nightingale*, 95–115.

6 Charles E. Rosenberg, *The Care of Strangers* (Philadelphia, University of Pennsylvania Press, 1983), 43–4, 213–15, 235.

7 Winfried Baumgart, *The Crimean War 1853–56* (London, Arnold, 1999), 16, 99–112, 107, 112–13, 121.

8 Neil Cantlie, *A History of the Army Medical Department*, 2 vols (Edinburgh, Churchill Livingstone, 1974), vol. 2, 187.

9 Sir George Bell, *Soldier's Glory* (Tunbridge Wells, Spellmount, 1991), 205.

10 Cantlie, *Army Medical Department*, vol. 2, 186–7.

11 Florence Nightingale, *Notes on Nursing* (London, Churchill Livingstone, 1980[1859]), 5–6; Guenter B. Risse, *Hospital Life in Enlightenment Scotland* (Cambridge University Press, 1986), 239.

12 Carl J. Pfeiffer, *The Art and Practice of Western Medicine in the First Half of the Nineteenth Century* (London, McFarland, 1985), 201–6.

13 A. E. Clark-Kennedy, *The London*, 2 vols (London, Pitman Medical Publishing, 1962–63), vol. 1, 40–1.

14 Brian Harrison, *Drink and the Victorians* (Pittsburgh, PA, University of Pittsburgh Press, 1971), 39–41.

15 Peter Stanley, *For Fear of Pain: British Surgery 1790–1850* (New York, Rudopi, 2003), 53–7; Charles E. Rosenberg, 'The therapeutic revolution', in Morris J. Vogel and Charles E. Rosenberg, *The Therapeutic Revolution* (Philadelphia, PA, University of Pennsylvania Press, 1979), 23.

16 Victor Bonham-Carter (ed.), *Surgeon in the Crimea* (London, Constable, 1968), 176–7.

17 Wellcome Institute (WI), Ms 8995/17.

18 Robert J. Graves, *Clinical Lectures on the Practice of Medicine* (2nd edn, 2 vols, Dublin, Fannin, 1848), vol. 1, 149–50, 155–6, 161; J. Cheyne, 'Medical Report of the Hardwicke Fever Hospital 1817', in *Dublin Hospital Reports*, 1 (1818), 25–6; Stanley, *Fear of Pain*, 53–7.

19 Zepherina P. Veitch, *Handbook for Nurses for the Sick* (London, 1870), 25–7, 30; Sister Casualty, 'A Reformation', in *St. Bartholomew's League News* (May 1902), 134–8; South, *Hospital Nurses*, 16.

20 Sister Mary Aloysius Doyle, 'Memories of the Crimea', in Maria Luddy (ed.), *The Crimean Journals of the Sisters of Mercy* (Dublin, Four Courts Press, 2004), 20.

21 Cantlie, *Army Medical Department*, 2, 188.

22 *Parliamentary Papers*, 1854–55, vol. 20, 8, 11–12; Surgeon-General T. Longmore, *Gunshot Injuries* (London, Longmans Green, 1877), 202.

23 Cantlie, *Army Medical Department*, vol. 2, 188; Doyle, 'Memories', 22–3.

24 Longmore, *Gunshot Injuries*, 202.

25 Longmore, *Gunshot Injuries*, 203–5. 215–18, 394–6.

26 Timothy Gowing, *A Voice from the Ranks* (Nottingham, privately printed, 1886), 71–2, 86–7; S. Terrot, *Reminiscences of Scutari Hospitals in Winter 1854–55* (Edinburgh, Andrew Stevenson, 1898), 62, 65; Doyle, 'Memories', 19–22.

27 Cantlie, *Army Medical Department*, vol. 2, 20, 23.

28 John Shepherd, *The Crimean Doctors*, 2 vols (Liverpool, Liverpool University Press, 1991), vol. 1, 194–200; vol. 2, 341–8, 518.

29 See Maling, 'American Nightingales', 56–57.

30 T. Holmes, *A System of Surgery* (4 vols, London, Parker and Son, 1860), vol. 1, 220; Longmore, *Gunshot Injuries*, 207–8, 230, 237, 239, 253–4.

31 Longmore, *Gunshot Injuries*, 417–21, citation on 418.

32 Longmore, *Gunshot Injuries*, 212–14, 399.

33 G. J. Guthrie, *Commentaries on the Surgery of the War*, 6th edn (London, Henry Renshaw, 1855), 415–16.

34 G. J. Guthrie, *Commentaries*, 617; Cantlie, *Army Medical Department*, vol. 2, 189–91; Stanley, *Fear of Pain*, 59–69.

35 South, *Hospital Nurses*, 10.

36 Terrot, 'Reminiscences', 63.

37 J. W. Fortescue, *A History of the British Army*, 13 vols (London, Macmillan, 1899–1930), vol. 13, 158–9.

38 F. Prochaska, *Women and Philanthropy in Nineteenth Century England* (Oxford, Faber, 1980), 3–4, 14, 17.

39 A. W. Kinglake, *The Invasion of the Crimea*, 9 vols (Edinburgh, Blackwood, 1891), vol. 7, 359–60, 363.

40 'Diary of Sarah Anne Terrot', in Robert G. Richardson (ed.), *Nurse Sarah Anne: With Florence Nightingale at Scutari* (London, John Murray, 1977), 105.

41 Orlando Figes, *The Crimean War* (New York, Henry Holt, 2010), 147–9; Florence Nightingale Museum (FNM) LMA/H02/ST/NC8/1.

42 K. Theodore Hoppen, *The Mid-Victorian Generation 1846-86* (Oxford University Press, 1998), 179–80; Fortescue, *British Army*, vol. 13, 169–71.

43 *Parliamentary Papers*, 1854–55, vol. 9, 264, 282–3; *Parliamentary Papers*, 1854–55, vol. 20, 3, 11–12, 14, 37.

44 Piers Compton, *Colonel's Lady & Camp Follower* (London, Robert Hale, 1970), 79–80, 83–4, 103, 110, 145–6.

45 FNM/LMA/H01/ST/NC8/1.

46 *The Lancet*, 13 January 1855, 53.

47 Carol Helmstadter, 'Shifting boundaries', in *Nursing Inquiry* 16, 2 (2009), 137–8.

48 See Maling, 'American Nightingales', passim.

49 Mother Francis Bridgeman, 'Mission of the Sisters of Mercy', in Luddy, *The Crimean Journals*, 139; Archives of the Sisters of Mercy, Bermondsey, Annals, 1854, 251.

50 WI/Ms/8995/78; Harrison, *Drink and the Victorians*, 37–63, 306–07; Abel-Smith, *Nursing Profession*, 9–10.

51 See for example British Library Additional Manuscripts (BL Add Mss) 43402 fols 3–6, 12, 13; Helmstadter and Godden, *Nursing Before Nightingale*, 107–8, 110–11.

52 Florence Nightingale, 'Notes on the Health of the British Army', in Lynn McDonald (ed.), *Florence Nightingale: The Crimean* War (Waterloo, ON, Wilfrid Laurier Press, 2010), 743.

53 Cantlie, *Army Medical Department*, vol. 2, 71–2, 89.

54 *Parliamentary Papers*, 1854–55, vol. 33, 329–31, 342; Fanny Taylor, *Eastern Hospitals and English Nurses*, 2 vols (London, Hurst & Blackett, 1856), vol. 1, 73–8, 114–15.

55 Terrot, 'Reminiscences', 37–40, 64–5, 68–9; Taylor, *Eastern Hospitals*, vol. 1, 203–4; *Parliamentary Papers,* 1854–55, vol. 33, 32.

56 *Parliamentary Papers*, 1854–55, vol. 20, 40; *Parliamentary Papers*, 1854–55, vol. 9 Part 1: 671, Part 2: 680; Cantlie, *Army Medical Department*, vol. 2, 59.

57 *Parliamentary Papers*, 1854–55, vol. 33, 329–31, 342.

58 WI/Ms 8994/117; BL Add Mss 43393 fol 128; *Parliamentary Papers*, 1854–55, vol. 33, 32–3.

59 BL Add Mss 43393 fol 64.
60 *Parliamentary Papers*, 1854–55, vol. 33, 32–3.
61 Terrot, 'Reminiscences', 102.
62 Doyle, 'Memories', 57–8 [emphasis original].
63 Helmstadter and Godden, *Nursing Before Nightingale*, 20.
64 Martin J. Wiener, *Reconstructing the Criminal* (Cambridge University Press, 1990), 16–33, 35–45; M. J. D. Roberts, *Making English Morals* (Cambridge University Press, 2004), 3–16.
65 Helmstadter and Godden, *Nursing Before Nightingale*, 20–2; Shepherd, *Crimean Doctors*, vol. 2, 428–9, 431–2.
66 See for example Shepherd, *Crimean Doctors*, vol. 1, 283, vol. 2; 428–9, 431–2.
67 Charles Bryce, *England and France Before Sevastopol* (London, John Churchill, 1857), 67–73, citation on 69–70.
68 Bermondsey Annals, 1854, 251, 278–9.
69 Taylor, *Eastern Hospitals*, vol. 1, 13, 37; vol. 2, 13–14, citation on 14.
70 Martha Nicol, *Ismeer or Smyrna and its British Hospital in 1855* (London, James Madden, 1856), 85–6.
71 Douglas Hill (ed.), *Letters from the Crimea* (Dundee, Dundee University Press, 2010), 60.
72 Anne Summers, *Angels and Citizens*, 30.
73 *Parliamentary Papers*, 1854–55, vol. 9, Part 3: 188.

2

American Nightingales: The influence of Florence Nightingale on Southern nurses during the American Civil War

Barbara Maling

Florence Nightingale, through her reported remodelling of nursing in the inadequate British army medical services in the Crimea, gave a degree of dignity to nursing as a profession in the 1850s. Nightingale's inspiration was felt throughout the western world including the antebellum South in the United States. Prior to the American Civil War (1861–65) Southerners shared many British Victorian values including the thoughts that caring for strangers outside of domestic confines was largely regarded as employment appropriate for individuals of the lower classes and preferably of the male gender. In the military, nurses were usually detailed or disabled soldiers who fitted within military hierarchies. Nevertheless, during the war, as manpower shortages, escalating casualties and patriotic ambitions overrode custom, a number of middle- and upper-class Southern white women pushed conventional boundaries. They rendered nursing care to strangers outside of the home and found in Nightingale a model for nursing legitimatisation and female heroism. The purpose of this chapter is to discuss and analyse the influence that Florence Nightingale had on Southern women providing nursing care to Confederate (Southern) soldiers during the American Civil War. Issues of class, gender, the status of nursing, and the need for women to give nursing care are considered within the context of the American Civil War and the influences of Florence Nightingale.

On the eve of the American Civil War (1861–65) people around the world admired Florence Nightingale as a heroine who reportedly revolutionised the inadequate British army medical services in the

Crimea.[1] Her iconic image was fostered by her prolific publications. In 1859 Nightingale published *Notes on Hospitals* concerning the correlations between the construction and management of hospitals and death rates.[2] Her book, *Notes on Nursing*, was published the same year and an American edition was released in 1860 just before the outbreak of the American Civil War.[3] According to Nightingale, *Notes on Nursing* was meant to 'give hints for thought to women who have personal charge of the health of others'.[4] Together, these writings and Nightingale's work in the Crimea provided some dignity to nursing as a profession. Her contributions and innovations would become increasingly important in the Southern United States where nursing strangers outside of the home and in hospitals was given little respect.[5]

Wars frequently usher in change and this was certainly the case during the American Civil War. In the early 1860s, the United States was a nation divided. It was split between the Northern states that fought for continuation of the Union and the South (the Confederacy) that sought separation and division of the United States. A bloody four-year war would ensue between the North and South that resulted in countless civilian casualties and a conservative estimated death rate of at least 600,000 soldiers.[6] Like the British in the Crimea, illness rather than injuries caused most mortality.[7] Disease ultimately killed two out of every three Confederate soldiers; thousands were left with significant disabilities.[8] Armies experienced illness, infirmities and deaths of previously unimagined scale in American history. The Civil War initiated a new era in not only battlefield medicine but nursing as well.

Although Nightingale never visited the United States, her humanitarian reforms as well as her name became a part of the change that occurred in Southern nursing during this new era. It is not unusual to find references to Florence Nightingale in letters, memoirs, diaries and newspapers of the time. Her name became synonymous with respected white nursing care providers who were, at times, referred to as 'Nightingales'. An American newspaper, *The New York Herald*, declared in 1864:

> During the Crimean War England produced a single Florence Nightingale, and the fame of her good deeds spread to the ends of the earth. Here all our

women are Florence Nightingales. Every hamlet produces at least one – every large city a hundred. They may be found in our hospitals, ministering like angels to the victims of war, succouring the sick and comforting the wounded, relieving the distressed and bringing peace to the dying.[9]

An 1866 text, *Women of the War*, noted: 'Many loyal women along the vexed border, and within the lines of the enemy, exhibited a more than human courage ... In the hospital, and amid the stormy scenes of war, they [women] surpassed the charity of Florence Nightingale, and repeated the humility and gentle sacrifices recorded of Mary in the sacred Scriptures.'[10]

In another instance Mary Chesnut, an affluent Southern woman, known best for her lengthy memoir about the war and her intermittent nursing activities wrote: 'Every woman in the house is ready to rush into the Florence Nightingale business.'[11] It is unclear in Chesnut's memoir if she fully understood that the 'Florence Nightingale business' was a model for nursing reorganisation based on a blending of concepts from religious sisterhoods, military hierarchies, Nightingale's understanding of medical theories and a belief that a woman's nature made her a more suitable care-giver than a man.[12] Nevertheless, it is evident that Chesnut held Nightingale in high esteem and shared with her some cultural values such as a woman's innate nature for nursing.[13]

The concept of nursing being 'natural' to women was embedded in nineteenth-century American culture where nursing was considered a domestic labour for women. Nursing was almost always home-based and rendered by female relatives or women of 'good moral character with references'.[14] According to Susan Reverby in *Ordered to Care*:

> In the world of early nineteenth-century America, more defined by death and debility than our own, almost every woman could expect to spend some part of her life caring for relatives or friends. Within the domestic boundaries of antebellum women's lives, nursing played an important part as caring and sacrifice become a poignant manifestation of female virtue.[15]

What would be different with the outbreak of the American War was the idea of respectable women providing genuine nursing care to strangers outside of the home.[16] During the mid-nineteenth century nursing care providers outside of domestic environments in America as well as those in Britain were given little esteem. Charles Dickens presented a stereotypical portrayal of a nurse in 1840s England in the creation of his character Sairy Gamp in *Martin Chuzzlewit*. Gamp was a gin-swigging, dispassionate character who cared little for patients who were dependent on her for care.[17] Gamp became a notorious typecast of incompetent and uncaring hospital nurses of the Victorian era. Nightingale even reported the dismissal of several working-class nurses from Crimean service for habitual drunkenness.[18]

Across the Atlantic in America, the standing of hospital nurses was no better. In the military, nurses were usually common soldiers who were detailed to this work or recovering themselves, who had no nursing education, and who fit within the lower echelon of military structures.[19] In the Southern United States hospital nurses included not only those from lower classes but enslaved African American men and women at the bottom of antebellum hierarchies.[20] Matters were complicated further in this era because care was given in hospitals that were filthy, crowded buildings where the destitute and chronically ill received minimal care if no other option was available to them.[21] Thus, when the Civil War erupted, women throughout America faced opposition to serving in military hospitals based on the prevailing nineteenth-century societal views about 'proper' behaviour. Hospitals were certainly not places where respectable white Southern women of the middle and upper classes would usually dare to enter.[22]

It was not just Southern women, but Northern women too who were bound by nineteenth-century customs. Northern women, however, had less difficulty in dealing with the disapproval of society than did their Southern sisters.[23] The North had re-examined gender assumptions more than a generation earlier, as women's rights advocates began to destabilise traditional understandings of men's and women's roles.[24] Although many Northerners were reluctant to fully support women in nursing roles outside of the home, the disruption of traditional roles generally made the mobilisation of female nurses more acceptable. For example, an affluent white woman, Dorothea Dix, was appointed 'Superintendent of Women Nurses' for the Union. Dix was an open admirer of Nightingale and achieved a degree of cultural authority she had seen Nightingale win during the Crimean War.[25] In addition to appointing a Superintendent of Women Nurses, the Union structured an official agency, known as the United States Sanitary Commission. One of the primary goals of the United States Sanitary Commission was coordinating the volunteer efforts of Northern women, including those serving as nurses.[26]

In contrast, the Confederacy never developed the equivalent of the US Sanitary Commission and Southern women struggled with the constraints of society. When respectable Southern women began to offer their labour in Confederate military hospitals, they undertook a dramatic departure from the traditional white Southern female role. At the time of the Civil War, the understandings of female and male roles in Southern hierarchies had not undergone the evolutionary changes that were taking hold in the North. Indeed, antebellum societal views and patriarchal hierarchy hampered elite white Southern women as they attempted to work outside the home.[27] In 1861, when Ada Bacot, a 27-year-old widow from an elite southern family in South Carolina, stated that she was considering nursing, a local minister told her father to dissuade her as, "twas [sic] scarcely a place for a lady'.[28]

The war, however, changed the status quo and necessitated a re-examination of values and resources. The Confederacy was an agricultural region that had neither the population nor means (both natural and industrial) to wage a long-standing war. Renowned Civil War historian, Shelby Foot, stated: 'I think that the North fought that war with one hand behind its back. If the Confederacy ever had come close to winning on the battlefield, the North simply would have brought that other arm out from behind its back. I don't think the South ever had a chance to win that war.'[29] In addition, most Civil War battles occurred on Southern soil, transforming the Southern home front into battlegrounds. Thus, the totality of warfare was direct as well as crucial for Southern Americans.[30]

Morbidity and mortality rates escalated and were so immense that they could not be borne by traditional pre-professional Southern nurses alone.[31] For example, during the three-day battle of Gettysburg in 1863 there were over 51,000 casualties.[32] During the same year the two-day battle of Chickamauga had an estimated 36,000 casualties.[33] Just as Nightingale's experiences in the Crimea had altered the British's view of acceptable nursing care-givers, traditional views of nursing came into question with patriotic ambitions and possible solutions to dwindling resources in the South. The war necessarily challenged the base of antebellum hierarchies compelling Southerners to rethink their most fundamental norms about their identities.

Defying the convention that being a military nurse was not an appropriate occupation for a woman, Mrs Fannie A. Beer accompanied her husband's Confederate battalion from Virginia to Tennessee, working in makeshift hospitals as a matron. Living in suboptimal conditions, she reportedly sought food and supplies on her own to care and feed Southern soldiers.[34] On one occasion a physician requested her help with emergency care on a battlefield. Beer wrote of her experience:

> Dr. McAllister silently handed me two canteens of water, which I threw over my shoulder, receiving also a bottle of peach brandy. We then turned into a ploughed field, thickly strewn with men and horses, many stone dead, some struggling in the agonies of death … The dead lay around us on every side, singly and in groups and piles; men and horses, in some cases, apparently inextricably mingled. Some lay as if peacefully sleeping; others, with open eyes, seemed to glare at any who bent above them … they [Union and Confederate soldiers] seemed mere youths, and I thought sadly of the mothers, whose hearts would throb with equal anguish in a Northern and a Southern home … Several badly wounded men had been laid under the shade of some bushes a little farther on; our mission lay here. The portion of the field we crossed to reach this spot was in many places slippery with blood. The edge of my dress was red, my feet were wet with it. As we drew near the suffering men, piteous glances met our own …'Water' was the cry … taking from my pocket a small feeding-cup, which I always carried for use in the wards, I mixed some brandy and water, and, kneeling by one of the poor fellows … tried to raise his head. But he was already dying … The next seemed anxious for water, and drank eagerly … A third could only talk with his large, sad eyes, but made me clearly understand his desire for water. As I passed my arm under his head the red blood saturated my sleeve and spread in a moment over a part of my dress. So we went on, giving water, brandy, or soup; sometimes successful in reviving the patient, sometimes only able to whisper a few words of comfort to the dying.[35]

Not deterred, Beer's returned from the battlefield to her nursing duties in a Confederate military hospital the next day. She cared for both Southern and Northern troops who had suffered injuries.[36]

For women, working in a military hospital, or in Beer's case on a battlefield, was a drastic departure from traditional female roles in the South. Nevertheless, *The Mobile Advertiser and Register* noted in June of 1861: 'All the poetical phrases which describe woman as a ministering angel, fail to convey the idea of the wonderful new reality now enacting before our eyes.'[37] At the same time, other publication columnists openly expressed concern about the challenge of hospital work to Southern women's images. One journalist in *The Southern Monthly Magazine* even discussed these concerns in relation to the work of Florence Nightingale in the Crimea. In 1862, the author warned against regarding Nightingale as an exemplary for women, writing: 'Many of her eulogists have forgotten to place due limitations on their recommendation of her example.' Further, ladies should satisfy themselves with 'making clothes for soldiers' and 'providing comforts and delicacies' as 'such services can be performed without a doubt of their propriety'.[38]

Nightingale's example in the Crimea brought into question what constituted 'proper' behaviour for women in the South. Some Southern elite, such as Mary Chesnut, ignored society's views and did what they thought best. Others were unwilling to push cultural boundaries and remained comfortable with the standard restrictions of society. Louisa H. A. Minor, a prosperous white slaveholding woman in Charlottesville, choose a traditional route while her sister, Betty, began to work as a nurse. Minor wrote:

> Find sister Betty has two convalescent soldiers … Dr Lewis and Mr Taylor … both of them belong to the 11th Miss. Regiment they seem to be gentlemen and add much to our little circle poor fellows my heart aches for them, when they talk of their far off homes and kindred and how they hope and watch for the time when they can return.[39]

For Louisa Minor, it was more acceptable to work within the confines of social norms or women's organisations. The furthest Louisa Minor ventured out of her home environment was to visit wounded troops in local military hospitals.

Despite societal concerns about proper employment for women, the Civil War was the first American conflict in which a number of prosperous Southern women provided care to strangers in military hospitals. With an increasing need for labourers as the war escalated, on 29 January 1862 (eighteen months after the onset of the war), a special Confederate Congressional Investigational Committee met and noted that they were 'deeply impressed with the inadequacy of the preparations and provision for sick soldiers'.[40] To remedy the situation, the committee suggested several changes, one of which was the establishment of a Confederate nursing corps, owing to the fact that, in the committee's words, 'Good nursing is of equal value to medical attention.'[41] In addition, on 27 September 1862, the Confederate Congress passed an Act which allowed each hospital to employ two matrons (who acted as head nurses and nursing supervisors), and as many nurses as might be needed for each ward.[42] Because of an available source of women and the appreciation for their talents within the home, those in charge of hiring these newest additions to the hospitals were instructed to '[give] preference in all cases to females where their services may best serve the purpose'.[43]

Following the Nightingale model, white nurses (often referenced as matrons) were 'to exercise superintendence over the entire domestic economy of the hospital, to take charge of such delicacies as may be provided for the sick, to apportion them out as required, to see that the food or diet is properly prepared, and to carry out all such other duties as may be necessary'.[44] Indeed, many of the qualifications for matrons reflected Nightingale's philosophies. First, requirements for the job of nursing care providers included a pleasant demeanour, ladylike behaviour, intelligence and a willingness to work hard. Further, personal letters of recommendations regarding the women's moral character were also required.[45]

With the change in the alignment of care-givers, conflicts followed as military surgeons and officers resented the intrusion of women into military affairs. According to Phoebe Pember, a woman from a prosperous South Carolina family who nursed at Chimborazo, a large Confederate hospital in Richmond, Virginia, 'matrons had no official recognition, ranking even below stewards from a military point of view'.[46] Pember also reported that a physician talking to a peer and well within her range of hearing, stated in, 'a tone of ill-concealed disgust, that "one of them had come"'. Later, Pember's presence was referred to as 'petticoat government'.[47]

While struggling with their identities and coming to grips with their changing roles, a number of elite white Southern women found in Nightingale a degree of legitimisation for female nursing outside of the home and a notion that a woman's moral and emotional attributes uniquely suited her for hospital work. References to Nightingale can be found in the diaries of four of the most famous Southern pre-professional nursing care providers: Mary Chesnut, Sally Tompkins, Kate Cumming and Phoebe Pember.

In her memoirs, Phoebe Pember casually speaks of Nightingale as if her name was part of everyday conversation. Travelling hundreds of miles from her home to provide care at Chimborazo Hospital, Pember wrote:

> The surgeon naturally thought that I had some experience, and would use the power the law of Congress gave me to arrange my own department; and I, in reading the bill passed for the introduction of matrons into hospitals, could only understand that the position was one which dove-tailed the offices of housekeeper and cook, nothing more. In the meanwhile the soup was boiling, and was undeniably a success from the perfume it exhaled. Nature may not have intended me for a Florence Nightingale, but a kitchen proved my worth.[48]

Sally Tompkins also mentioned Nightingale in her memoirs. After the first Battle of Manassas in 1861, Tompkins established her own private hospital in Richmond Virginia, the capital of the Confederacy, and was the only woman to be commissioned as an officer in either the army of the Confederacy or the Union.[49] It is not known if Tompkins directly modelled her hospital after recommendations made by Nightingale. Nevertheless, like the hospitals Nightingale reorganised in the Crimea, Tompkins's hospital developed a reputation for low mortality rates, cleanliness, and a 'blend of compassion and tight discipline'.[50] Although Tompkins used men and slaves in the care of soldiers in her hospital,[51] it seems that she may have agreed with Nightingale's philosophies of the gender division of labour, with nursing best suited to a woman's nature. After the war she commented: 'Sometimes I read about others in my profession – Florence Nightingale, Clara Barton and two writers turned nurse, Louisa M. Alcott and Walt Whitman, the latter most disturbing.'[52]

Mary Chesnut, a member of the privileged and educated slave-owning class of the Confederate South who socialised with the South's most elite including the president of the Confederacy, Jefferson Davis and his wife, refers to fellow nursing providers as 'Nightingales' in her memoirs.[53] Examples include: 'I had only encountered Mrs. Web, our Florence Nightingale, at her hospital on 12th Street and there she is the center of sweet charities and a bright sample of all the Christian virtues.' When referring to Sally Tompkins, Chestnut wrote: 'A rose by any other name – that is, our Florence Nightingale – Sally Tompkins. Went to her hospital today.'[54]

Chesnut's examples of fellow nurses such as Web and Tompkins may have drawn her to nursing duties. After 'fainting fits' in a Richmond Hospital, Chesnut stated that she deemed it wise to, 'do my hospital work from the outside', by raising supplies.[55] Later, however, she returned to intermittent nursing duties until the war ended in 1865. Chesnut did not seem to fear for her propriety or the propriety of older nurses, but it was evident that she held some class and gender values of the antebellum South. She commented that she did not like to see younger ladies, particularly unmarried women, exposed to the scrutiny and the comments of common soldiers, who too often showed insufficient respect for female delicacy stating: 'I cannot bear young girls to go to hospitals, wayside or otherwise.'[56] Chesnut was, of course, referring to white upper- and middle-class women in her memoirs.

A vigorous upholder of a woman's right to work as a nurse was a single, Scottish-born Southerner, Kate Cumming. Cumming's own family opposed her work despite the fact that two of her sister's female in-laws had nursed with Florence Nightingale in the Crimea.[57] Undaunted, she entered service with the Confederate Army of Tennessee in April 1862 and immediately encountered some hostility from the men around her. Writing about the incident in her memoirs she stated that there was, 'a good deal of trouble about the ladies in some of the hospitals of this department. Our friends here have advised us to go home, as they say it is not considered respectable.'[58]

Cumming's family may have questioned the propriety of her new position, but the possibility of alleviating some of the terrible suffering she had witnessed and the model of Florence Nightingale reinforced her determination. 'It seems strange', she wrote, 'that the aristocratic women of Great Britain have done with honor what is a disgrace for their sisters on this side of the Atlantic to do.'[59] Sharing with Nightingale the belief that nurses required a strong moral character and nursing knowledge, Cumming stated after the battle of Shiloh in April 1862 and faced with close to 11,000 Confederate casualties:

> We have men for nurses ... they are detailed from the different regiments, like guards. We have a new set every few hours. I cannot see how it is possible for them to take proper care of the men, as nursing is a thing that has to be learned and we should select our best men for it – the best, not physically, but morally.[60]

In summary, the circumstances of the American Civil War including manpower shortages, escalating casualty rates and patriotic motivations necessitated the re-evaluation of using white females in nursing roles. Female nurses such as Sally Tompkins may have moulded the care they provided on recommendations outlined by Nightingale including the importance of care provided by women of good moral character, gender division of labour, and the importance of diet and clean and well ventilated environments. Despite some liberties, many Southern women, like Louisa Minor, struggled with their identities and remained tied to traditional customs. In fact, there is little documentation that Nightingale's influence was enough to overcome Southern culture during the war or at its termination for many Southerners.[61] Nevertheless, the image of Florence Nightingale as a saviour of the British army was prevalent for literate white women. Nightingale's example and accomplishments played a part in the thinking of women such as Pember, Cumming, Chesnut and Tompkins, influencing them to temporarily overcome societal restrictions inherent in Southern values.

Recognised as a respectable woman of high social standing, Nightingale had, through her actions and her widely read *Notes on Nursing*, established legitimacy for female nursing outside of the home. Although nineteenth-century feminism, at the onset of the American Civil War, exerted little impact in the South, the notion that a woman's moral and emotional attributes uniquely fitted her for nursing gained momentum during the war. This view was certainly fuelled by need as the majority of Civil War battles occurred on southern soil and as an agricultural society the South lacked natural resources or the sheer number of people required for an extended conflict. Nevertheless, numerous middle- and upper-class Southern women braved the frowns of those around them and negotiated difficult cultural boundaries to give care to those in need. Providing a degree of dignity to nursing, women found a model for female heroism in Nightingale that might have been as Phoebe Pember stated 'inappropriate under different circumstances'.[62]

Notes

1 Mark Bostridge, *Florence Nightingale: The Making of an Icon* (New York, Farrar, Straus and Giroux, 2008). Mark Bostridge is a Gladstone Memorial Prize Winner from Oxford University. His biography of Florence Nightingale is well researched and respected. Bostridge references a wealth of unpublished material, including previously unseen family papers, to throw new light on Nightingale's extraordinary accomplishments as a woman and iconic figure in the nineteenth century.

2 Sarah Southall Tooley, *The Life of Florence Nightingale* (New York, Cassell and Company, Ltd, 1914), 276; Florence Nightingale, *Notes on Hospitals*, 3rd edn (London, Longman, Green, Longman, Roberts, and Green, 1863), p. v (preface). In 1859 Florence Nightingale published *Notes on Hospitals*. The basis for this publication was a paper she prepared for the British Social Science Association. Her book investigated the influences and correlations that hospital construction and management had on mortality rates. In 1863 *Notes on Hospitals* was reprinted in a larger edition. Nightingale opens *Notes on Hospitals* with: 'It may seem a strange principle to enunciate as the very first requirement in a hospital that it should do the sick no harm.'

3 Florence Nightingale, *Notes on Nursing: What It Is and What It Is Not*, Introductions by Dunbar and Dolan (New York, Dover Publications, Inc., 1969). The first American edition of *Notes on Notes* was published by D. Appleton and Company in New York. Another reference concerning Nightingale's publication of the American version of *Notes on Nursing* is in Susan Reverby, *Ordered to Care: The Dilemma of American Nursing, 1850–1945* (New York and Cambridge, Cambridge University Press, 1987), 44.

4 Nightingale, *Notes on Nursing*, iv (preface).

5 Reverby, *Ordered to Care*, 41.

6 James McPherson, *Battle Cry of Freedom: The Civil War Era* (New York, Ballantine Book, 1988). McPherson's account of the American Civil War is considered a classic by many. Written in a clear and intellectual manner, it won the Pulitzer Prize shortly after publication. For other classic references on the American Civil War, see S. Foote, *The Civil War: A Narrative, Fort Sumter to Perryville* (New York: Vintage Books, 1986); S. Foote, *The Civil*

War: A Narrative, Fredericksburg to Meridian (New York: Vintage Books, 1986); and S. Foote, *The Civil War: A Narrative, Red River to Appomattox* (New York, Vintage Books, 1986).

7 John Shepherd, *The Crimean Doctors*, 2 vols (Liverpool, Liverpool University Press, 1991), vol. 1, 194–200; vol. 2, 341–8 and 518.

8 Wyndham Blanton, *Medicine in Virginia in the Nineteenth Century* (Richmond, VA, Garrett & Massie, Inc., 1933), 291–7.

9 *The New York Herald*, Tuesday Edition, #10.062, 15 April 1864.

10 Frank Moore, *Women of the War* (Hartford, CT, S. S. Scranton & Co., 1866), 17–18.

11 Mary Chesnut, *Mary Chesnut's Civil War*, ed. C. Vann Woodward (New Haven, CT, Yale University Press, 1981), 85.

12 Lynn McDonald, *Florence Nightingale: the Crimean War* (ONT, Wilfrid Laurier University Press, 2010); and Barbara Dossey, *Florence Nightingale: Mystic, Visionary, Healer* (Springhouse, PA, Springhouse Corporation, 2000). There are numerous references written on Florence Nightingale. The above list is by no means complete.

13 Chesnut, *Mary Chesnut's War*, 85, 161 and 530.

14 Charles Rosenberg, *The Care of Strangers: The Rise of America's Hospital System* (New York, Basic Books Inc., 1987), 15–46.

15 Reverby, *Ordered to Care*, 11.

16 Carol Green, *Chimborazo: The Confederacy's Largest Hospital* (Knoxville, TN, The University of Tennessee Press, 2004), 44–6; Richard Hall, *Women on the Civil War Battlefront* (Lawrence, KS, University Press of Kansas, 2006), 18–24; Drew Faust, *Mothers of Invention: Women of the Slaveholding South in the American Civil War* (Chapel Hill, NC, The University of North Carolina Press, 1996), 92.

17 Charles Dickens, *Martin Chuzzlewit*, Oxford World Classics, reprinted with foreword notes by Margaret Cardwell (Oxford, Oxford University Press, 2011), 265, 269, 270–9, 313 and 333; Donald Hawes, *Who's Who in Dickens* (London, Routledge, 1998), 84–6.

18 Brian Abel-Smith, *A History of the Nursing Profession* (London, Heinemann, 1964), 8–9. See also Carol Helmstadter, 'Class, gender and professional expertise: British military nursing in the Crimean War', in this book, regarding the drinking habits of British society and government nurses in the late nineteenth century.

19 Green, *Chimborazo*, 41–63.

20 James Brewer, *The Confederate Negro: Virginia's Craftsmen and Military Laborers, 1861–1865* (Tuscaloosa, AL, The University of Alabama Press, 1969), 95–130.

21 Reverby, *Ordered to Care*, 22–6.

22 Jane Schultz, *Women at the Front: Hospital Workers in Civil War America* (Chapel Hill, NC, The University of North Carolina Press, 2004), 50.

23 Elizabeth Fox-Genovese, *Within the Plantation Household: Black and White Women of the Old South – Gender and American Culture* (Durham, NC, The University of North Carolina Press, 1988); Catherine Clinton, *The Plantation Mistress: Women's World in the Old South* (New York, Pantheon Books, 1982).

24 Schultz, *Women at the Front*, 49.

25 Thomas J. Brown, *Dorothea Dix New England Reformer* (Boston, MA, Harvard University Press, 1998).

26 William Maxwell, *Lincoln's Fifth Wheel: The Political History of the United States Sanitary Commission* (New York, Longmans, Green & Co., 1956). The US Sanitary Commission was modelled after the Royal or British Sanitary Commission. Influenced by Nightingale, the British Sanitary Commission's goal was to see that better care was provided for soldiers and to press the English government to live up to its responsibilities for wounded British soldiers. These goals were shared by the US Sanitary Commission, which was an official agency of the United States government (created by legislation and signed by President of the United States, Abraham Lincoln), on 18 June 1861. It coordinated the volunteer efforts of women who wanted to contribute to the war effort of the Union states during the American Civil War. Preaching the virtues of clean water, good food, and fresh air the US Sanitary Commission pressured the Army Medical Department to improve sanitation, build large well-ventilated hospitals, and encourage women to join the newly created nursing corps.

27 Clinton, *The Plantation Mistress*; George Rable, *Women and the Crisis of Southern Nationalism* (Urbana, IL, University of Illinois, 1989); Schultz, *Women at the Front*. There are numerous references that address traditional antebellum views related to Southern women in service related jobs outside of the home. It should be noted that there is significant dispute among references concerning the actual number of Southern women who provided nursing care during the American Civil War.

28 Ada Bacot, *Confederate Nurse*, ed. Jean V. Berlin (Columbia, SC, University of South Carolina Press, 1994), 56.

29 Shelby Foote quoted in Kenneth Lauren Burns' documentary, *The Civil War*, 1990.

30 McPherson, *Battle Cry of Freedom*. McPherson is given as a reference in this chapter although hundreds of resources are available and confirm that most of the fighting during the American Civil War took place on Southern soil. War action in the South created many hardships for Southerners as their homes were transformed into battlefronts.

31 McPherson, *Battle Cry of Freedom*, 478–89.

32 Stephen W. Sears, *Gettysburg* (New York, Houghton Mifflin Company, 2004), 226, 239–40, 350–1, 467–9.

33 McPherson, *Battle Cry of Freedom*, 674–5.

34 Hall, *Women on the Civil War Battlefront*, 33–4.
35 Fannie A. Beers, *Memories: A Record of Personal Experience and Adventure during Four Years of War*, Kindle edn, 23 March 2011 (Philadelphia, J. B. Lippincott, 1888), 152–7.
36 Beers, *Memories*, 157.
37 *The Mobile Advertiser and Register* (1862), 11 June.
38 *The Southern Monthly Magazine* (1862), May.
39 *The Minor Diary* (1861), 18 and 24 August. This unpublished short diary is located in the *Minor Records* at the Albert and Shirley Small Library, University of Virginia, Charlottesville, Virginia, USA.
40 T. N. Waul, 'Special Report of the Committee appointed to examine into Quartermaster's, commissary and Medical Departments', 29 January 1862, US War Department, *War of the Rebellion: A Compilation of the Official Records of the Union and Confederate Armies* (Washington, DC, Government Printing Office, 1880–91), series 4, vol. 1, 883.
41 Horace Cunningham, *Doctors in Gray: The Confederate Medical Service* (Baton Rouge, LA, Louisiana State University Press), 73.
42 Cunningham, *Doctors in Gray*, 73.
43 Cunningham, *Doctors in Gray*, 72–3.
44 Phoebe Pember, *A Southern Woman's Story*, ed. George C. Rable (Columbia, SC, University of South Carolina Press, 2002), 15.
45 Green, *Chimborazo*, 50.
46 Pember, *A Southern Woman's Story*, 4.
47 Phoebe Pember, 'Reminiscences of a Southern hospital: By its matron', *The Cosmopolite* 1, 1 (January 1866), 70–89. The first page of Pember's memoir notes that it was copyrighted in 1865 by T. C. DeLeon in Maryland.
48 Pember, 'Reminiscences of a Southern hospital', 70–89.
49 John Coski, 'Stroll through the streets or through the collections to meet the women of wartime Richmond', *The Museum of the Confederacy Magazine* (spring 2010), 18–21.
50 Coski, 'Stroll through the streets', 19.
51 Keppel Hagerman, *Dearest of Captains: A Biography of Sally Louisa Tompkins* (Richmond, VA, Brandylane Publishers, 1996), p. 32. In her memoirs, Tompkins recognised the help of soldiers and gave brief references concerning the utilisation of black labour to assist her in nursing duties. Tompkins wrote that she had help from 'My faithful helpers … Phoebe, my beloved Mammy, and also from the two Betsy's'. Explaining how hard her African American staff worked, Tompkins noted that they laboured 'long hours at grim and dirty work, assisted by one steward'.
52 Hagerman, *Dearest of Captains*, 72.
53 Chesnut, *Mary Chesnut's Civil War*, 85, 161 and 530.
54 Chesnut, *Mary Chesnut's Civil War*, 661.
55 Chesnut, *Mary Chesnut's Civil War*, 372.

56 Chesnut, *Mary Chesnut's Civil War*, 668.
57 Kate Cumming, *Kate: The Journal of a Confederate Nurse*, ed. Richard Harwell (Baton Rouge, LA, Louisiana State University Press, 1998), xii.
58 Kate Cumming, *A Journal of Hospital Life in the Confederate Army of Tennessee: From the Battle of Shiloh to the End of the War* (Louisville, KY, Morgan and Company, 1866), 44.
59 Cumming, *A Journal of Hospital Life in the Confederate Army of Tennessee*, 44.
60 Cumming, *The Journal of a Confederate Nurse*, 16.
61 Faust, *Mothers of Invention*, 107 and 109.
62 Pember, *A Southern Woman's Story*, 90.

3

Traversing the veldt with 'Tommy Atkins': The clinical challenges of nursing typhoid patients during the Second Anglo-Boer War (1899–1902)

Charlotte Dale

The decades following the Crimean War witnessed a burgeoning of personal narratives relating accounts of nurses who ministered to combatants in the Franco-Prussian and Anglo-Zulu wars.[1] From these, the general public could vicariously experience the working lives of those who travelled far and wide to care for the common working-class soldier, immortalised by Rudyard Kipling in the early 1890s as 'Tommy Atkins'.[2] By the time of the Second Anglo-Boer War in 1899, nurses could access the sphere of war as part of the Army Nursing Service, the Army Nursing Service Reserve, or as civilian nurses employed locally in South Africa.[3] Such nurses, not only as professional practitioners, but also as women, wished to prove their ability to survive the hardships of war on an equal footing with their male counterparts as 'real citizens'.[4] Nurses frequently relocated to wherever 'Tommy' required skilled care provision across the South African veldt: the wide-open rural spaces where battle often took place. This chapter examines the challenges faced by nurses caring for the thousands of soldiers suffering as a result of the typhoid epidemics that infected the ranks of the army. Many of the nurses' personal testimonies detail how the contemporary army medical service was deficient in meeting the complex care needs of those suffering from typhoid fever and how greater numbers of nurses were required to care for the sick and wounded in times of war and peace.[5]

Civilian nurses in the sphere of war

Owing to a shortage of nurses within the regular Army Nursing Service and the Reserve, hundreds of civilian nurses were hastily enrolled for service in South Africa.[6] Reports of ever-increasing numbers of soldiers afflicted by typhoid fever led many civilians to join the ranks of the Reserve or to find their own means of accessing the sphere of war. One such nurse was New Zealand born Emily Peter, who had undergone nurse training at the Westminster Hospital in 1891 before working as a private nurse.[7] Although the New Zealand government did not officially recruit nurses for military service, many nurses, including Peter, volunteered with private funding. Typhoid fever, also known as enteric fever at the time of the Anglo-Boer War was one of the key reasons cited by British nurse Eleanor Laurence, who had decided as early as 1883 that she would obtain the Royal Red Cross award, for enlisting:

> I couldn't stand it any longer; all my friends were going off to the front; and, though many people said the war would be over before they landed, we kept hearing accounts of how bad the enteric was, and that the nurses were being overworked, so I felt I must at least offer to lend a hand.[8]

The personal testimonies of Reserve nurse Edith Hancock who trained at St Bartholomew's in London, Emily Wood of the Glasgow Infirmary who joined the Scottish Red Cross Hospital and Kate Driver, a South African born nurse who joined the Natal Volunteers in support of British troops are also examined here.[9]

When the nurses arrived in South Africa they were faced with having to adapt to life under canvas and exposure to the dangerous wildlife including snakes, scorpions and tarantulas.[10] These, however, were not the only difficulties that civilian nurses would face as they travelled widely to various stationary and base hospitals. Nurses soon found that the clinical care they were to deliver was not primarily to the wounded in battle as some had expected, but to the malnourished and exhausted soldiers who had fallen victim to the epidemics of typhoid fever.[11]

Clinical challenges: the typhoid epidemic

In times of war armies have fought campaigns not only against the enemy, but also against the damaging presence of disease.[12] As Kevin Brown, author of *Fighting Fit: Health Medicine and War in the Twentieth Century* states: 'War and typhoid, often known as enteric fever, were old companions.'[13] During the Anglo-Boer War military medical historians Richard Gabriel and Karen Metz assert that 6,000 men died from enemy fire while a further 16,000 died from disease, predominantly typhoid and dysentery.[14] A vaccine had been developed by Almroth Wright, the Professor of Pathology at Netley Military Hospital in Southampton, initially trialled in 1897 on the inmates of a 'lunatic asylum' in Kent.[15] Despite the availability of a vaccine, Phillip D. Curtain states that less than 4 per cent of the British army was inoculated, perhaps owing to suspicions voiced by army doctors and the sometimes violent and adverse side effects of the vaccine.[16] As a consequence, Gabriel and Metz claim that 74,000 soldiers experienced enteric and dysentery, with over 8,000 dying from enteric fever alone.[17] Thus, the nursing of patients with typhoid was to comprise the greater part of the nurses' work in South Africa, with the Anglo-Boer War subsequently described by medical historians as 'the last of the typhoid campaigns'.[18]

Typhoid fever had traditionally been confused with typhus fever (a louse-borne disease), owing to certain similarities in disease aetiology. It was eventually identified, via post-mortem examinations, that in the body of a typhoid sufferer the Peyers glands within the intestines were invariably diseased, unlike those with typhus and that it was contracted through drinking contaminated water, or from the excretions of those already infected.[19] The first symptoms of typhoid fever would typically present as general weakness, headache, chills, loss of appetite and a disorder of the stomach and bowels. This was recognised as the 'invasion' stage, occurring during the first or second weeks of infection and coinciding with a rash of red spots on the trunk. With typhoid fever, the nurses' initial concern was the risk of haemorrhage in the bowels, liable to occur during the second to fourth week of the illness. Following this, the primary concern was the possible perforation of the bowel, which could occur because of constant ulceration, reducing bowel lining to the thickness of paper.[20]

If perforation occurred the outcome of typhoid fever was usually death. In 1899 Dr J. K. Watson detailed the condition and presentation of a typhoid patient for the education of nurses:

> There is great muscular weakness, and the pulse is almost or quite imperceptible … and passes his urine and faeces under him. His lips are parched and covered with crusts (sordes), and the tongue is dry and glazed. The abdomen is probably distended, from accumulation of flatus. Breathing is irregular, and the 'cheyne-stokes' type of respiration may be present. Bed sores are very apt to form.[21]

The nursing care described in contemporary textbooks like Watson's demanded 24-hour care provision. In critical cases nurses were required to monitor temperature precisely and hourly via the axilla, taking five to ten minutes to register accurately, as this was indicative of haemorrhage.[22] The symptomatic treatment of diarrhoea would have been primarily with oral opium, or delivered by enema if combined with starch, while acetate of lead, sulphuric acid, or chalk and iron were sometimes used.[23] Those suffering from diarrhoea would have required careful monitoring of pressure areas and the regular changing of bed linen as contemporary accounts stated typhoid patients often defecated up to seventeen or eighteen times a day.[24] Bedsores were accordingly a risk, therefore regular repositioning, powdering the back with zinc and starch before rubbing with spirit or egg whites to harden the skin were frequent and time-consuming methods of prevention.[25] Nursing typhoid patients required knowledgeable trained nurses who had been educated as to the rationale for symptomatic treatment and the precepts of 'careful nursing'.[26] Careful sanitation and 'careful nursing' were recognised as requisite to the recovery of typhoid patients at this period.[27] Therese Meehan discusses how careful nursing was developed during the nineteenth century with a key aim to relieve distress by keeping all 'patients as clean and comfortable as possible, administering food, fluids and palliatives'.[28] Moreover, careful nursing necessitated a considerable complement of capable trained nurses to administer this care to the increasing numbers of soldiers infected with typhoid fever.

During the Anglo-Boer War two serious typhoid epidemics occurred in the besieged garrisons at Ladysmith and Bloemfontein, with claims that there were no fewer than 5,000 hospital cases and often up to forty deaths per day.[29] The epidemics were caused not solely by deficient sanitation, but also by a neglect of basic hygiene with troops observed to obtain drinking water from streams and rivers contaminated by the carcasses of dead horses.[30] At Ladysmith, Kate Driver remarked that the whole camp 'reeked of dysentery and enteric' owing to an 'erratic' water supply, and that 'disinfectants were very scarce'.[31] Queen Victoria's own surgeon, Frederick Treves detailed in his account of working on the veldt, *The Tale of a Field Hospital*, that, 'The water is the colour of pea-soup, and when in a glass is semi-opaque and a faint brownish colour. The facetious soldier, as he drinks it, calls it "khaki and water".'[32] The problem of how to address this crisis was considered by Dr Leigh Canney who had previously served with the army in Egypt. Canney believed a Royal Water Corps was necessary to ensure 'approved' water was always available to protect soldiers from typhoid, which he called the 'destroyer of armies'.[33] However, this was not to occur during the Anglo-Boer War.

Edith Hancock, writing to her family about the typhoid epidemic, stated that Bloemfontein was a 'death trap' and that, 'one cannot grasp the amount of Enteric that is amongst our troops ... The medical work to be done out here is tremendous, but they are all sick[.] I have not seen any wounded yet.'[34] Trained nurses such as Hancock were essential to nurse the 'tremendous' numbers of sick. Owing to the high prevalence of typhoid fever, historian Anne Summers asserts that efficient nursing was paramount to the successful recovery of those infected as:

> the damage done, a large and experienced nursing staff was essential to the care of gastro-enteric sufferers. Patients needed food and medicine; to be kept clean; to be kept in bed; to be kept from getting dehydrated; to be kept apart. In short, they needed constant attention and supervision; and in the end, successful nursing was largely a matter of numbers.[35]

In spite of this, large numbers of nurses were not available to provide 'constant attention' and 'successful nursing'.[36] At Kroonstadt, Emily Wood was required not only to complete her own nursing duties but also those of the orderlies whom she found to be inadequately trained to meet the complex care needs of typhoid patients.[37]

The male orderlies who served during the war came from various backgrounds and included trained orderlies of the Royal Army Medical Corps (RAMC), the St John Ambulance (SJAB) volunteers and convalescent soldiers who were often recruited to assist on the wards.[38] The trained RAMC orderlies were the elite as the SJAB orderlies had only undergone five lectures on nursing.[39] The orderlies were required to work long arduous hours and were severely under-manned, and although many such as the RAMC orderlies were excellent care providers the ever-increasing numbers of sick found them to be insufficient in number.[40]

Driver consequently recorded in her diary that typhoid patients 'needed the best nursing that could be given, and [that] there were so few to nurse them'.[41] The 'best nursing', as discussed by Driver, necessitated 'special' individual nursing and 24-hour care provision. Eleanor Laurence commented specifically upon the nurse's role in the successful recovery of typhoid patients acknowledging that it was, 'day and night work for us the first two or three days; as each man seemed to need individual nursing if he was to have any chance of pulling round'. But she was happy to do this as, 'we can feel we are actually saving the lives of some of these men by sheer hard nursing, and that is good enough for me'.[42] Prior to the universal introduction of intravenous therapy for the replacement of fluid and the administration of medications, fluids were administered orally or in the case of those patients who could take nothing by mouth, by enema.[43] Carol Helmstadter and Judith Godden state that nurses would have given one to two ounces of fluid every one to two hours, administering a variety of nutritive mixtures.[44] In extreme cases some attempts were made to provide fluids via naso-gastric tubes or by 'transfusion' of saline, but nurses in the personal testimonies did not discuss such practices.[45] The feeding of patients and the provision of oral fluids was therefore especially necessary at night and formed a core part of nursing care.[46] The journal, *Nursing Notes* considered how the dearth of trained nurses alongside the intensive nature of clinical work impacted on those nursing typhoid patients with, 'many themselves fallen victims … and more have been utterly overdone by heavy work and the heart-breaking feeling that, work as hard as they might, they were insufficient in numbers to cope with the rush of cases'.[47]

The boundaries of practice: deficiencies in the army medical system

Insufficient numbers meant that nurses in South Africa were over-worked and overburdened owing to the intensive regime of nursing those with typhoid fever. Nurses were required at the bedside throughout the day and night, moving the patient to prevent bed sores, keeping him clean, monitoring his temperature, pulse and respiration rate, and providing him with regular nourishment. Many nurses recounted how they were required to work all night as well as all day caring for those too sick to be left with untrained orderlies.[48] SJAB orderly W. S. Inder observed the problems that consequently occurred when the 'typhoid monster raised its head', and how all systems of working were 'rudely hustled'.[49] Inder stated that a 'fever case takes as much nursing and attention as would be needed for twenty wounded, and the attendant was lucky who escaped the terror himself'.[50]

It was a frequent complaint of the civilian nurses that army nurses delegated too many nursing tasks to male orderlies, risking the lives of those in their care. However, since the period of the Crimean War, army nurses had been employed for the principal purpose of supervision. Florence Nightingale concluded in her *Subsidiary Notes as to the Introduction of Female Nursing into Military Hospitals in Peace and in War* that, 'Nobody ever contemplated giving to a Nurse the entire charge of a number of sick in a Military General Hospital. It is no part of good Hospital nursing to do so. With proper Orderlies, a Nurse can very well attend to sixty or seventy sick.'[51] Emily Peter described the neglect of a typhoid patient for whom Peter and another nurse had been providing 24-hour care to and raised concerns regarding the capabilities of some orderlies to provide skilled nursing. Peter stated that:

> We did work so hard to save him for his mother, and to think that he should be killed after all. Nurse Cameron told me Sister Bond did not go on as I did, but gave her orders to the orderly and left him to his tender mercies most of the time. Hundreds were murdered through carelessness and ignorance.[52]

It is apparent that Peter believed her young typhoid patient, when left to the ministrations of the 'ignorant orderlies', was 'simply murdered' for he had been making a promising recovery prior to Peter's relocation to another camp. Peter's accusation of 'murder' was perhaps a case of personal sensationalism as there are no recorded official concerns. However, it was recognised that some untrained male orderlies were 'quite unfit to be left in charge of enteric patients' following accounts of their feeding bread and butter to those whose intestines were severely damaged, resulting in death.[53] As a consequence of anxieties raised over the standards of care provision a Royal Commission was sanctioned in 1901 to investigate and report on the care and treatment of the sick and wounded.

Peter evidently believed that the current army system in which army nurses supervised and delegated tasks to orderlies, some of whom lacked the requisite training, was deficient.[54] Yet Summers points out that nurses of the Reserve tended to be more biased in their criticisms against male orderlies, a bias perhaps owing to the fact that female nurses held no authority over orderlies, a prevalent theme featuring in many nurses' testimonies, which may have been used as a vehicle in the arguments for trained nurses to be given authority in the future.[55] Nevertheless, although some nurses' do proffer critical accounts of the work of the orderlies, many also testify that not all orderlies were inadequately trained for their role, nor were they all uncaring.[56] Many of the RAMC trained orderlies were excellent at their work but were hindered by the complex way the system was run, alongside the fact that the Corps was undermanned, necessitating the recruitment of untrained convalescent soldiers to nurse the sick.[57] *The Nursing Record* mirrored this sentiment asserting that female nurses 'existed somewhat under sufferance, and in numbers totally insufficient to carry out nursing as it is understood in civil hospitals', stating further that the 'so-called trained orderlies are as a matter of fact, not in the least competent, from the training point of view, to do the work they are called upon to undertake'.[58] Irrespective of whether orderlies were competent or not, such statements were used to support arguments that trained nurses should be employed in greater numbers in times of war and to be involved in the training of orderlies in times of peace.

The civilian nurses also perceived the army hospitals as not being up to the standard of civilian hospitals in the United Kingdom. A civilian nurse, maintaining her anonymity by using the pseudonym Sister X in her published memoirs, found working at the College

Hospital in Maritzburg to be 'very tiresome', claiming that it was impossible 'to get anything done, as we, in our civil hospital had been accustomed to have them done as a matter of routine'.[59] Laurence had been anxious to observe the conditions within the army hospitals, but on visiting the Military Hospital in Natal she found the wards to be dirty and untidy, with food from previous meals left on patients' lockers and covered with flies. Laurence was surprised at this, considering typhoid fever to be rife in the camp and she believed the state of the hospital to be 'a great source of danger'.[60] Deficient sanitary precautions were accordingly a key concern of nurses. On arrival at the No. 1 Stationary Field Hospital at Modder Spruit Peter soon discovered that:

> There is no water for anything; the patients simply have their faces and hands washed in water that is quite green, got out of holes somewhere near the camp. Body lice abound everywhere, there is no water to wash the bedpans, and the tins they drink out of are rinsed twice a day in this same dirty water.[61]

The shortage of water was also apparent in Bloemfontein with the result that patients remained covered with 'pediculi, far worse than in a receiving room in the East end'.[62] The scarcity of water risked the further spread of infection by cross-contamination. Sister X claimed certain orderlies omitted to obtain fresh water to wash each patient and that when one patient thanked her for making him 'feel washed', Sister X asked why he didn't always:

> 'Well, it is this way, Sister,' chimed in a fellow-sufferer, 'they won't be bothered to get fresh water each time, so they wash us all in the same water – such a drop too!'[63]

Yet a dearth of water was a frequent consequence of the mobile nature of military nursing on the veldt. Some nurses recorded their dismay at discovering how easily staff members were risking the spread of typhoid by sharing equipment between patients.[64] Peter stated that it was impossible to obtain anything for the patients, 'no towels to sponge a man, you have to borrow the towel of another who is lucky enough to have one of his own, if you want to do that'.[65] One soldier nursed by male orderlies could not understand how more patients at a hospital in Wynberg did not contract typhoid, as they all 'had to drink milk out of the same glass, and have our temperatures taken with the same thermometer as the enteric patients, the thermometer being taken out of the mouth of an enteric case and put, unwashed, straight into the mouth of a wounded man'.[66] Canadian nurse Georgina Fane Pope remarked that 'a field hospital for 100 is being used for 700 and there is one horn medicine glass for the whole hospital'.[67]

Yet all these extreme accounts may have related more to the unexpected exigencies of war than examples of outright neglect or ignorance of the principles of germ theory. By this period trained nurses were aware of the methods of antisepsis, with textbooks detailing the dangers of putrefactive changes to wounds and the substances that could be used to inhibit them, namely antiseptics: – *anti*, against; *sepsis*, putrefaction.[68] The precepts of antisepsis first advocated by Lister in the 1860s were routinely followed in civilian practice, yet in times of war inadequate supplies including antiseptic agents, combined with hospital overcrowding and care delivery by some who had not received the same education as trained nurses, further risked cross-infection.[69] Laurence, when reflecting on receiving thirty patients at short notice, observed that in London she would have thought it a 'heavy day' if six or eight patients were admitted to a ward where everything would have been ready at hand with 'several well-drilled nurses to help'.[70] In South Africa, it is apparent that the exigencies of war often meant that routine and acknowledged good practice was not always possible and that nurses were required to adapt to the situation at hand. Peter further attributed inadequacies regarding the dearth of medical equipment to the fact that everything was 'badly done' in the army, with items left to 'rot' in the stores, owing to inefficiency in distribution.[71] Moreover, inadequate transport facilities for the transfer of supplies, owing in part to the vast size of South Africa and the derailment of British supply trains by Boer insurgents, further hindered the work of the already strained RAMC.[72]

Fighting for their food and stimulants

With neither definitive nor an effective treatment regime identified for typhoid fever, it was still common practice in 1899 to treat typhoid with stimulants and by antipyretic methods.[73] It would be another forty-nine years before the discovery of the antibiotic chloramphenicol to prove effective against this disease, thus doctors during the

Anglo-Boer War were often faced with failure.[74] It was perhaps owing to this fact, that the administration of stimulants and the provision of 'careful nursing' became the recognised remit of the nurse, with many medical men identifying skilled nursing care as key to the successful recovery of typhoid patients.[75] However, the effectiveness of this nursing care relied upon the availability of provisions on the veldt and sufficient staff to perform nursing duties.

Stimulants were a key element in the care of typhoid and while some nurses could obtain abundant supplies, many were left with insufficient quantities. Laurence, on night duty at the privately funded Princess Christian Hospital in Natal, was able to give her patients ample supplies of milk and brandy, some of whom were prescribed ten ounces per day.[76] Yet out on the veldt, nurses were sometimes forced to fight the establishment in order to obtain stimulants. This was due in part to inadequately managed medicine distribution, combined with the army's routine dilution of brandy for the sick. When Peter questioned how to ensure all her patients would receive their prescribed stimulants she was informed by the head of her hospital to:

> Put less water in it myself, what good was that when I did not know how much was in it already; and when 8 oz. were ordered I did not get 8 oz. when part of it was water.[77]

Peter was aware that patients were disadvantaged in their recovery. However, she claimed that although typhoid patients in other wards were dying at a rate of three, sometimes five per night, she only lost one. This, she stated, was due to her personal fight against the authorities for her patients' right to prescribed food and stimulants, which made her unpopular within camp. This direct conflict with authority does not fit with the stereotypical subordinate nurse of the Victorian period who was trained to display 'implicit obedience' to the doctor.[78] Peter appears to have considered her care provision as a matter of autonomous decision-making, placing her patients' welfare before complete obedience to authority.

Many of the nurses personal experiences of the care provided by the army medical services left much to be desired, recognising the inefficiencies, inadequacies and the 'red tape' which restricted care delivery across the veldt. Reserve nurse Emily Andrews went so far as to state that: 'The work here is hard & there is enough red tape to give every man a yard to hang himself & two yards for each woman.'[79] The personal testimonies of nurses caring for the 'Tommies' in South Africa demonstrate some of the deficiencies of the fledgling army medical services. It could be argued that the itinerant nature of medical and nursing care provision meant that where the nurses were based and what equipment was available to her determined the standard of care that she could deliver. Yet it must be acknowledged that during siege periods rations and supplies were generally scarce, and obtaining milk and stimulants for typhoid cases was a continual challenge.[80]

Nurses working in privately funded hospitals observed that the requisite equipment for efficient nursing care was often abundant. Nevertheless, on the vast veldt where many of the stationary military hospitals were required to relocate, the lines of communication were often broken and the provision of stimulants was therefore dependent upon those in charge of the army medical services stores. Inequality of supplies distribution was uncovered within some military hospitals with accounts of one army major instructing all medical comforts be stopped – including the brandy used for typhoid fever – to be subsequently siphoned off to his civilian friends, yet official records stated that they had been consumed by patients.[81] The British Red Cross Society were aware of the 'gross abuse' of their gifts with items supplied for the sick and wounded discovered to have been consumed within the 'Medical Officers Mess after urgent demands' on the behalf of patients.[82]

Conclusion

The deficient medical care noted by the civilian nurses did not go unacknowledged. It was apparent that the inadequate distribution of equipment resulted in varying standards of care provision, depending where typhoid patients were nursed in South Africa. The itinerant nature of nursing work at that time meant that nurses were in a prime position to observe these disparities. In time, the British public became aware of the Tommies' suffering as a result of the reports of William Burdett-Coutts, a prominent Member of Parliament who was invited to South Africa to observe the work of the army medical services. Burdett-Coutts criticised the army medical arrangements in *The Times* and in his book, *The Sick and Wounded in South Africa:*

What I Saw and Said of Them and the Army Medical System.[83] He remarked that the requisites for the successful recovery of typhoid patients were clearly lacking:

> On that night (Saturday, the 28th of April) hundreds of men to my knowledge were lying in the worst stages of typhoid, with only a blanket and a thin waterproof sheet … between their aching bodies and the hard ground, with no milk and hardly any medicines, without beds, stretchers or mattresses, without linen of any kind, and without a single nurse amongst them … and with only three doctors to attend on 350 patients.[84]

Civilian doctor Francis E. Fremantle, from Guy's Hospital London, believed that Burdett-Coutts was exaggerating the severity of the situation, but added that he himself had observed many typhoid patients lying out on the veldt with only blankets and waterproof sheets.[85] Civilian nurses also witnessed typhoid patients having to endure substandard conditions. Edith Hancock stated that she found 'every available place' taken up with the sick and that the beds and mattresses were 'divided up so as to make them go further but a great many are still on the floor with one blanket & an overcoat'.[86] In Kroonstadt, Pope observed 'a hundred Tommies [*sic*] lay in filth on the floor in their clothes & one died as we stood there', overcrowding and inadequate care was rife.[87] Nevertheless, Lieutenant-Colonel Ryerson, who was affiliated to the Red Cross, believed that the army had been beset by great difficulties with regard to transportation and the availability of food for troops, considering that approximately 100,000 soldiers and 'twenty thousand camp-followers' were 'thrown' into South Africa, followed by a swift outbreak of typhoid fever hospitalising up to a thousand men a day.[88] In Ryerson's opinion the RAMC 'rose to the occasion' admirably, but added the caveat that the medical organisation in general was by no means unflawed and would necessitate 'readjustment' once the war was concluded.[89]

A Royal Commission was soon appointed. Its findings confirmed that both the military and medical authorities had not been able to anticipate in advance the eventual scale of the war and the impact this would have on their preparations, which had left them insufficiently organised with regard to staff and equipment.[90] It was also evident that high-standard nursing care delivered by trained nurses was imperative to the continued health and fitness of the army in times of both war and peace.[91] Wartime nursing enabled trained nurses to demonstrate their expertise and to be recognised as essential primary care providers and as educators of orderlies. Charlotte Searle claimed that 'even the most prejudiced army doctor' was able to admit by the end of the war that trained nurses were essential within military hospitals and, as in civilian practice, the nursing should be 'largely left to women who are trained', not to male orderlies.[92] The result was a reformation of the army medical services and the establishment of the Queen Alexandra's Imperial Military Nursing Service (QAIMNS) in 1902 to replace the small cohort of the Army Nursing Service, who had been forced to rely heavily on civilian nurses.[93] Female nurses were to be integral in the planning for nursing care during wartime, forming part of an Advisory Nursing Board, with the aim that in future military campaigns adequate care provision would have a permanent and regulated place.[94] Following the cessation of hostilities in South Africa many nurses enrolled into the QAIMNS with Sidney Browne as the first Matron-in-Chief.[95] Eleanor Laurence's one experience of wartime nursing gained her the much-coveted Royal Red Cross. She reflected that, should there be another war, the suffering of soldiers would be lessened if the relevant services had already been organised in times of peace.[96] The widespread reforms of the army medical services and the newly established QAIMNS were intended to address such problems. In twelve years' time, these newly organised services would be put to the test on a worldwide scale.

Notes

This chapter is based on chapter 7 'The last of the typhoid campaigns', in Dale's PhD thesis, 'Raising professional confidence: The influence of the Anglo-Boer War (1899–1902)' on the development and recognition of nursing as a profession.

1 Anne Summers, *Angels and Citizens: British Women as Military Nurses 1854–1914* (London, Routledge & Kegan Paul, 1988). Narratives including the experiences of Anne Thacker, *The Narrative of my Experiences as a Volunteer Nurse in the Franco-German War of 1870–1* (London, Abbott, Jones & Co. (1897); Florence Lees, *In a Fever Hospital before Metz* (1873); Louisa McLaughlin and Emma Pearson, *Our Adventures During the War of 1870*. www.nursing.manchester.ac.uk/ukchnm/archives/militarynursing/ouradventures.pdf (accessed 6 February 2013).

2 Angela Woollacott, *On Her Their Lives Depend: Munitions Workers in the Great War* (California, University of California Press, 1994), 6.
3 Anonymous, 'Army nursing notes', *The Nursing Record and Hospital World* 24, 635 (2 June 1900), 437.
4 Summers, *Angels and Citizens*, 204.
5 Edith Hancock, Correspondence with Superintendent Sidney Browne (23 May 1900) Army Medical Services Museum; ANR, 'Our Foreign Letter Chieveley, Natal', *The Nursing Record* 24, 637 (16 June 1900), 483; Anonymous, 'War notes', *Nursing Notes: A Practical Journal for Nurses* 23, 151 (1 July 1900), 91.
6 At the time of the Anglo-Boer War there were fewer than 200 nurses in both the ANS and ANSR. Lee Holcombe, *Victorian Ladies at Work Middle-Class Working Women in England and Wales 1850–1914* (Devon, David & Charles Holdings Ltd, 1973), 82.
7 Joan Woodward and Glenys Mitchell, *A Nurse at War: Emily Peter 1858–1927* (New Zealand, Te Waihora Press, 2008).
8 Eleanor Laurence, *A Nurse's Life in War and Peace* (London, Smith, Elder & Co, 1912), 17.
9 Emily Wood, Boer War nurse's journal, MS. 6034 Wellcome Library; Keiron Spires, 'Edith Hancock and Kate Driver', http://boerwarnurses.com/main/index.php/nurses-databases (accessed 24 July 2013); Kate Driver, *Experience of a Siege: A Nurse Looks Back on Ladysmith* (South Africa, Ladysmith Historical Society, 1994).
10 Laurence, *A Nurse's Life*, 219; Driver, *Experience of a Siege*, 17.
11 Mrs Bedford Fenwick, 'Enteric stalks the British army', *The Nursing Record* 26, 675 (9 March 1901), 181.
12 G. C. Cook, 'Influence of diarrhoeal disease on military and naval campaigns', *Journal of the Royal Society of Medicine* 94 (2001), 95–7, 95; Maire A. Connolly and David L. Heyman, 'Deadly comrades: war and infectious diseases', *The Lancet Supplement* 360 (2002), 23–4, 23; Mark Harrison, *Medicine and Victory British Military Medicine in the Second World War* (Oxford, Oxford University Press, 2004), 92.
13 Kevin Brown, *Fighting Fit: Health, Medicine and War in the Twentieth Century* (Gloucestershire, History Press, 2008), 17.
14 Richard A. Gabriel and Karen S. Metz, *A History of Military Medicine, Vol. II: From the Renaissance through Modern Times* (London, Greenwood Press, 1992), 217.
15 Gabriel and Metz, *A History of Military Medicine*, 144; Oscar Craig and Alasdair Fraser, *Doctors at War* (Co. Durham, The Memoir Club, 2007), 18. Netley Hospital was the military hospital where Queen Victoria had assisted in laying the foundation stone and where the Army Medical School was also located. Historically, Netley has been referred to as the 'cradle of the Army Nursing Service, as it was the original headquarters and depot

when the service was officially established in 1881. The demolition of Netley commenced in 1966 – Elizabeth Haldane, *The British Nurse in Peace and War* (London, John Murray, 1923), 164, Ian Hay, *One Hundred Years of Army Nursing The Story of the British Army Nursing Services from the time of Florence Nightingale to the present day* (London, Cassell and Company, 1953), 37, Juliet Piggott, *Queen Alexandra's Royal Army Nursing Corps* (London, Leo Cooper Ltd, 1975), 18; Anonymous, 'Netley Hospital', www.qaranc.co.uk/netleyhospital.php (accessed 6 February 2013).

16 Francis E. Fremantle, *Impressions of a Doctor in Khaki* (London, John Murray, 1901), 210–11; Summers, *Angels and Citizens*, 208; Philip D. Curtin, *Disease and Empire The Health of European Troops in the Conquest of Africa* (Cambridge, Cambridge University Press, 1998), 209; Brown, *Fighting Fit*, 22–3.

17 Gabriel and Metz, *A History of Military Medicine*, 217.

18 Jan Bassett, *Guns and Brooches Australian Army Nursing from the Boer War to the Gulf War* (Melbourne, Oxford University Press, 1997), 19; Daniel Low-Beer, Matthew Smallman-Raynor and Andrew Cliff, 'Disease and death in the South African War: Changing disease patterns from soldiers to refugees', *Social History of Medicine* 17, 2 (2004), 223–45, 223.

19 A. P. Stewart, 'Typhoid fever', *British Medical Journal* 2, 985 (15 November 1879), 795; Laurence Humphry, *A Manual of Nursing Medical and Surgical* (London, Griffin, 1898), 118–20; R. Moorehead, 'William Budd and typhoid fever', *Journal of the Royal Society of Medicine* 95 (2002), 561–4; Deborah Brunton, 'Dealing with disease in populations', in Deborah Brunton (ed.), *Medicine Transformed Health, Disease and Society in Europe 1800–1930* (Manchester, Manchester University Press, 2004), 180–210, 190.

20 C. J. Cullingworth, *Manual of Nursing Medical and Surgical* (London, Churchill, 1889), 27; Watson, *A Handbook for Nurses*, 234; T. E. Hayward, 'A Lecture to nurses on typhoid fever', *Nursing Notes* 22, 137 (1 May 1899), 61–3, 61.

21 J. K. Watson, *A Handbook for Nurses* (London, Scientific Press, 1899), 234.

22 Eva C. E. Luckes, *General Nursing* (London, Kegan Paul, Trench, Trubner & Co., Ltd, 1898), 147, 294.

23 Watson, *A Handbook for Nurses*, 238.

24 Lieut-Colonel G. Sterling Ryerson, *Medical and Surgical Experiences in the South African War Being addresses to the Toronto Clinical Society and Canadian Medical Association* (1900), 10 Army Medical Services Museum (AMS).

25 Luckes, *General Nursing*, 58; Watson, *A Handbook for Nurses*, 240.

26 For a full discussion of 'careful nursing', see Therese Connell Meehan, 'Careful nursing: a model for contemporary nursing practice', *Journal of Advanced Nursing* 44, 1 (2003), 99–107.

27 T. E. Hayward, 'A lecture to nurses on typhoid fever', *Nursing Notes* 22, 136

(1 April 1899), 47–8, 48; Thomas Pakenham, *The Boer War* (London, Time Warner, 1992), 382; Mary T. Sarnecky, *A History of the U.S Army Nurse Corp* (University of Pennsylvania Press, 1999), 36.

28 Meehan, 'Careful nursing', 100.

29 Arthur Conan Doyle, *The Great Boer War* (London, Smith, Elder & Co., 1900), 370; Gabriel and Metz, *A History of Military Medicine*, 217; Curtin, *Disease and Empire*, 209.

30 W. S. Inder, On active service with the SJAB, South African War, 1899–1902 (Whitefish, MT, Kessinger Publishing, 2009), 55.

31 Driver, *Experience of a Siege*, 20.

32 Frederick Treves, *The Tale of a Field Hospital* (London, Cassell & Co., 1900), 4.

33 Leigh Canney, 'Typhoid in the army', *The Times*, no. 36540 (1901), 8; Leigh Canney, 'Typhoid the destroyer of armies and its abolition opinions of the military, medical and general press The House of Commons August 17th 1901', *The Times* (London, 1901) E5256, V 9.661.

34 Hancock, Correspondence (23 May 1900), AMS.

35 Summers, *Angels and Citizen*, 209.

36 Anonymous, 'The nursing of our soldiers', *Nursing Notes* 23, 147 (1 March 1900), 33.

37 Wood, Boer War nurse's journal (21 June 1900), MS. 6034 Wellcome Library.

38 Charlotte Searle, *The History of the Development of Nursing in South Africa 1652–1960 A Socio-historical Survery* (South Africa, Struik, 1965), 194.

39 Sir William Stokes, 'A visit to the General Hospital Ladysmith', *British Medical Journal* 1, 2060 (16 June 1900), 1495.

40 Dora Harris, Manuscript Diary (14 May 1900) 1976-11-17 NAM; Arthur Conan Doyle, 'The epidemic of enteric fever at Bloemfontein', *British Medical Journal* 2, 2062 (7 July 1900), 49–50.

41 Driver, *Experience of a Siege*, 23.

42 Laurence, *A Nurse's Life*, 162 and 178.

43 Noha Barsoum and Charles Kleeman, 'Now and then, the history of parental fluid administration', *The American Journal of Nephrology* 22 (2002), 284–9, 288; Carol Helmstadter, 'Early nursing reform in nineteenth-century London: A doctor-driven phenomenon', *Medical History* 46, 3 (2002), 325–50, 326; Carol Helmstadter and Judith Godden, *Nursing before Nightingale, 1815–1899* (Surrey, Ashgate Publishing Ltd, 2011), 118.

44 Helmstadter and Godden, *Nursing before Nightingale*, 37.

45 George Lynch, *Impressions of a War Correspondent* (London, Newnes Ltd, MCMIII), chapter 1, no page number accessed via Project Gutenburg at archive.org/stream/impressionsofawa21661gut/pg21661.txt_(22 December 2012), NB, Contemporaneously the 'infusion' of fluids was referred to as

transfusion, which is now used to describe the transfer of blood products. Edward H. Benton, 'British surgery in the South African War: The work of Major Frederick Porter', *Medical History* 21, 3 (1977), 275–90, 287–88.

46 Helmstadter and Godden, *Nursing before Nightingale*, 118.

47 Anonymous, 'War notes', 91.

48 Hancock, Correspondence (18 May 1900) AMS; Sister X, *The Tragedy and Comedy of War Hospitals* (New York, E. P. Dutton, 1906), 96; Laurence, *A Nurse's Life* 162; Woodward and Mitchell, *A Nurse at War*, 90.

49 Inder, *On Active Service*, 92–3.

50 Inder, *On Active Service*, 92–3.

51 Florence Nightingale, *Subsidiary Notes as to the Introduction of Female Nursing into Military Hospitals in Peace and in War. Presented to the Secretary of State for War (Thoughts submitted as to an eventual Nurses' Provident Fund)* (London, Harrison & Sons, 1858), 133.

52 Woodward and Mitchell, *A Nurse at War*, 92.

53 Anonymous, 'War notes', 91.

54 Woodward and Mitchell, *A Nurse at War*, 92–3.

55 Summers, *Angels and Citizens*, 332.

56 Nursing Sister M. S. Barwell, Minutes of Evidence (30.07.1900) Report of the Royal Commission Appointed to Consider and Report upon the Care and Treatment of the Sick and Wounded during The South Africa Campaign: Presented to both Houses of Parliament by Command of Her Majesty (London, HMSO, 1901), 82.

57 Searle, *The History of the Development of Nursing* 185; Christopher Schmitz, '"We too were soldiers": The experiences of British nurses in the Anglo-Boer War, 1899–1902', in Gerard J. DeGroot and Corinna Peniston-Bird (eds), *A Soldier and a Woman: Sexual Integration in the Military* (Harlow, Pearson Education Ltd, 2000), 49–65, 56.

58 Anonymous, 'War notes', *The Nursing Record* 23, 152 (1 August 1900), 105.

59 Sister X, *The Tragedy and Comedy*, 6.

60 Laurence, *A Nurse's Life*, 147.

61 Woodward and Mitchell, *A Nurse at War*, 94.

62 Anonymous Sister, 'Army nursing notes', *The Nursing Record* 24, 635 (2 June 1900), 437.

63 Sister X, *The Tragedy and Comedy*, 123.

64 Laurence, *A Nurse's Life* 261–2.

65 Woodward and Mitchell, *A Nurse at War*, 93.

66 Anonymous, 'Army nursing notes', *The Nursing Record* 25, 648 (1 September 1900), 174.

67 Georgina Fane Pope, Correspondence with Superintendent Sidney Browne (29 May 1900) 16/1956–5 AMS.

68 Watson, *A Handbook for Nurses*, 114.

69 Joseph Lister, 'On the antiseptic principle in the practice of surgery', *The Lancet* 90, 2299 (21 September 1867), 352–6.

70 Laurence, *A Nurse's Life*, 167–8.

71 Woodward and Mitchell, *A Nurse at War*, 90.

72 Eric Taylor, *Wartime Nurse One Hundred Years from the Crimea to Korea 1854–1954* (London, ISIS, 2001), 67; Brown, *Fighting Fit*, 16.

73 NB, Antipyretic methods included: tepid sponging, cold bathing and the administration of salicylic acid. Jan R. McTavish, 'Antipyretic treatment and typhoid fever 1860–1900', *Journal History Medical Allied Science* 42, 4 (1987), 486–506, 505–6.

74 Brown, *Fighting Fit*, 18.

75 A. Knyvett Gordon, 'Notes on practical nursing', *The Nursing Record* 26, 674 (2 March 1901), 165; Watson, *A Handbook for Nurses*, 238; Humphry, *A Manual of Nursing*, 120.

76 Laurence, *A Nurse's Life*, 165.

77 Woodward and Mitchell, *A Nurse at War*, 90.

78 Eva C. E. Luckes, *Lectures on Nursing: Lectures on General Nursing, Delivered to the Probationers of the London Hospital Training School for Nurses*, 4th edn (London, Paul, Trench, 1892), 11; Christopher J. Maggs, *The Origins of General Nursing* (London, Croom Helm, 1983), 29; Eva Gamarnikow, 'Nurse or woman: Gender and professionalism in reformed nursing 1860–1923', in Pat Holden and Jenny Littlewood (eds), *Anthropology and Nursing* (London, Routledge, 1991), 110–29, 111; Anne Marie Rafferty, *The Politics of Nursing Knowledge* (London, Routledge, 1996), 29.

79 Emily Andrews, Correspondence with Superintendent Sidney Browne (20 June 1900) 16/1956–12 AMS.

80 Anonymous Bloemfontein Sister, 'Army nursing notes', *The Nursing Record* 24, 632 (12 May 1900), 376.

81 Pakenham, *The Boer War*, 354; Peter Prime, *The History of the Medical and Hospital Service of the Anglo-Boer War 1899 to 1902* (Anglo-Boer War Philatelic Society, 1998), 14.

82 G. Bonham-Carter, Extract from report received from Mr G. Bonham-Carter Assistant Commissioner to the Red Cross Society, Capetown, 15 September 1900, British Red Cross Museum and Archives WAN/15/8/17 Stores and Supplies.

83 William Burdett-Coutts, 'Our wars and our wounded', *The Times* 36179 (27 June 1900), 4.

84 William Burdett-Coutts, *The Sick and Wounded in South Africa: What I Saw and Said of Them and of the Army Medical System* (London, Cassell & Co., 1900), 19.

85 Fremantle, *Impressions of a Doctor*, 241, 388.

86 Hancock, Correspondence (23 May 1900), AMS.

87 Pope, Correspondence (29 May 1900) 16/1956–5 AMS.

88 Ryerson, *Medical and Surgical Experiences*, 21 AMS.

89 Ryerson, *Medical and Surgical Experiences*, 22 AMS.

90 Anonymous, 'The Royal Commission on South African Hospitals', *British Medical Journal* 1, 2091 (26 January 1901), 236.

91 Anonymous, 'War notes', 91.

92 Searle, *The History of the Development of Nursing in South Africa*, 202.

93 Summers, *Angels and Citizens*, 220–3.

94 Summers, *Angels and Citizens*, 220–3.

95 Summers, *Angels and Citizens*, 218.

96 Laurence, *A Nurse's Life*, 311.

Part II

Industrial war

4

'This fiendish mode of warfare': Nursing the victims of gas poisoning in the First World War

Christine E. Hallett

On 22 April 1915, German troops stationed behind defensive trenches just East of Ypres in Belgium opened 6,000 canisters of chlorine gas, allowing their contents to drift across no man's land to the allied trenches opposite.[1] Their action marked the start of an escalating and destructive form of chemical warfare, which came to be seen as a defining characteristic of the First World War. Both sides experimented with increasingly destructive compounds with which to kill and disable their enemies.[2] The earliest poison gases were 'drift gases' – heavier than air, and capable of travelling across land when carried by the wind;[3] they acted as lung irritants, asphyxiating their victims. Later weapons were deployed via 'gas shells' fired into enemy trenches.[4] On 13 July 1917, the Germans used dichlorethylsulphide, or 'mustard gas', for the first time. Its effect was to scorch the airways, violently inflame the eyes, and burn the skin.[5] Chemical warfare became a field which tested the ingenuity of both prize-winning scientists and strategists.[6] As chemical weapons became increasingly sophisticated, the means for protecting those exposed barely kept pace. The result was that casualty clearing stations (CCSs) on the Western Front found themselves inundated with large numbers of severely damaged men, who arrived en masse in what were referred to as 'rushes'.[7] As these small field hospitals struggled to cope, they moved large numbers of still-critical casualties onto hospital trains and barges and, hence, 'down the line' to base hospitals on the coast of Northern France, which, in their turn, found themselves struggling with waves of seriously ill patients.

This chapter focuses on the hitherto unexplored work of those allied nurses who were based in CCSs and base hospitals on the Western Front, and casts light on the hidden nature of nursing work. It also explores the idea that working with the victims of poison gas permitted nurses to identify themselves as significant participants in the allied war effort. Alongside their medical colleagues, nurses were able to implement life-saving, emergency interventions. But they were also uniquely positioned – and uniquely skilled – to offer the supportive care that would permit long-term survival. And in addition to claiming such significance for their work, nurses were also able to present themselves as important actors operating close to the 'front lines' of war and, sometimes, putting their own lives at risk.

Historical research in this field has focused on the role of physiological and medical science in developing both chemical weapons themselves and defensive responses to them. The work of Steve Sturdy highlighted the roles of the Royal Society's Physiology (War) Committee and the Chemical Warfare Medical Committee, using the example of research and innovation in gas warfare as a case study to illustrate the point that 'war itself [was] an experimental enterprise'. In this 'war of invention ... victory would go to the side that first developed the technical means of breaking through the enemy's defences'.[8] This chapter takes a very different approach to the allied response to gas warfare, by focusing on an aspect of the historical record that has never before been considered. It examines the day-to-day clinical interventions of nurses and explores the claims they made in their personal writings, textbooks and journal articles for the significance of their work with gas casualties. Whilst never presented as open claims for recognition, many these writings were couched in terms of quiet confidence; they reveal a belief that nursing interventions were an important element of the war effort.

Material for this study was obtained from the writings of nurses. Among the more personal texts are diaries, letters and autobiographical accounts held at the Imperial War Museum, London; the Archive of the Army Medical Services Museum, Aldershot (QARANC Collection); the Maryland Historical Society, Baltimore, USA; the Australian War Memorial, Canberra; and the Alexander Turnbull Library, Wellington, New Zealand. Among nurses' professional writings are articles in nursing journals, and material from the most influential text book of war nursing published in Britain during the war: Violetta Thurstan's *A Text Book of War Nursing*. These are placed alongside medical journal articles that discuss the scientific bases for treatments. The mention of nursing is conspicuous by its absence in medical journals, where the convention was to write in the passive voice, giving the impression that the actors – the executors of care and treatment – were the mere ciphers of medical decision-making. A reading of nurses' own writings reveals that, while they did adopt the passive role of 'observer' when reporting on major scientific decisions – such as the most effective chemical treatments and the design of gas masks – their own work was punctuated by rationales for treatment and care, considering, for example, how to keep asphyxiated patients alive; how to enable them to breathe most easily; how to alleviate their suffering; and how to support their physiological systems to enable full recovery. The effectiveness of nursing interventions in both saving lives and promoting quality of life was further enhanced by the morale-raising presence of female nurses in the so-called 'zone of the armies'.[9] When nurses wrote of the dangers they faced from gas warfare, they perceived themselves not only as the healers of the most cruel wounds of war, but also as brave participants in the allied war effort.

Chemical warfare on the Western Front

The release of chlorine gas at the so-called Second Battle of Ypres in April 1915 was coordinated by German military meteorologists, who had studied the prevailing wind conditions for several weeks prior to the attack. Although allied military intelligence had identified a number of strange canisters in the German trenches three weeks before the assault, the element of surprise – an element that would never again be present – was still powerful. The chlorine gas is believed to have killed approximately 1,000 French and Algerian soldiers, disabling 4,000 others, and permitting the Germans to penetrate the allied lines along a 6-km front.[10] Over the course of the next three and a half years, several thousand men were to die of gas poisoning.[11]

One anonymous nurse-writer, stationed in a hospital in Furnes,

Belgium, described the helplessness of the military medical services in the face of the new weapon:

> Our hospital soon became a shambles, the theatre a slaughterhouse. We started working that day, April 23rd, and we never stopped for about two weeks … Gas had been used in the trenches for the first time that day. There they lay, fully sensible, choking, suffocating, dying in horrible agonies. We did what we could, but the best treatment for such cases had yet to be discovered, and we felt almost powerless.[12]

Writings such as these illustrate how powerless nurses felt in the spring of 1915, as they faced chemical warfare for the first time. And this powerlessness was accompanied by extreme pressure of work, which made it difficult for nurses to evaluate the ways in which their traditional skills might be adapted to cope with this extraordinary and unforeseen emergency. Their indignation at the indiscriminate destructiveness of poison gas resonates through their writings. Sister Ellen Cuthbert of the Australian Army Nursing Service felt that it was 'on seeing such cases as these that one feels the injustice of this war. It is not war – just murder',[13] while one British nurse referred to chemical weaponry as 'this fiendish mode of warfare'.[14]

A gas attack could place CCSs under great pressure. As Violetta Thurstan commented: 'this emergency strains the resources of the staff to the uttermost, as the men are generally very ill indeed when they arrive'.[15] The most destructive feature of chlorine gas was its action as a lung irritant. Direct contact could also damage the delicate tissues of the eyes, causing temporary – or sometimes permanent – blindness. George Adami described the appearance of gas casualties. They were, invariably, 'weak and semi-stuporose, with bloodshot eyes and hacking cough'.[16] Bromine and phosgene were used from late 1915 onwards.[17] Like chlorine, they acted as lung irritants, burning the surfaces of the deepest lung tissues, and causing both suffocation and heart failure.[18] Mustard gas, used from 1917 onwards, created horrific chemical burns, dissolving in both the skin and the mucus membranes lining the respiratory tract, and causing blistering and the rapid destruction of vast swathes of tissue. Lewisite had a 'universal' action on all tissues, dissolving in them, burning and releasing toxic M-1 oxide; it was known by allied troops as the 'dew of death'.[19]

The allies deployed two responses to the Germans' use of chemical weaponry: they mobilised gas attacks of their own and they devised a range of devices to protect their troops. But all too often, particularly in the early years of the war, gas masks were unavailable, proved ineffective or were donned too late, resulting in mass casualties. One of the most disturbing sights of the war was of lines of blinded men each with a hand on the shoulder of the patient in front of him, being led by an orderly, which were so graphically depicted in John Singer Sargent's painting: *Gassed*.[20]

Work with lung-damaged patients in casualty clearing stations and base hospitals

One of the earliest reports of the treatment of gas-poisoning cases on the Western Front was offered by three medical officers based in a CCS. They wrote of 685 cases, treated between 2 and 7 May, 1915. Their failure to mention the contribution of nursing staff to the care and treatment of these patients is notable, given that the remedies they recommend clearly required close one-to-one care involving the positioning of patients, the administration of emetics, stimulants and oxygen and the promotion of rest and sleep.[21] The authors, J. Elliot Black, Elliot Glenny and J. W. McNee, began by distinguishing between two groups of patients: one group of about 120, who, upon arrival at the CCS seemed in imminent danger of death from asphyxiation; and the remainder, whose conditions were not so critical. Of the first group, thirty-three died, among whom were many of the older patients. The overall death rate among those victims who managed to reach the CCS was approximately five per cent, although this only accounted for deaths in the acute phase of the poisoning. The authors acknowledged that many more deaths from bronchitis would have occurred at the base, while the study took no account of even later deaths association with chronic lung damage.

Patients exhibited classic symptoms of lung congestion; the damage caused by the toxic gas led to the effusion of lymph, which collected in the airways, slowly drowning the man.[22] Patients were 'making agonizing efforts to breathe, clutching at their throats, and tearing open their clothes'. They were cyanosed and exhausted: their faces and hands were 'of a leaden hue', and a light frothy fluid was escaping from the mouths and noses of the worst cases (the ones who did not recover).[23]

Nursing journals were quick to pick up on reports of gas poisoning. In May 1915, an article in *The Nursing Times,* referred to J. S. Haldane's work for the War Office in identifying the gases used in early 1915, and explained how post-mortem examinations had revealed that patients killed by the earliest toxic gases had died of acute bronchitis.[24] One account of the pulmonary symptoms experienced by men 'gassed' on Hill 60 was included in the 15 May 1915, issue of *The Nursing Times*:

> Their faces, arms, hands, were of a shiny, grey-black colour, with mouths open and lead-glazed eyes, all swaying slightly backwards and forwards trying to get breath. It was the most appalling sight; all these poor black faces struggling, struggling, for life, what with the groaning and noise of the efforts for breath … The effect the gas has is to fill the lungs with a watery, frothy matter, which gradually increases and rises, till it fills up the whole lungs and comes up to the mouth; then they die. It is suffocation; slow drowning, taking in some cases one or two days. Eight died last night out of the twenty I saw, and most of the others I saw will die; while those who get over the gas invariably develop acute pneumonia. It is without doubt the most awful form of scientific torture.[25]

The plain language used in *The Nursing Times* contrasts with the scientific reporting of Black *et al.* The symptoms described are essentially the same, but the language used is almost entirely devoid of jargon or scientific terms; it is also much more emotive. The description is, nevertheless, precise, and offers a clear rationale for the treatments implemented. Although medical language is dropped, the adherence to medical explanations is rigorous.

Black and his colleagues noticed that those who recovered passed through three stages: 'the asphyxial stage'; 'the quiescent or intermediate stage'; and 'the bronchitic stage'.[26] If the patient could be 'brought through' the asphyxial stage, he was likely to recover, but having survived and fallen into a deep sleep, he generally became acutely ill again within half a day, as the bronchitic stage – characterised by acute inflammation of the airways, often associated with infection – set in.[27] Staff in CCSs would try to clear surviving patients to the base hospitals before the bronchitic phase began.

The scientific team deduced that, because most patients died of acute lung congestion, the main aims of treatment must be: '1. To expel the excessive secretion from the lungs by emetics and stimulating expectorants; 2. To diminish the secretion; 3. to support the failing heart and reoxygenate the blood.'[28] The meeting of these aims required the implementation of multiple treatments by nurses. They gave emetics (particularly salt and water) in an attempt to reduce congestion, and then remained with their gasping and vomiting patients.[29] They gave stimulating expectorants (usually ammonium carbonate), and then supported their patients as they expelled copious, frothy secretions from their lungs. They also administered oxygen through face masks – often with great difficulty, as patients found it almost impossible to tolerate the masks.[30] In order to attempt to reduce the secretions in the lungs, some CCSs administered atropine, or attempted venesection.[31] Heart failure was combated with pituitary extract.[32] Milder cases were given steam inhalations, impregnated with benzoin, and cases suffering from the most extreme emotional distress were given opium.[33] Violetta Thurstan commented on the wide variety of measures prescribed by medical officers, ranging from old-fashioned remedies, such as 'cupping' to heroic treatments, such as strychnine.[34]

As hundreds of men staggered, or were carried, into their CCSs, nurses worked fast to combat the effects of toxic gases. Each patient was placed in whatever position of rest, calm and quiet most seemed to help him – not easy in the reception hut of a busy CCS or field hospital. Some were allowed to rest in an upright position to assist the breathing; others were placed on their sides, to permit the drainage of fluid from the mouth and nose.[35] Agnes Warner, a Canadian nurse, based at a mobile unit in Belgium, commented that 'the nursing is awfully hard, for they cannot be left a moment until they are out of danger'.[36]

Julia Stimson, matron of American Base Hospital 21, located on Rouen Race Course, commented that a lot of the gassed men who came into her hospital 'cough and cough continuously, like children with whooping cough', adding:

We had a very bad case the other night who had not slept one hour for cough nights or days, and whose coughing paroxysms came every minute and a half by the clock. When finally the nurses got him to sleep, after

87

rigging up a croup tent over him so that he could breathe steam from a croup kettle over a little stove that literally had to be held in the hands to make it burn properly, they said they were ready to get down on their knees in gratitude, his anguish had been so terrible to watch. They said they could not wish the Germans any greater unhappiness than to have them have to witness the sufferings of a man like that and know that they had been the cause of it.[37]

Such writings illustrate the extent to which nurses struggled to treat gas poisoning, and demonstrate their willingness to pour great effort into their work. They infused that effort with a sense of moral purpose, explicitly blaming their 'enemies' for the suffering caused by gas warfare, and positioning themselves as significant participants in an allied war effort, fighting on the side of 'right'.

Within three months of the first chlorine gas attacks a routine treatment had been 'evolved from experience'.[38] This involved placing patients in a current of fresh air (either out of doors or close to an open window); providing adequate warmth, using blankets and hot water bottles; offering a salt and water emetic if the patient had not already vomited, ammonium carbonate, or some other expectorant, oxygen inhalation, opium and pituitary extract (in cases of obvious heart failure).[39] Measures to combat lung damage evolved slowly and nurses found themselves constantly challenged by new weapons and innovative treatments; their personal writings suggest that, as their expertise in this field expanded, their confidence grew.

The care of damaged eyes

One of the features of bromine was its tendency to irritate the conjunctiva to the point where the eyes could simply not be opened.[40] Most patients suffered from both photophobia and the sealing of the eyelids with dried secretions. Both symptoms could be alleviated by bathing with a sterile solution of sodium bicarbonate.[41] In severe cases the eyes were bathed frequently and covered with a compress of gauze soaked in the bathing solution.[42] Australian nurse, Ellen Cuthbert, based in Abbeville, described how gas-damaged eyes required treatment every two to three hours, and could take several weeks to recover.[43] Ellen McClelland, similarly, described how the eyes of mustard gas victims required 'constant attention'.[44] Frequent, careful swabbing prevented dangerous and damaging infections in eyes that were already badly damaged. Violetta Thurstan offered the following detailed advice to those nursing the victims of mustard gas poisoning:

> The patients are practically blind for the time being, as the pain and photophobia (shrinking from light) are intense … The best immediate treatment has been found to be a thorough irrigation of the eyes with a 1 per cent solution of bicarbonate of soda, followed by drops of castor oil poured into the eye. A wet lint compress wrung out of a solution of bicarbonate of soda placed over the eyes (and lightly bandaged round the forehead only) serves the double purpose of protection from the light and neutralisation of the gas, which is acid, on the eyelids and surrounding parts … Actual blisters may be dressed with boracic ointment or boracic vaseline, as in the case of burns.[45]

Such careful and intricate work could be particularly difficult at times of overcrowding; and the earliest gassed patients rarely arrived in small numbers. American nurse, Helen Dore Boylston, who was based with the Harvard Unit in Northern France described how 'two hundred gassed cases came down last night. Poor wretched things. And we had no beds for them. Had to put stretchers on the floor. And they were so uncomplaining about it. One said to me, as I was bathing his eyes while he lay on the floor, "It's jolly good to be here sister".'[46] While Boylston's main aim seems to be to convey a sense of the uncomplaining and generally sunny nature of the British 'Tommy', it is possible that this particular patient was experiencing some relief that he had sustained a chemical 'wound' rather than a potentially more permanently damaging bullet, or shrapnel, injury. His relief was, almost certainly, due to the fact that he had survived and was now safe in a military hospital well behind the front lines.

In fact, patients with gas-damaged eyes experienced intense anxiety, and emotional care was an important feature of the nurse's role. Julia Stimson described how one of her nursing staff spoke to her of the gas-poisoned cases in her ward:

> Of the sixty-four new stretcher cases we got in last night, all have bandaged eyes. They are the worst gassed men I have ever seen. I've done nothing but irrigate eyes all the morning. One man discovered that he could see a little

when I got his lids opened and his eyes washed out, and he burst out 'Oh, sister, I can see, and I am not going to be blind after all, am I?' Then I realized what an agony of fear there must be in the minds of those sixty-four motionless men, not one of whom had even whimpered – so since then I've been saying to each one that he was sure to see after a while, for you know if they live they nearly all do get back their sight … But think what they have been suffering![47]

The care of gas-damaged eyes was one of the most intricate and time-consuming elements of the nurses' work. When gassed patients arrived in large 'rushes', during assaults on the Western Front, much time had to be devoted to eye-care, as nurses recognised that lasting damage need not take place, as long as toxic chemicals were removed promptly and infection was avoided.

The care and treatment of burns

Compounds such as mustard gas and lewisite caused particularly cruel symptoms. They dissolved in the skin, producing deep and traumatic burns, which induced shock and caused intense pain. Nurses were obliged, initially, to heighten these symptoms, by removing all the patients' clothing; washing affected areas with kerosene or gasoline (in the case of mustard gas) or oils, hot water and soap (in the case of lewisite); rubbing dry and rinsing again with hot water.[48] In order to halt the effects of the chemicals, it was necessary to remove them from the body within three minutes – something which could rarely be achieved, which meant that patients arrived in CCSs with extensive burns.

Even after their conditions had been stabilised, and they had been transferred to base hospitals, patients' burns required continuing attention. One volunteer-nurse related her experiences in a base hospital:

I was sent to Ward 4B … The patients in that particular ward seemed very ill and the wounds looked awful. They were all patients who had been gassed in France and it was the VAD's duty to look after those who were unable to bear bandages on their pouring wounds and therefore were put straight into baths. We had to sit by them and keep the water at an even temperature, bring their meals and look after them.[49]

The chemical burns which were caused by mustard gas and lewisite were among the most complex wounds of war, requiring constant attention. They posed a serious infection risk and had to be handled using a strict aseptic technique. They also caused intense pain, leaving their patients in great need of both analgesia and emotional support.

Total nursing care

Sister Ellen Cuthbert of the Australian Army Nursing Service, referred to 'these gassed boys' who she considered were 'such wonderfully patient fellows ... laying back there quite helpless being fed and looked after'.[50] It was the helplessness of their patients that made the work of nurses so onerous. Blind, breathless and debilitated, these patients were unable to do so much as feed themselves, and coping with such disability in a crowded and busy CCS, where there were so many other wounded and shocked patients requiring immediate attention, was not easy. On transport services, such as hospital trains and barges, where conditions were overcrowded and airless, such work was especially difficult. Sister Millicent Peterkin described how the overcrowding of patients on board a hospital barge could lead to a dangerously unhealthy atmosphere, in which nurses themselves could feel quite 'gassed'.[51]

Gas-poisoned patients were often still severely debilitated following their arrival at base hospitals. Any attempt at exertion could result in severe breathlessness. Their fundamental needs were met by nurses and volunteers, who spent much of their time feeding, washing and toileting helpless patients. The administration of food and fluids was as important as – if not more so than – the giving of medical treatments, and could mean the difference between recovery and death or permanent lung damage.

Rehabilitative care

Nurses and volunteers commented on the fact that one of the most deplorable features of gas poisoning was the long-term damage it caused to the lungs.[52] One medical officer commented that one of his patients found it impossible to walk at more than two miles per hour without experiencing breathlessness. He concluded that the damage caused by the toxic gas had led to lung fibrosis, a condition which carried an extremely poor prognosis.[53] This supposition was confirmed by an Australian medical officer, who examined several gas-poisoned soldiers on their return from active service in 1918 and 1919. Many had been wounded at Ypres in 1917, or in Northern France, during the period of mobile warfare between April and November, 1918. He noted that many had persistent lesions, which caused cough and breathlessness on exertion, and concluded that these patients were likely to suffer very long term effects of their wounding and were also now highly prone to tuberculosis.[54] Indeed, the treatment recommended for such patients was similar to that adopted in tuberculosis sanatoria: a regime of gradually increasing exercise in the fresh air.[55]

In the early 1920s, large numbers of ex-servicemen were still suffering from persistent chronic bronchitis and/or emphysema, characterised by breathlessness upon exertion, palpitations and a severe cough, which was worse in the morning, and became troublesome in the winter months.[56] Violetta Thurstan commented that in many cases, the patient 'may never be the same man again, subject to severe bronchitis and fit for very little work'.[57] Nurses throughout the Western world were caring for the victims of gas poisoning on the medical wards of general hospitals for many decades after the armistice.

Self-protection

The earliest 'gas masks' were only partially effective. A piece of muslin, laced with thiosulfate, was tied over the mouth and nose. The chemical was effective in neutralising the effects of toxic gases, but the device was hardly efficient. Supplies were, initially, poor and some troops found themselves being advised, in the event of a gas-attack in which they had no protective mask, to use a urine-soaked gauze and cotton-wool dressing held over the nose and mouth.[58] Eventually, a range of increasingly effective but highly dehumanising gas masks were devised, beginning with all-enveloping gas hoods, which had the disadvantage that they made the wearer clumsy and ineffective, and progressing to fairly efficient masks, which nevertheless still reduced their wearers to 'goggle-eyed imbecile frogs'.[59]

Kate Evelyn Luard, a member of the Queen Alexandra's Imperial Military Nursing Service Reserve based in a field hospital in Northern France, wrote of her experience of nursing medical officers who had been experimenting with the earliest protective gas masks:

> This afternoon the medical staffs of [two] divisions have been trying experiments in a barn with chlorine gas, with and without different kinds of masks soaked with some antidote such as lime. All were busy coughing and choking when they found the A.D.M.S. of the —Division getting blue and suffocated; he'd had too much chorine, and was brought here, looking very bad, and for an hour we had to give him fumes of ammonia till he could breathe properly. He will probably have bronchitis. But they've found out what they wanted to know – that you can go to the assistance of men overpowered by the gas, if you put on this mask, with less chance of finding yourself dead too when you got there. They don't lose much time finding these things out, do they?[60]

Caring for casualties close to the front lines – particularly in CCSs – meant that nurses placed themselves at risk of gas poisoning.[61] By 1917, effective measures had been put in place to protect them. Julia Stimson described the preparation that was given to nursing sisters at the 'gas school' at a nearby training camp, prior to embarking on a 'tour of duty' at a CCS. They were first taught how to put on their gas masks – a complex procedure, which involved fitting clamps over the nose and inserting a breathing tube into the mouth. She continued: 'They then have to learn how to breathe just through the mouth without choking or what is worse, Miss Cuppaidge said, without dribbling.'[62] Once their masks had been properly adjusted, the nurses were put into a room filled with tear gas for five minutes. If they experienced any eye irritation, their masks were further adjusted, before they were taken to a practice trench, where they were exposed to a variety of gases. Their practical training was accompanied by theoretical instruction on the toxicity of gases. Eventually, Miss Cuppaidge returned to the base hospital 'smelling like the dickens, but ... entirely unafraid of gas and quite prepared to guard against it'.[63]

Nurses were acutely aware that they had chosen to place themselves in danger close to the front lines of battle. Many seemed proud to be putting themselves at risk in order to 'play their part' in the war. Writers such as Claire Tylee and Trudi Tate have commented on the pervasive influence of British war propaganda, and it is clear that most nurses were heavily influenced by the belief that the war as a fight of 'good against evil'.[64] The use of chemical weaponry by the German army strengthened this perspective, which does not appear to have been modified by any awareness that the allies turned the same weapons on the Germans. In May 1915, the *British Journal of Nursing*, in characteristically outspoken style, raged against German methods:

> Neither horror nor indignation describes the feeling of civilised human beings at Germany's method of warfare. The poisoning by gas of brave men ready for a fair fight; the shooting of prisoners, the poisoning of wells, the murder of women and children on the high seas, and the gloating of armed men over the deaths of the defenceless has made so deep an impression on brain and heart that we are now quite certain of victory. The right to live is at stake, and we mean to secure that God-given right at all costs.[65]

The editorial deliberately juxtaposes the honourable British soldier ('ready for a fair fight') with the 'gloating' Germans, who use underhand methods – including poisons of various types – and therefore cannot possibly win. It offers both a remarkable example of the receptivity of the nursing profession to the propaganda of the war years and an indication of their assertive belief in the significance of their work. By saving the lives of poisoned soldiers and by exposing themselves to the dangers of poisoning, nurses were able to position themselves as significant participants in the allied war effort – however invisible their clinical efforts might have been in the writings of others.

Conclusion: saving lives and fighting the allied cause

Chemical warfare on the Western Front resulted in multiple, severely damaged casualties. Matron Julia Stimson, referred to it as 'at one and the same time the refinement of science and civilization, and of hideous barbarism'.[66] Caring for the victims of chemical warfare was extremely labour-intensive. Nurses treated and dressed wounds, swabbed eyes and administered oxygen and stimulants. Because patients were, initially, so severely disabled, nurses had to offer total patient care and meet all of their blind, breathless and pain-wracked patients' needs, from hygiene to feeding and toileting. Nurses removed patients' contaminated clothing, cleansed their skin of toxic substances, administered oxygen, inhalants and stimulants, offered food and fluids, and provided the calm, reassuring environment that would permit healing. A reader examining the medical journal articles of the time could be excused for believing that either the doctors themselves, or some unknown – perhaps even invisible – assistants were providing both the care and the treatment that enabled patients to survive and regain their health. Only one medical author actually acknowledged the importance of nursing interventions, and then only by pointing out, in a brief concluding comment, that: 'warmth and good nursing might pull a man through'.[67] An examination of nurses' own writings reveals not only the intricacy of their work, but also their sense of themselves as significant participants in the war. Allied propaganda encouraged them to view themselves as protagonists fighting on the side of 'good'. When one British nurse referred to the use of toxic gas as 'this fiendish mode of warfare', she was undoubtedly expressing the view that she and other nurses were an integral part of the fight against such evil.

Notes

1 Gerard Fitzgerald, 'Chemical warfare and medical response during World War I', *American Journal of Public Health* 98, 4 (April 2008), 611–25, 611; Laurence Sondhaus, *World War One: The Global Revolution* (Cambridge, Cambridge University Press, 2011), 131–2; Mark Harrison, *The Medical War: British Military Medicine in the First World War* (Oxford, Oxford University Press, 2010), 56.

2 In the autumn and winter of 1915, bromine and phosgene began to replace chlorine as the preferred methods of killing. A paper by Leonard Hill, published in December 1915 suggested that German scientists had been experimenting with poison gases for years before the war: Leonard Hill, 'An address on gas poisoning. Read before the Medical Society of London', *British Medical Journal* 2 (4 December 1915), 801–4, 801. See also, Martin Goodman, *Suffer and Survive* (London, Simon & Schuster, 2007); Edward M. Spiers, *Haldane: An Army Reformer* (Edinburgh, Edinburgh University Press, 1980).

3 Hill, 'An address on gas poisoning', 801. On the toxicity of chlorine gas, see also, Thomas Aitchison, 'Gas poisoning', *The British Medical Journal* 2 (25 September 1915), 488.

4 Mark Harrison states that gas shells were first used during the Somme offensive in the second half of 1916: Mark Harrison, *The Medical War: British*

95

Military Medicine in the First World War (Oxford, Oxford University Press, 2010), 107.

5   Sir Wilmot P. Herringham, 'Gas poisoning', *The Lancet* 195, 5034 (21 February 1920), 423–4, 423.

6   On the various types of gas used, see T. E. Sandall, 'The later effects of gas poisoning', *The Lancet* 200, 5173 (21 October 1922), 857–9, 857. On the winning of Nobel Prizes for Chemistry by the inventors of poisonous gases, see Goodman, *Suffer and Survive*, 275.

7   Christine Hallett, *Containing Trauma: Nursing Work in the First World War* (Manchester, Manchester University Press, 2009), 16.

8   Steve Sturdy, 'War as experiment. Physiology, innovation and administration in Britain, 1914–1918: The case of chemical warfare', in Roger Cooter, Mark Harrison and Steve Sturdy, *War, Medicine and Modernity* (Stroud, Sutton Publishing, 1998), 65–84: quotations on 74–5. On the allied response to chemical warfare, see also L. F. Haber, *The Poisonous Cloud: Chemical Warfare in the First World War* (Oxford, Clarendon Press, 1986); Steve Sturdy, 'From the trenches to the hospitals at home: Physiologists, clinicians and oxygen therapy, 1914–30', in John Pickstone (ed.), *Medical Innovations in Historical Perspective* (Basingstoke, Macmillan, 1992), 104–23.

9   The 'zone of the armies' refers to an area, with a width of about 10 km, behind the front line trenches, within which no women, or other civilians, were allowed. Casualty clearing stations, the first points in the lines of evacuation where nurses were permitted to work, were situated at approximately this distance until the later years of the war.

10 Fitzgerald, 'Chemical warfare and medical response', 611.

11 T. J. Mitchell and G. M. Smith, *History of the Great War Based on Official Documents: Medical Services* (Uckfield, West Sussex, The Naval and Military Press Ltd with the Imperial War Museum; facsimile of book first published 1931), 111.

12 Anonymous, *A War Nurse's Diary: Sketches from a Belgian Field Hospital* (New York, The Macmillan Company, 1918), 98–9. On the earliest victims of gas poisoning, see also, Anonymous, Column, *The British Journal of Nursing* 54 (1 May 1915), 368.

13 Sister Ellen Cuthbert; Nurses' Narratives, Butler Collection; AWM41/958; Australian War Memorial, Canberra, Australia.

14 Anonymous, 'The passage of a dudshell through the Western Front, Or, some experiences of an army nurse in the late war'; Nurses' accounts; QARANC Collection, Army Medical Services Museum, Aldershot, 27.

15 Violetta Thurstan, *A Text Book of War Nursing* (London, G. P. Putnam's Sons, 1917), 167.

16 J. George Adami, *War Story of the Canadian Army Medical Corps* (London, Colour Ltd and the Roll's House Publishing Co Ltd, for the Canadian War Records Office, 1918), unpaginated.

17 Alice Fitzgerald commented in November 1916 that the Germans were using 'a new kind of gas, invisible and very deadly': Alice Fitzgerald, unpublished memoirs, incorporating War Diary; Alice Fitzgerald Papers, Maryland Historical Society, Md HR M2633; Md HR M 2634; entry for 10 November.

18 J. Elliot Black, Elliot T. Glenny and J. W. McNee, 'Observations on 685 cases of poisoning by noxious gases used by the enemy', *The British Medical Journal* (31 July 1915), 165–7, 165.

19 On the introduction of lewisite towards the end of the war, see Fitzgerald, 'Chemical warfare and medical response', 613.

20 The painting is available in the Imperial War Museum, London. On its significance, see Santanu Das, *Touch and Intimacy in First World War Literature* (Cambridge, Cambridge University Press, 2005), 1–5.

21 Black, Glenny and McNee, 'Observations on 685 cases of poisoning', 165–7.

22 Hill, 'An address on gas poisoning', 802; Herringham, 'Gas poisoning', 423.

23 Black, Glenny and McNee, 'Observations on 685 cases of poisoning', 165.

24 Anonymous, 'Asphyxiating gases in war', *The Nursing Times* XI, 523 (8 May 1915), 549. See also, Anonymous, Column, *British Journal of Nursing* 54 (1 May 1915), 368.

25 Anonymous, 'Gas poisoning', *The Nursing Times* XI, 524 (15 May 1915), 585. Hill 60 was an area of rising ground (literally 60 metres above sea level) in the northern part of the Western Front, which was held by the Germans. The allied forces made repeated, unsuccessful attempts to capture it during the early years of the war.

26 Black, Glenny and McNee, 'Observations on 685 cases of poisoning', 165–7.

27 On the symptoms of chlorine gas poisoning, and the shift from asphyxiating to bronchitic symptoms, see: Hill, 'An address on gas poisoning', 802. Towards the end of 1918, the conditions of these men could be further complicated by their susceptibility to the so-called 'Spanish influenza': Anonymous, Column, *The British Journal of Nursing* 61 (19 October 1918), 232.

28 Black, Glenny and McNee, 'Observations on 685 cases of poisoning', 165.

29 Black and his team, along with most medical officers on the Western Front, prescribed emetics because of the obvious relief they appeared to offer. However, Sir Wilmot Herringham commented after the war that it was later discovered that emetics caused more harm than good because they induced exhaustion: Herringham, 'Gas poisoning', 423.

30 Thurstan, *A Text Book of War Nursing*, 168. The most effective apparatus for administering oxygen was invented by J. S. Haldane: Herringham, 'Gas poisoning', 424. See also, Goodman, *Suffer and Survive*, 268–306; Hill, 'An address on gas poisoning', 804.

31 On the use of venesection in toxic gas poisoning, see E. A. Schafer, 'Treatment of chlorine gas poisoning', *The British Medical Journal* 1 (27 May

1916) 774; A Stuart Hebbelthwaite, 'The treatment of chlorine gas poisoning by venesection', *The British Medical Journal* 2 (22 July 1916), 107–9; W. Hale White, 'The treatment of chlorine gas poisoning by venesection', *The British Medical Journal* 2 (29 July 1916), 159.

32 Black, Glenny and McNee, 'Observations on 685 cases of poisoning', 166. See also, J. D. Mortimer, 'The treatment of gas poisoning', *The Lancet* 185, 4789 (12 June 1915), 1262.

33 Black, Glenny and McNee, 'Observations on 685 cases of poisoning', 166. On the range of treatments for victims of asphyxiating gases, including the use of artificial respiration, see also, Hill, 'An address on gas poisoning, 804.

34 Thurstan, *A Text Book of War Nursing*, 167. The term 'heroic' is used here to indicate the risky nature of the treatment.

35 Black, Glenny and McNee, 'Observations on 685 cases of poisoning', 166.

36 Agnes Warner, *My Beloved Poilus* (St John, New Brunswick, Barnes and Co. Ltd, 1917), 111.

37 Julia Stimson, *Finding Themselves. The Letters of an American Army Chief Nurse at a British Hospital in France* (New York, The Macmillan Company, 1927), 79–80.

38 Black, Glenny and McNee, 'Observations on 685 cases of poisoning', 166.

39 Black, Glenny and McNee, 'Observations on 685 cases of poisoning', 166.

40 Hill, 'An address on gas poisoning', 801.

41 Violetta Thurstan recommended this and drops of castor oil: Thurstan, *A Text Book of War Nursing*, 167.

42 J. M. Lazenby, 'The treatment of irritant gas poisoning', *The British Medical Journal* 2 (28 September 1918), 342. On the use of 'alkaline douches' see also, Sir Wilmot P. Herringham, 'Gas poisoning', *The Lancet* 195, 5034 (21 February 1920), 423–4, 424.

43 Cuthbert; AWM41/958; Australian War Memorial.

44 Sister Ellen McClelland; Nurses' Narratives, Butler Collection; AWM41/1000; Australian War Memorial, Canberra, Australia.

45 Thurstan, *A Text Book of War Nursing*, 191–2.

46 Boylston, Helen Dore, *'Sister': The War Diary of a Nurse* (New York, Ives Washburn, 1927), 29. The care of blinded patients is discussed by Julie Anderson, who observes that gassed soldiers' anxieties were associated with the fear of emasculation and childlike dependency which blindness brought. See Julie Anderson, *War, Disability and Rehabilitation in Britain: Soul of a Nation* (Manchester, Manchester University Press, 2011).

47 Stimson, *Finding Themselves,* 79–80.

48 Fitzgerald, 'Chemical warfare and medical response', 613.

49 Ruth Manning, *Three ms diaries*; 4763; 80/21/1; Imperial War Museum, London.

50 Cuthbert; AWM41/958; Australian War Memorial.

51 Sister Millicent Peterkin, *Work on a Hospital Barge in France*; Nurses' Accounts; Archive of the Army Medical Services Museum, Aldershot (QARANC Collection).

52 Interview transcript: Florence Le Lievre, interviewed by Jane Tolerton and Nicholas Boyack, 15 May 1988; OHInt – 0006/50; Alexander Turnbull Library, Wellington, New Zealand; Rebecca West, *War Nurse: The True Story of a Woman Who Lived, Loved and Suffered on the Western Front* (New York, Cosmopolitan Book Corporation, 1930), 70.

53 Walter Broadbent, 'Some results of German gas poisoning', *The British Medical Journal* 2 (14 August 1915), 247.

54 On the risk of contracting tuberculosis following gassing, see also: Harold Vallow, 'The later effects of gas poisoning', *The Lancet* 200, 5175 (4 November 1922), 985.

55 Anonymous, 'The after-effects of gas poisoning' [relating the findings of Captain S. O. Cowen in the *Medical Journal of Australia,* 1 November 1919], *The Lancet* 195, 5031 (31 January 1920), 273–4.

56 Sandall, 'The later effects of gas poisoning', 857–9. See also, W. N. Abbott, 'Sequelae of gas poisoning', *The British Medical Journal* 2 (1938), 597. Some physicians were sceptical about the long-term effects of gas poisoning. See, for example, Adolphe Abrahams, 'The later effects of gas poisoning', *The Lancet* 200, 5174 (28 October 1922), 933–4.

57 Thurstan, *A Text Book of War Nursing*, 169.

58 Sir Wilmot Herringham also commented on how the eye-pieces in the earliest gas-masks would shatter: Herringham, 'Gas poisoning', 424.

59 Fitzgerald, 'Chemical warfare and medical response', 616. On the 'insidious nature of chlorine' and the need for effective masks, see also, Edward Bigg, 'Notes on three cases of chlorine gas poisoning', *The Lancet* 188, 4851 (19 August 1916), 341. On the earliest gas masks, see Anonymous, Column, *The British Journal of Nursing* 54 (8 May 1915), 383.

60 Anonymous [Evelyn Kate Luard], *Diary of a Nursing Sister on the Western Front 1914–1915* (Edinburgh and London, William Blackwood and Sons, 1915), 268–9.

61 One well-known description of gas-poisoning can be found in the memoirs of Elsie Knocker: The Baroness de T'Serclaes, *Flanders and Other Fields* (London, George G. Harrap and Co. Ltd, 1964), 99–100. The *Nursing Times* also contains an example of a field hospital, in which nurses were poisoned by gas shells: Anonymous, Column [Quoting from a letter to the *Australasian Nurses' Journal*] *Nursing Times* (16 February 1918), 205.

62 Stimson, *Finding Themselves*, 52–4.

63 Stimson, *Finding Themselves*, 54. The *Nursing Times* carried a number of images of nurses wearing gas masks during the war years. See, for example, issues of 6 May 1916, 536; 3 August 1918, 812; and 12 May 1917, 574.

64 Claire Tylee, *The Great War and Women's Consciousness: Images of Militarism and Womanhood in Women's Writings, 1914–64* (Houndmills and London, Macmillan, 1990), 252; Trudi Tate, *Modernism, History and the First World War* (Manchester, Manchester University Press, 1998), 41–62.

65 Anonymous, Editorial, *The British Journal of Nursing* 54 (15 May 1915), 423.

66 Stimson, *Finding Themselves*, 94–5.

67 Hill, 'An address on gas poisoning', 804.

5

Health, healing and harmony: Invalid cookery and feeding by Australian nurses in the Middle East in the First World War

Kirsty Harris

On 6 August 1915, the No. 3 Australian General Hospital opened its wards to wounded and sick soldiers on the Greek island of Lemnos in the Mediterranean Sea. Owing to an administrative error, the hospital's equipment had not arrived and the female nurses of the Australian Army Nursing Service (AANS) nursed men from Gallipoli on the ground and in the open air. With food supplies compromised, Staff Nurse Nellie Pike recollected:

> We kept ourselves alive by the Red Cross issue of Ideal Milk, tins of coffee *au lait*, [and] Huntley and Palmer biscuits. We, in turn, kept our patients alive by the same means plus soup made from dried cubes and cooked over an open outdoor fire in a dixie, bully beef, army biscuits, salty bacon, badly cooked porridge, prunes, rice and straw.[1]

The Australian Imperial Force (AIF) first engaged en masse with the enemy in the First World War in the campaign for the Dardanelles commencing 25 April 1915 and ending in evacuation some nine months later. For Australian Army nurses working on hospital ships in the Mediterranean Sea and in Egypt and Greece during this period, feeding soldiers suffering malnutrition and disease was a significant part of their workload and inventive solutions were necessary in countries overflowing with casualties, and short on food and water supplies. This chapter explores the feeding of hospital patients at a time when invalid foods, cookery and the serving of the food were all the domain of the ward nurse. Owing to poor army field rations, many soldiers suffered malnutrition on the battlefield, and the trained AANS nurses spent much time in their wards cooking invalid foods to feed their patients. Invalid feeding offered as much as wound treatment to return soldiers to health. It illustrates one of the crucial roles that nurses played in the health of the allied troops as food was often the only medical treatment for diseases, providing comfort and aiding faster recovery.

Invalid food practices in hospitals in the early twentieth century have not captured the imagination of contemporary Australian nursing historians. This may be due to a lack of available primary sources in Australian public repositories on pre-war hospital diets and invalid cookery. Few of the secondary sources written by historians include information on this topic. The only Australia-wide nursing history covering this period, Bartz Schultz's *A Tapestry of Service*, contains no information on invalid cookery although Kirsty Harris's book, *More than Bombs and Bandages*, redresses this omission with some discussion.[2] Thus, this chapter, using standard historical inquiry techniques, uses these scant resources to illustrate the Australian-wide picture.[3]

In contrast, for wartime memories, there exists a rich and growing body of work. These sources discuss Australian First World War military nurses, including those who served outside the AANS. They include descriptive analysis of AANS diaries written during the war as well as letters sent home, and later interpretation of the nurses' published recollections. Most publications have examined soldiers' trauma and illness combined with the administrative side of deploying the AANS and the postings of the nurses, the gender issues of wartime history, the adventures of nurses during the war, or centred on the biographical.[4] To add further context, soldiers and medical officers' views are included in this chapter to demonstrate nursing activities unrecorded by the nurses themselves. For a medical view, I have relied on the *Official Medical History* of the war written by A. G. Butler, a serving Australian Army medical officer.[5] Other available primary source materials include a range of diaries, the short transcripts of more than one hundred AANS interviews conducted by a senior matron at the end of the war and held at the Australian War Memorial, and letters published in newspapers – sources that are contextually limited due to editing.[6]

In the primary material available from the war period, perceptions are that invalid cooking was a safe subject to record; censors would be unlikely to remove it and most readers of letters and memoirs could easily understand the topic. While Australian military nurses were providing these treatments, and it was of such consequence to the nurses they included it in their writings, invalid cookery is a neglected topic; secondary sources do not often mention the topic, let alone discuss it. For example, the official medical war history does not mention invalid food. Marianne Barker in her popular history *Nightingales in the Mud* takes account of food supply problems for nurses and patients but does not discuss invalid food and diets and their application. Jan Bassett's scholarly *Guns and Brooches*, which admittedly covers six wars, also gives little attention to First World War food problems, and then again only for the nurses themselves, not for their thousands of patients.[7] The natural tendency to focus on traumatic surgery and illnesses peculiar to the war such as gas attack and trench feet, has led historians to overlook the more mundane yet no less pressing problems such as patient foods and diet.

There is no doubt that the domestic service origins of this work, and the possibility of labelling nurses as servants, has led authors and researchers investigating nurses' work to exclude the topic. In addition, earlier war historians may have considered it typical 'women's work' rather than a learned and important skill. Indeed, nursing historians have not seen it as an important skill to discuss or record, even though invalid cookery training continued in hospitals for Australian nurses for many decades after the war. However, domestic tasks such as cooking take on new importance when seen as part of a larger system of restoring men's health or curing them during wartime; it becomes a vital component of the medical service system of saving lives and returning men to the front.

In the first decade of the twentieth century, leaders in the field of dietetics in Europe and North America began to reveal discoveries about the value of invalid foods.[8] However, with no professional dieticians existing in Australia at the declaration of war in 1914, the main source of information on this topic, readily available in American and Canadian nursing circles, is missing. This presents great difficulty for the Australian historian, given the developing scientific nature of invalid cookery at the time and inclusion in nursing curricula.[9]

There appear to be no copies publicly available of one Australian source that might have revealed this developing nature before the war.[10] Australian nursing association journals did publish articles on diets such as an outline of different food groups in 'Dietetics' in the Victorian journal *Una* in September 1914.[11]

While the question of food seems commonplace as a nursing activity, military nurses who had many more sick, than wounded, patients often struggled to feed the men and even find the right foods to cook. Unlike civilian patients, often soldiers were severely malnourished and dehydrated when they arrived at hospital.[12] For patients staying in hospital for long periods, in this era before antibiotics and intravenous drips, hospital food was of vital importance; patients required food and fluids for recovery from all illnesses and surgery. Most patient survival was due to the nursing they received, not the medical treatment or surgery given by doctors, and invalid foods were a key part of nursing. Invalid cookery and foods provided by nurses therefore provided the means for 'curing' patients, a function seen as more prestigious than nurse 'caring'.[13]

The diaries, letters and papers of the nurses show how the differing environments of the war and foreign countries and foods contributed to making this role more important and challenging than at home. War altered standardised methods and ritualised practice in invalid food.[14] Invalid cookery required significant time and daily nursing effort, thus omitting discussion of this topic would indicate that historians are only examining part of nurses' military working lives. An analogy would be discussing surgery without mentioning the necessary anaesthesia. Invalid cookery continued to be important in hospitals up to the 1960s in western countries. It is still vital in the developing world, owing to malnutrition and disease brought about by poverty, war and famine, and the lack of medical facilities to replace fluids and nutrition.[15] As it is also important in bariatric treatments, in laparotomy and intestinal post-surgical treatments, and post removal of nasogastric tubes, it would be a crucial omission not to highlight its importance during a major conflict of the twentieth century.[16]

This chapter is divided into four parts. First is an exploration of what nurses learned about invalid foods in civilian hospitals and through their training courses pre-war. Then, three areas are identified: food for healing, food for health and food for harmony, showing how military nurses' work changed during the war.

Pre-war training

By the close of the nineteenth century, 'sickroom cookery' and hospital diets had become synonymous. By the outbreak of the war in 1914, invalid cookery, which included knowing how to prepare and serve a variety of invalid food and drinks to patients, was an important part of the training programme and working lives of Australian professional nurses.[17] Specialist courses on invalid cookery became available to hospital nurses, and some hospitals included the subject in their basic nursing course.[18] Articles to support nurses in their education were being published before the war but, as the first Australian nursing textbook did not appear until 1935, Australian nurses during 1900–20 often used British textbooks such as Stewart and Cuff's *Practical Nursing* to guide their learning in invalid food practices.[19] Trained nurses were required to gain a certificate in invalid cookery before graduation and they grew familiar with cooking broths, poultry, fish, meats, eggs, light puddings such as blancmange, and jellies.[20] As convalescence was slow and patients were often hospitalised for months, nurses had to manage their patients' food needs from the worst of their illness through to convalescence. Nurses, or often their female probationers (nurses in training), prepared these invalid foods as well as breakfasts and suppers for their patients in their ward pantries, cooking over a range or multiple gas rings. Most pantries had hot water on tap that also allowed drinks to be prepared.

Nurses fed very ill patients according to a prescribed diet of foods set by a doctor.[21] For the most seriously ill, the usual recommendation was a milk diet. A more variable diet was a 'fluid' diet, meaning that nurses could offer any kind of fluid such as barley-water, lemon-water, strained coffee, broth and beef tea but no solid food.[22] Nearly all of these liquids required preparation or cooking. For convalescing patients it was necessary to give them 'light' or 'bland' food. Light diets were often named after their major ingredient such as 'chicken', and a diet such as this in Australia usually included steamed white meat, eggs, soup, spinach, well-boiled onions and sometimes potatoes and stewed fruit.[23] There were also special diets designed to maximise recovery from surgery, and from specific diseases such as pneumonia, dysentery or typhoid.[24] Typhoid fever victims had the most carefully controlled and recorded diet, as doctors believed any solid food was likely to cause complications such as a perforated bowel.[25]

Warfare greatly affected the work of nurses particularly in the sphere of invalid cooking. Australian military nurses working overseas in 1915 did not have the benefit of trained probationers to carry out this work and therefore had to take it up themselves or train their male orderlies in the work. On the Greek island of Lemnos, food for staff and patients alike was poor and inadequate when the nurses first arrived. The quantity of food increased as time went on, but the quality did not significantly improve. Such issues therefore increased the workload of nurses and their ward staff.

Hospital nurses were used to feeding 'poor' patients in Australia. Initially, although there is a lack of significant discussion in the primary source material in the early months of the Gallipoli campaign, it appears that military nurses considered all feeding requirements for malnourished soldiers to be similar until they realised that their patients had very different needs. During 1915, the nurses of No. 2 Australian General Hospital (AGH) at the Ghezireh Palace Hotel, Cairo tended nearly ten thousand patients, with one of the three most common issues being digestive complaints ranging from the subacute 'gippy tummy', indigestion and food poisoning to cholera, typhoid, gastroenteritis and epidemic diarrhoea.[26] Continued malnutrition emphasised the importance of diet in hospital and thus the importance of the military nurses' work.

Nurses often had to cook food on a small primus stove or similar; this might have been a constructed mud oven outdoors if the ward consisted of tents. Usually, the primus was the only means of boiling water, cooking food and making all hot drinks. It was also utilised for sterilising equipment. Nurses missed their built-in kitchen facilities. At No. 1 AGH at Heliopolis in Egypt, nurses such as Margaret Brown remembered experiencing the 'laborious cooking of Bengers, arrowroot, eggs & so on over a blue-flame oil stove in the unventilated & electric-lit service room of an enteric ward'.[27] With a stove able to take only one large pot at a time, the nursing staff had to prioritise its use to meet their patients' needs. One nurse recalled 'it took some

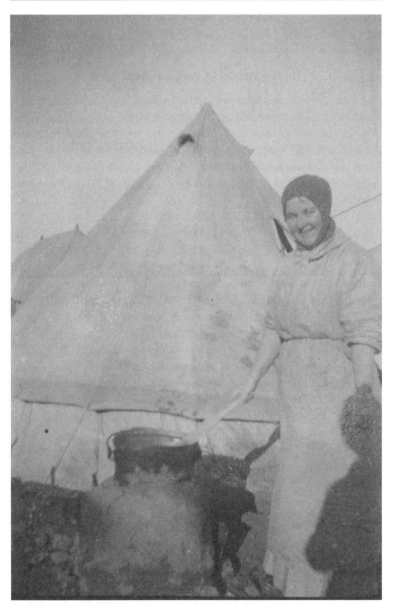

5.1 Staff Nurse Edith Rush, stirring pea soup outside a tent on Lemnos Island during the Gallipoli Campaign, 1915

calculation and work to poach 80–100 eggs on a primus in a short time'.[28]

Healing: food as medical treatment

The first aspect to consider is food for healing. The number of troops affected by disease elevated the importance of food in the First World War in this pre-antibiotic era. During the war, the allied troops in the east suffered more from dysentery than any other disease, and I use this disease to illustrate the role food played in treating it. By August 1915, of the Australian troops on Gallipoli, 77 per cent were emaciated and anaemic – which in turn made them 'just skin and bone; hands, arms, and legs covered with septic sores; [and] ill with dysentery'.[29] Dysentery had a devastating effect on gastro-intestinal status of the troops. On arrival at hospital, nurses reported many as looking like walking corpses – haggard, ragged boys in a wretched condition – too weak with starvation to walk.[30]

Both nurses at sea and on land used whatever appropriate foods were available to them. Doctors recommended a diet consisting of albumin-water, rice-water, or light meat broth, and then arrowroot and cornflour. Sister Ella Tucker's dysentery patients on the hospital ship *Gascon* on its way to Malta from Lemnos faced the standard dietary treatment: 'water arrowroot was the main article of food this trip, had 96 patients in my ward, and they were nearly all query enteric & dysentery, our tin milk was getting short, the majority of the patients were sea sick'.[31]

At Lemnos, fresh milk was not available immediately so nurses used all kinds of condensed and powdered milks until proper supplies arrived. Sister McLean at the Choubra Infectious Diseases Hospital, Cairo, wrote in a letter home:

> All our worst patients are fed mostly on Red Cross foods, such as glaxo, Benger's and Mellin's foods. When they are too bad to take the milk they get here we give them nothing else but glaxo and alb. water, and they improve wonderfully on it; when well enough they have Benger's and malted milk.[32]

Nurses in Egypt and Malta were able to take patient specimens and have them assessed for the presence of dysentery. If staff noticed any relapsing symptoms, they decreased the diet immediately. On the other hand, when convalescence set in, these patients had toast, custard, mashed potato and steamed white fish, or one of the light diets previously mentioned added to their meals – whatever food would give the patient additional nourishment.

Health: food for recovery

Providing food for health and recovery was a most important role for nurses, as the condition of soldiers arriving from the battlefield was often distressing. The second aspect shows how both doctors and nurses believed food was an essential component for their patients' well-being and consequently how vital invalid cookery was in the war effort.[33]

The First World War occurred at a time when medicine could contribute far less than it can now to successful recovery from illness. Thus, good nursing and an appropriate diet had far greater importance. A key factor for military nursing staff was each soldier's nutritional condition when they arrived for medical treatment. Field rations, or lack of an appropriate variety, directly affected the condition of men, and left them greatly susceptible to disease and debility.[34] However, there was little knowledge of general nutrition in 1915; Australian nurses learnt from nursing journal articles in 1914 that food might contain 'proteids, carbohydrates, fats, salts and water'. There was no mention of vitamins.[35] Hospitals trained nurses in dietetic management of their cases, not the nutrition that their patients actually required.[36] This was the purview of doctors and they learnt many lessons in 1915 such that 'much of the flux at Gallipoli was due to irritation – food *per se*'.[37] Australian medical staff were unaware until after the campaign that the rations supplied on Gallipoli were deficient in vitamins B and C and were largely indigestible.[38]

It was obvious that nurses receiving patients in their wards thought the army 'practically starved' the soldiers.[39] The 'hard' ration scale in the field for the Australian Imperial Force (AIF) included bully beef (corned or pickled beef), hard biscuits, jam, cheese and bacon.[40] However, flies or sand often blanketed the food and the bacon was often rancid. Thus, the food meant to keep the troops healthy in fact contributed to their ill health. The monotonous rations, or lack of them, therefore directly affected the nursing of soldier patients already challenged by disease, septic wounds, extremes of climate and delays in reaching hospital. Only a month into the Gallipoli campaign Sister Janey Lempriere, with Anglo-Boer war experience, wrote in a letter home of the Australian men she saw: 'They look like men who have had a great nervous shock, from wounds & exposure & want of food. It will take weeks of nursing to cure them.'[41]

Sometimes injured soldiers went up to four days without food before evacuation by sea.[42] The limited food and drink available during the voyage back to medical centres contributed to the soldier's stress. Sister Jean Bisset, on board a hospital ship on the ferry service between the Dardanelles and Lemnos, received patients who had been lying unfed for two days on shore after the big attack in early August. She wrote: 'They were all young fellows, with dreadful wounds, and were all so thankful to get into a bed and have something to drink … it is pitiful to see how eager they are for it.'[43]

Men evacuated from the battlefields always needed fluids urgently to treat dehydration from haemorrhage, the sweat of battle and shock.[44] Nothing sustained them more than the administration of artificial warmth, most effectively delivered through hot drinks.[45] An unknown AANS nurse wrote about her experiences when she first arrived at Lemnos in August 1915:

> Two days after 600 more freshly wounded and sick arrived, taxing our hospital to its utmost, so … all kinds of condensed and liquid milks (fresh milk unobtainable) and broths made for the patients till we could get our proper supplies. In those early days … water almost unobtainable, only enough to make tea, as the condensers were not yet in working order, so our supply was very small.[46]

For those that could drink, nursing staff provided a variety including tea, coffee, cocoa, Bovril or hot soup that 'warmed them quicker than all our steam pipes could manage'.[47] Hot tea with plenty of sugar was the preference of most soldiers, although hospitals in Egypt did have access to ice to cool drinks.[48]

Although military hospital kitchens provided meals for ambulatory patients, in their small and often makeshift ward pantries, the nurses prepared and cooked small meals such as special diets for the very sick cases and light diets, thus imitating their home practices.[49] One medical officer's diary indicates that this food included jelly, puddings and beef tea.[50] Eggs played a vital role in the invalid diet, as they could be prepared in many ways.

As well as honing their cooking skills, military nurses became logistical experts, crossing and redefining usual occupational boundaries and limits.[51] Obtaining invalid foods in the military was not just a case of going to the hospital kitchen and requesting items. They commonly negotiated the army's requisition system, the vagaries of supply from local shopkeepers and farmers in foreign countries and the Red Cross's distribution system to provide their patients with what they considered suitable food in appropriate quantities.[52] Designated invalid food was not always available. The provision of foods suitable for invalids varied enormously and often depended upon local availability. Nurses frequently commented on the quality, which ranged across 'not specially good', and 'unsuitable for the sick'.[53] For example, food in Egypt suitable to the Australian/European palate was difficult to find and the local foodstuffs such as 'buffalo butter' caused many complaints.[54] Coaxing patients to eat such food was all part of nursing work. Margaret Aitken reported the trials of finding appropriate food: 'The food supply at first was very bad especially for Medical cases, everything tinned – bread awful, uneatable at times, water very scarce.'[55] Bully beef and biscuit were wholly unsuitable for sick men and often gave them violent colic.[56]

Cultural differences in patient treatment were evident in the provision of invalid foods. Many Australian nurses had never travelled outside Australia, and then often only to other English-speaking countries and lacked understanding in how other nationalities lived. For Cecil Wray, forty-five Greek dysentery patients in her ward were a big problem, as they 'wouldn't keep to their diet'; the patients sourced and ate yoghurt, as per their own cultural norms.[57]

The British, Australian, Canadian and New Zealand nurses who served on hospital and transport ships in the Aegean and Mediterranean Seas had to deal with any shortfalls in their food supplies, which was difficult with no local shops or place to trade until they reached shore. On the hospital ship *Gascon* off Cape Helles, Hilda Samsing complained of:

> the way the steward will not get enough food for the milk diets, either he is at fault or the patients are robbed of their rice & oatmeal, so I had him up

before the O.C. The amount of food the ship gives is not enough to keep …
on, except to the ordinary diets.[58]

Nurse Ellen Barron kept Bovril, coffee and bread and butter for her
patients, and was astounded how badly wounded men wanted to eat:

'Butter,' they would cry, 'butter. I haven't tasted butter for four months.'
They would eat and eat, and enjoy it, and afterwards when I saw their
wounds I gasped, and wondered, not only that they could eat, but in some
cases how it was they were alive.[59]

Sometimes the supplies on the ships ran out, owing to constant
demand. The large number of patients to feed was a change from
civilian practice. Individual nurses looked after hundreds of men
with only the assistance of male orderlies, untrained in cookery. It
was a stressful situation for nurses when patients depended on food
for their recovery.

Lack of supplies meant lack of food and nourishment for patients;
lack of invalid food supplies meant nurses having to use their initiative.[60] Nurses became logistical experts, requisitioning items from the
Quartermaster and his staff who had control of the kitchen, cooks,
food and feeding.[61] There were issues with the supply system. Esther
King at Luna Park hospital in Cairo could get no rations for her new
patients for twenty-four hours:

Consequently there was severe shortage. One day in going off duty I left
only 60 patients in my ward and next morning there were 140 and the food
for 60 had to do for the 140 men. There was so much trouble though we
reported the matter even as far as the O.C.[62]

Sometimes, improvisation was required. As Sister Rachel Pratt had
no green vegetables on Lemnos, she looked to nourish her patients by
serving each a bottle of stout.[63]

Harmony: the morale-boosting impact of food

Nurses used food in their hospital wards to promote harmony and to
comfort men. Integrating caring and curing was particularly important to nurses.[64] Military nursing staff were encouraged to keep up
the men's morale and often used what Butler called 'psychophysical
tonics', such as food and cooking to cheer to their patients especially

on occasions such as birthdays, national holidays and Christmas.[65] Letitia Moreton helped give her patients at Maadi Hospital in Egypt 'a very nice little Xmas. A very nice dinner, roast turkey, chicken, ham, plenty vegetables, plum pud, claret cup, beer, soft drinks, sweets etc. They did enjoy it, poor things.'[66]

Although many soldiers' diaries contain no reference to their hospital stay, those that do refer to hospital food in positive terms. Light Horse trooper Ion Idriess, recovering at the Egyptian Government Hospital, Alexandria in September 1915, illustrates this in his post-war book: 'Same doctors, same smiling nurses, same good old tucker.'[67] Letters home contain more comments, mainly reiterating that hospital food was 'good'. Private J. C. Philpot became a patient at No. 2 AGH at Ghezireh in Cairo in August 1915 and after fifteen weeks in the trenches wrote in a letter to a friend that the 'food and beds are first class'.[68] Likewise, Chas Taylor at Hayat Convalescent Hospital, Egypt in September thought the meals 'better food – what ho!' after living on biscuits and jam. However, he found his stomach rejected the food for 'being so rich. I have been on a light diet for a couple of days, as the other did not agree with me.'[69] This amply illustrates the need for invalid foods.

For patients, food was a key ritual in their day and men looked forward to meals as a welcome break, a positive distraction that broke the monotony of long periods in hospital. It rated high in importance alongside sleep when they were away from the battlefront. The ritual of meals provided opportunities for sociability as well as nourishment. Convalescing patients often enjoyed light diets, as they usually contained none of the foodstuffs found in the field.[70]

Doctors favoured alcoholic medical comforts in the nineteenth century, and used them mainly as stimulants.[71] However, by the advent of the First World War, doctors had supposedly discarded the use of alcohol and Dr Butler, the official medical historian, stated that: 'Alcohol had little place, if any, in the treatment of wounded men.'[72] Evidence suggests otherwise. While the army officially prohibited the provision of alcohol to patients except on the signed prescription of a medical officer, sisters working close to the front knew differently, with brandy often used as a stimulant for those affected by the cold, influenza, or to mask the bad taste of medicine.[73] The list of rationed 'medical comforts' stored on one ship sailing from Australia for medical use in convalescent diets, included ale (1,440 bottles), brandy (300 bottles), champagne (300 pints), stout (1,440 bottles) and port wine (450 bottles).[74]

Sometimes, those nurses who could cook well spoilt their patients with additional offerings such as custard or stewed fruit that might perhaps tempt them to eat and thus build them up. These efforts to make their wards 'a home' give importance to a nursing activity often downplayed as simply being traditional women's work.[75]

Queenie Avenell recorded in one of her letters home in 1915 that her soldiers particularly appreciated eggs in their diet and the eggflips she made were deemed by soldiers 'very acceptable after bully beef'.[76] However, edible eggs could be difficult to obtain. In his war diary, Australian surgeon Claude Morlet at Luna Park hospital reflects his stress in trying to cope with the first influx of wounded from Gallipoli and his sympathy for the lot of the soldier: 'Imagine trying to keep the peace single-handed among 400 men, convalescent and slightly wounded, when only 300 eggs were obtainable for their tea!'[77] Private John Hampson at No. 1 AGH at Heliopolis in early June experienced the poor quality of eggs available to hospital staff in Egypt. Out of the first eight eggs served to him, 'only one was good'.[78]

The frequent lack of food variety bored patients. Nurse Lilian Coomer at No. 1 Australian Auxiliary Hospital in Luna Park recalled that there was plenty of food but it was mostly chicken and 'the boys very soon tired of it'. Military nurses appreciated any additional supplies such as jam, tinned fruit and meat extract.[79] Much desired extras such as cocoa, sweetened condensed milk and chocolate came from assorted lines of supply including the Red Cross societies of many countries including Australia and Britain, in Christmas tins donated by patriotic funds and in parcels from families. In some locations, the extras were necessities. Elsie Eglinton working at the Citadel Hospital, Cairo also found members of the Red Cross Society a great help: 'It's lovely to come on duty at night and find great bowls of beef jelly and mutton broth and all kinds of nourishment for our patients at night, made by these ladies.'[80]

As matrons did not permit nurses to visit stores or kitchens, military nurses sought to provide the 'boys' with additional foodstuffs from outside the official systems.[81] Like Australian soldiers, clever at what they termed 'legitimate scavenging', the nurses' resourcefulness in adding vegetables and fruit to the basic diet of their patients was outstanding. Sometimes the nurses helped themselves – an easier solution than negotiating in a foreign language with foreign currency. Often this 'acquisition' aspect of their work, presented as 'surprises' for the men, generated much conviviality and sociability on the wards as well as aiding their patients' recovery.

Conclusion

The extent of malnourishment among soldiers meant that the military nurse's role of acquiring supplies, cooking for, and feeding, their ward patients played a more crucial part in improving the health of soldiers than it did for civilian patients in Australia. Food was a major component of medical treatments of the time; and Australian Army nurses had to manage debilitated patients requiring conflicting diets in a physical environment where the right foods or sufficient food were difficult to obtain, as was cooking in the bulk quantities required. Using their initiative and any means available, nurses physically and mentally rebuilt the health of the soldiers so they could again 'march on their stomachs'.

Food provided by nurses in the war environment of Egypt and Greece in 1915 demonstrated the nurses' adaptability and ingenuity with both acquiring and cooking food for their patients. Military nurses saw food not just as an agent for healing but also as an aid to creating harmony and happiness in their wards. The nurses' use of food to provide comfort and boost morale highlights their understanding of the psychosocial needs of their soldier patients. Increasing our understanding of invalid food feeding adds to our knowledge of military history as it shows the complexity of the military nurses' work at a time when the emphasis lay on wounded soldiers rather than the sick.

Notes

1 Nellie Pike in John Laffin, *Digger – The Legend of the Australian Soldier* (Melbourne, Macmillan Australia, revd edn, 1986), 64.

2 Bartz Schultz, *A Tapestry of Service – The Evolution of Nursing in Australia*, Volume I Foundation to Federation 1788–1900 (Melbourne, Churchill Livingstone, 1991); Kirsty Harris, *More than Bombs and Bandages, Australian Army Nurses at Work in World War I* (Newport, NSW, Big Sky Publishing, 2011).

3 Australian hospital histories also neglect the topic. Out of a sample of twenty books, the only histories that directly mention invalid cookery are K. S. Inglis, *Hospital and Community – A History of the Royal Melbourne Hospital* (Melbourne, Melbourne University Press, 1958) and J. Frederick Watson, *The History of the Sydney Hospital from 1811 to 1911* (Sydney, W. A. Gullick, Government Printer, 1911). In both cases, the entry was brief.

4 Jan Bassett, *Guns and Brooches – Australian Army Nursing from the Boer War to the Gulf War* (Melbourne, Oxford University Press Australia, 1992); Rupert Goodman, *Our War Nurses, The History of the Royal Australian Army Nursing Corps, 1902–1988* (Brisbane, Boolarong Publications, 1988); Joy Damousi and Marilyn Lake (eds), *Gender and War – Australians at War in the Twentieth Century* (Melbourne, Cambridge University Press, 1995); Beverley Kingston, *My Wife, My Daughter and Poor Mary Ann* (Melbourne, Nelson, 1975); Patsy Adam-Smith, *The Anzacs* (Melbourne, Thomas Nelson Australia Pty Ltd, 1978); Marianne Barker, *Nightingales in the Mud – The Digger Sisters of the Great War 1914–1918* (Sydney, Allen & Unwin, 1989); Janet Butler, *Kitty's War* (St Lucia, Queensland, University of Queensland Press, 2013); Melanie Oppenheimer, *Oceans of Love – Narrelle – an Australian Nurse in World War I* (Sydney, ABC Books, 2006); Ruth Rae, *Veiled Lives* (Burwood, NSW, The College of Nursing, 2009).

5 A. G. Butler, *Official History of the Australian Army Medical Services 1914–1918, Volume III – Special Problems and Services* (Canberra, Australian War Memorial (hereafter AWM), 1943), chapter X.

6 AWM, Canberra, AWM41/1072, 'Interviews containing accounts of Nursing experiences in the AANS'. Butler commissioned 128 interviews by Matron Kellett in 1919.

7 Bassett, *Guns and Brooches*.

8 Frederick W. Clements, *A History of Human Nutrition in Australia* (Melbourne, Longman Cheshire, 1986), 64.

9 Alfred Hospital, Melbourne, 'Rules, etc. for nurses under training, 1884', 7, 'Schedule A, Examination Paper'; Eva Lückes, *General Nursing*, 8th edn (London, Kegan Paul, Trench, Trübner & Co. Ltd, 1910 [1884]), 291, 297; Kathryn McPherson, *Bedside Matters – The Transformation of Canadian Nursing, 1900–1990* (Toronto, Oxford University Press, 1996), 113.

10 W. A. Osborne, *A Primer of Dietetics* (Melbourne, W. Ramsey & Co., 1910).

11 Outline of different food groups in 'Dietetics', *Una – The Journal of the Royal Victorian Trained Nurses' Association* (hereafter cited as *Una*), XII, 7 (30 September 1914), 215.

12 An AIF member in France, in J. N. I. Dawes and L. L. Robson, *Citizen to Soldier - Australia before the Great War Recollections of Members of the First A.I.F.* (Melbourne, Melbourne University Press, 1977), 204.

13 See McPherson, *Bedside Matters*, 77.

14 McPherson, *Bedside Matters*, 85.

15 See, for example, Barbara A. Parfitt, *Working Across Cultures: A Study of Expatriate Nurses Working in Developing Countries in Primary Health Care* (Developments in Nursing and Health Care) (Aldershot, Avebury, 1998). Oral rehydration therapy is a modern invalid food. See references such as World Health Organization, *The Treatment of Diarrhoea - A Manual for Physicians and Other Senior Health Workers*, 4th revd edn (2005), listed at http://en.wikipedia.org/wiki/Oral_rehydration_therapy.

16 'Prospective, randomized, controlled trial between a pathway of controlled rehabilitation with early ambulation and diet and traditional postoperative care after laparotomy and intestinal resection', http,//knowledgetranslation.ca/sysrev/articles/project51/Delaney2003.pdf, (accessed 1 January 2013); www.livestrong.com/article/310868-soft-diet-list-for-intestinal-surgery/ (accessed 1 January 2013).

17 Anonymous, 'The invalid's tray in summer', *Una* VII, 9 (30 November 1909), 143; Patricia Gwillim, BA (Hons), 'The History of Nursing at the Royal Melbourne Hospital 1846-1951', 9, in University of Melbourne Archives, RVCN, Box 99, Industrial papers 1911-1964, citing Melbourne Hospital 56th Annual Report, 1902-3; E. I. Curwood, OH183, J. S. Battye Library of West Australian History, Oral History Programme; an interview by Miss Vicky Hobbs, 27 October 1975, 8; Anonymous, 'RVTNA Medical Exam June 1910 and Answers', *Una* IX, 7 (30 September 1911), 150; Anonymous, 'Dietetics', *Una* XII, 7 (30 September 1914), 215.

18 Laurel Dyson, *How to Cook a Galah: Celebrating Australia's Culinary Heritage* (South Melbourne, Lothian Books, 2002), 101; Helen Gregory, *A Tradition of Care - A History of Nursing at the Royal Brisbane Hospital* (Brisbane, Boolarong Publications, 1988), 51; Elizabeth Burchill, *Australian Nurses since Nightingale 1860-1990* (Melbourne, Spectrum Publications, 1992), 38; Curwood, OH183, 8.

19 Anonymous, 'Dietary of the sick room', *Una* I, 1 (April 1903), 16-20; Anonymous, 'Dietetics', 215; See, for example, Maude Earle, *Sickroom Cookery and Hospital Diet, with Special Recipes for Convalescent and Diabetic Patients* (London, Spottiswoode & Co., 1897); Isla Stewart and Herbert E. Cuff, *Practical Nursing*, 3rd edn (Edinburgh and London, William Blackwood and Sons, 1911), 6, 394; Eva Lückes, *General Nursing*. The first Australian book was Gwendolin N. Burbidge, *Lectures for Nurses*, 2nd edn (Sydney, Australasian Medical Publishing Company, 1939 [1935]), which contains a lecture on diets for specific diseases but no discussion of nutritional values.

20 Anonymous, 'Savory broths and meat jellies for the sick', *Una* XV, 9 (30 November 1917), 285.

21 Anthea Hyslop, *Sovereign Remedies – a History of Ballarat Base Hospital, 1850s to 1980s* (Sydney, Allen & Unwin Australia Pty Ltd, 1989), 169.

22 Anonymous, 'Dietary of the sick room', 16–20; Anonymous, 'Dietetics', 215; W. Spalding Laurie, 'Diet in typhoid fever', *The Australian Medical Journal* (27 June 1914), 1627.

23 See for example, Anonymous, 'Savory broths and meat jellies for the sick', 285.

24 Anonymous, 'RVTNA Medical exam June 1910 and answers', 150; 'New books', *Una* (29 June 1918), 112.

25 For example, Anonymous, 'Detail nursing in case of typhoid fever', No. 2 examination paper answer, *Una* (28 February 1914), 324; W. Spalding Laurie, 'Diet in typhoid fever', *The Australian Medical Journal* (27 June 1914), 1627; Anonymous, 'Best answers to medical paper', *Una* (28 February 1917), 377.

26 Butler, *Official History, Vol III, Statistics of the War*, table 58.

27 Miss M. K. Brown, AWM, Canberra, AWM41/948, 2–3.

28 AWM, Canberra, AWM27/373/61, *No. 14 Australian General Hospital* (no date, no author), 3.

29 A. G. Butler, *Official History of the Australian Army Medical Services 1914–1918, Volume I – Gallipoli, Palestine and New Guinea*, 2nd edn (Canberra, AWM, 1938), 352.

30 Hope Weatherhead. in Muriel E. Clampett, *My Dear Mother* (Melbourne, Muriel Clampett, 1992), 147.

31 Sister Ella Jane Tucker, diary 26 September 1915, AWM, Canberra, AWM41/1053.

32 Sister McLean, letter to Mrs Peters, Rose Park in 'Red Cross needs', *The Register* (16 December 1915), 6.

33 Sister I. I. Lindsay in Butler, *Official History*, vol. III, 557–8.

34 See, for example, Bill Gammage, *The Broken Years – Australian Soldiers in the Great War* (Canberra, Penguin Books Ltd, 1975), 187.

35 'Dietetics' in *Una* XII, 7 (30 September 1914), 215.

36 'New books', in *Una* (29 June 1918), 112. Later journal articles suggest that Australian nurses learnt from 1917 onwards that traditional diet lists were now out of vogue and nurses should know physiological and food chemistry and be able to work out diets on a caloric basis.

37 A .G. Butler, *Official History of the Australian Army Medical Services 1914–1918, Volume II – The Western Front* (Canberra, AWM, 1940), 584 fn.

38 Butler, *Official History*, vol. II, 583.

39 Blodwyn E. Williams, AWM, Canberra, AWM41/1057; Hope Weatherhead in Clampett, *My Dear Mother*, 147.

40 'Narrative Account of No. 26 Amb. Train, Sister H. Chadwick', AWM, Canberra, AWM41/953, 2; 'Food value of cheese', *Una* XIII, 10 (30 December 1915), 322.

41 Sister Janey Lempriere, papers, Alfred Hospital Nursing Archives, letter 20 May 1915, 4.

42 Alice E. B. Kitchen, diary 9 August 1915, MS 9627 MSB 478, State Library of Victoria (hereafter SLV); Anonymous, 'Nurse's Letter', *Sydney Morning Herald* (17 November 1915), 14.

43 Jean Bisset, 'Letter from Sister Bisset', *Una* XIII, 11 (29 January 1916), 346.

44 Butler, *Official History*, vol. II, 345.

45 Butler, *Official History*, vol. II, 343.

46 Anonymous, 'Extracts from Letters' *Una* XVI, 2 (30 April 1918), 39.

47 Jean Bisset, 'Letter from Sister Bisset', dated 13 August 1915, *Una* XIII, 11 (29 January 1916), 346; Sister R. A. Kirkcaldie, *In Gray and Scarlet ...* (Melbourne, Alexander McCubbin, 1922), 95; Patrick M. Hamilton, OBE, *Riders of Destiny, The 4th Australian Light Horse Field Ambulance 1917–1918 – An Autobiography and History* (Melbourne, Mostly Unsung Military History Research and Publications, 2nd edn, 1996), 66–7.

48 Butler, *Official History*, vol. II, 345.

49 First Major, 'In Praise of the Primus', in *The Kia Ora Coo-ee* (June 1918), Egypt, 2; AWM, Canberra, AWM41/965, Sister Elfreda M. Doepke, 4.

50 Springthorpe, *Diary of the War*, 69.

51 McPherson, *Bedside Matters*, 100.

52 Butler, *Official History*, vol. III, 501, 693.

53 AWM, Canberra, AWM41/1072, Kellett interview no. 54, Miss Helen Keith; AWM, Canberra, AWM41/1072, Kellett interview no. 17, Miss Victoria E. Drewett; Gertrude Davis in Patsy Adam-Smith, *Australian Women at War* (Melbourne, Thomas Nelson Australia, 1984), 28; AWM, Canberra, AWM41/1072, Kellett interview no. 3, Miss Marie Bass, 1; AWM, Canberra, AWM41/1072, Kellett interview no. 10, Miss I. A. Burns.

54 Suzanne Brugger, *Australians and Egypt, 1914–1919* (Melbourne, Melbourne University Press, 1980), 28.

55 AWM, Canberra, AWM41/937, Margaret Aitken, 2; on Lemnos. Similar sentiments by Sister Hope Weatherhead in Clampett, *My Dear Mother*, 147.

56 Butler, *Official History*, vol. I, 249.

57 AWM, Canberra, AWM41/1062, Sister Wray. At No. 50 British General Hospital, Salonika.

58 AWM, Canberra, AWM PR 85/374, 'Papers of Sr H. Samsing, AANS', diary, 29 July 1915.

59 'A nurse's experiences. With the wounded off Gallipoli', *Brisbane Courier* (20 November 1915), 6.

60 Matron Cornwell in 'Magnificent story of the Australian army nurses', *The Leader*, Melbourne (2 May 1931), 42.

61 Butler, *Official History*, vol. II, 369.
62 AWM, Canberra, AWM41/992, Sister E. W. King.
63 R. Pratt, 'Nursing at Lemnos – August–December, 1915' *Reveille* 6, 12 (1 August 1933), 42.
64 McPherson, *Bedside Matters*, 95.
65 Butler, *Official History*, vol. II, 465–6; Australian War Memorial, Canberra, AWM41/937, Margaret Aitken, 2. Psychophysical tonics were environmental remedies such as food, warmth and bedding.
66 AWM, Canberra, AWM/2/DRL 0097, Letitia Moreton, letter 9 January 1916.
67 Ion L. Idriess, *The Desert Column* (Sydney, Angus & Robertson Ltd, 1933), 26 (accessed 6 February 2013), at www.epubbud.com/read.php?g= BQEYL48U&tocp=3.
68 'Letters from our boys', *Wyalong Advocate and Mining, Agricultural and Pastoral Gazette* (22 September 1915), 2.
69 'A few cold feet', *Molong Express and Western District Advertiser* (30 October 1915), 3.
70 Corporal Geebung, 'Hospital memories', *The Kia Ora Coo-ee* (15 August 1918), 17; Adam-Smith, *The Anzacs*, 81; 'With the Australians', *Ballarat Courier* (6 December 1915), 3.
71 Schultz, *A Tapestry of Service*, 120 citing Mrs Leila Murray, 1906, 'Notes on my acquaintance with Prince Alfred Hospital', *Australasian Nurses' Journal* (15 May 1906), 154–9.
72 Butler, *Official History*, vol. II, 345.
73 Graham Wilson, 'Everything on its belly', *Sabretache* 41, 3 (1 September 2000), 20; 'Poultice' [author], 'A trooper's opinion of a medico', *Vulamend Souvenir*, No. 2 Australian Stationary Hospital, AIF (December 1914 to July 1919), in University of Melbourne Archives, 20; Matron Bessie Pocock diary, 4 January 1916, copy in possession of author; Doris Grylls (née Eastwood), OH224, interview for the Oral History Programme by Chris Jeffery, 9 August 1977, JS Battye Library of West Australian History, Perth, 6.
74 Wilson, 'Everything on its belly', 20, citing Neville Tregarthern, *Sea Transport of the AIF*, Naval Transport Branch, Melbourne, undated, 98–9.
75 See discussion in McPherson, *Bedside Matters*, 35.
76 Queenie Avenell, *Letters of Sister E .F. Avenell, 1915–1917*, MS 12567, Box 3409/8, SLV, letter 14 September 1915, Heliopolis.
77 Geoffrey Morlet, *Eyes Right, The Life of Claude Morlet, DSO, Eye Surgeon and Soldier* (Adelaide, Lythrum Press, 2007), 74.
78 'An Australian hero', *Riverine Herald* (16 September 1915), 3.
79 AWM, Canberra, AWM41/1072, Kellett interview no. 11, Miss L. Comber; Springthorpe, *Diary of the War*, 69.
80 AWM, Canberra, AWM PR 86/068, E. A. Eglinton, 36, letter 23 May 1915; Sister Olive Haynes, letter to my dear Nell, 28 April 1915, in Margaret Young

(ed.), *We Are Here, Too* (Adelaide, Australian Down Syndrome Association Incorporated, 1991), 38.

81 Tilton, *Grey Battalion*, 55, 289; 'Magnificent story', 42; AWM, Canberra, AWM/PR/86/068, Eglinton, 86, letter 8 October 1916; AWM, Canberra, AWM25/509/5, memo E. M. McCarthy, Matron-in-Chief, British Expeditionary Force, 26 September 1917 to Matron, 3 AGH.

6

Eyewitnesses to revolution: Canadian military nurses at Petrograd, 1915–17

Cynthia Toman

Sir Edward Kemp, Minister of the Overseas Military Forces of Canada, wrote in 1919 that 'it is impossible to divorce the Medical Services from the rest of the military machine which it serves'.[1] It was also impossible to divorce the Medical Services from the political machine that it served as an embedded part of the armed forces. Political alliances were not always clear or consistent during the First World War, and Russia had a particularly uneasy relationship with other Allied countries. This was partially due to Russian heritage along its shifting western boundary, and partially due to the presence of highly valuable oil and copper resources located near its border with Germany. In spite of close familial relationships between the monarchs of both countries, England worried that Russia would leave the Western alliance and align itself with Germany.

England was particularly sensitive to Russian demands for Allied support and responded by establishing a joint Anglo-Russian hospital unit at Petrograd. The hospital opened in January 1916, intentionally staffed by nurses from the Dominions. The hospital was situated in the Palace of Grand Duke Dimitri, complete with ballrooms, reception rooms, and state apartments converted into wards. It became an atypical working environment for four Canadian Army Medical Corps (CAMC) nurses, compared to tented hospital facilities on the European Western Front where nurses frequently complained of the cold, rain and mud. These four nurses, known by military rank and title as nursing sisters, served brief periods at the Anglo-Russian Hospital from November 1915 to the fall of 1917: Dorothy Macleod Penner Cotton, Edith Tilley Hegan, Lucy Gertrude Squire and Mabel Lindsay.

Dorothy Cotton is the best known of the four, partly owing to her 'distinguished Montreal military family' background, partly because she served the longest with the hospital (two periods of six–eight months duration), and mostly because she left written accounts and photographs about the experience.[2] She prepared three formal reports for the CAMC and published an account in the *Canadian Nurse* (1926), as well as writing a diary and letters which her family kept.[3] In Cotton's own words, '[The Anglo-Russian Hospital] was undertaken as a "political entente" between the British and Russian Governments. The Dominions contributed generously to the funds, and representatives [personnel] were sent from Canada, Australia and South Africa.'[4] The Canadian government donated £10,000 'thus to express Canadian appreciation of valour and heroism of Russian armies'.[5]

Canadian scholar David Mackenzie suggests that individual experiences can challenge the way we think and write about war. [6] In particular, he refers to Douglas McCalla's argument that established stories and images tend to 'dominate understanding long after research has called them deeply into question' and there is 'a need to retell the story on a different basis altogether'.[7] The Anglo-Russian Hospital, as seen through Cotton's experiences, provides a window into seldom-acknowledged aspects of military nursing work – the politics and diplomacy of wartime caregiving – which appear contradictory to traditional accounts that portray medical and nursing services as neutral and either very heroic or merely supportive work compared to real soldiers (men) in the field.

There is a paucity of historical research regarding military nursing as enabling state agenda during wars. Historian Katie Pickles explored gendered imperialism in the context of the Imperial Order Daughters of the Empire (IODE), a national federation of women founded in Canada during 1900 and incorporated as a charitable organisation in 1901. The IODE declared its purpose as promoting patriotism, loyalty, service, and in particular, strengthening Canada's national ties to the British Empire.[8] Pickles argues that women participated in distinctly gendered forms of female imperialism, based on perceived maternal capabilities, as in nurturing and caring activities.[9] Jeffrey Reznick examined the culture of caregiving within the context of Britain and the First World War, with one focus on 'how soldiers, their caregivers and the public made sense of the war in the context of healing sites used to sustain manpower for battle as well as mass support for the war effort'.[10]

Another body of literature focuses on the intersection of war, relief efforts for both soldiers and civilians, and voluntary [non-military] organisations. John Hutchinson, for example, provides a critique of national Red Cross societies and how they enabled war.[11] Julia Irwin traced the involvement of four American Red Cross nurses involved with relief work following the First World War, concluding that,

> The avowedly humanitarian nature of U.S. nurses' assistance projects served as valuable cultural diplomacy. Their provision of voluntary expert assistance to remedy local health issues, coupled with efforts to nurture local professionals, helped legitimize the spread of U.S. cultural and political influence by masking the more violent and aggressive aspects of American empire and defining U.S. influence in the world as a force for good.[12]

Heather Jones studied humanitarian aid to prisoners of war, pointing out that reciprocity was a key to the aid provided, 'in terms of both reciprocal reprisals and reciprocal privileges allowed to captives. States copied each other's prisoner treatment and, to a certain degree, punishments.'[13] Jones argues that: 'Ultimately, the war's unleashing of nationalised aid efforts based on reciprocity also served to undermine the neutral, international humanitarian approach.'[14] Rebecca Gill compared the British National Aid Society and the Friends' War Victims Relief Fund during the Franco-Prussian War (1870–71) in one study and examined British relief agencies during the South African War (1899–1902) in another.[15] In arguing that 'compassion' had boundaries, Gill suggests that relief organisations 'were far from being examples of no strings giving. New imperial relationships were enacted or aspired to, shared values cultivated and obligations of loyalty and friendship anticipated.'[16]

This chapter extends the scholarship by examining the nature of military nurses' work as a form of gendered imperialism, as politically situated, and as diplomatically sensitive. While enlistment was voluntary for Canadian nurses, once enlisted, they were paid professionals and completely embedded within the armed forces – calling their presumed neutrality into question. Analysis of Cotton's accounts with the Anglo-Russian Hospital clearly suggests that she was very aware of her position as the main Canadian representative in this diplomatic mission. She revelled in opportunities to mingle with the royal family of Tsar Nicholas II as well as other prominent people, recorded her perspectives of the Russian revolution from the vantage point of hospital windows overlooking streets where events were taking place, and finagled her way into prisons, refugee camps and a field hospital on the southern Russian front by using her social and political connections. Military nurses like Cotton enabled political alliances that partially kept Russia from becoming allied with Germany during the First World War.

Canada's nursing sisters and the Anglo-Russian Hospital

Four CAMC nursing sisters served at the Anglo-Russian Hospital between its founding in November 1915 and closure in January 1918. Initially, Dorothy Cotton was the only Canadian appointed but while on leave to Canada in 1916 (after the death of her two brothers in France), the CAMC appointed Edith Hegan and Gertrude Squire as replacements during her absence. Mabel Lindsay joined Cotton upon her return to Petrograd in January 1917 as Hegan and Squire rejoined units in England and France in May 1917.

Edith Hegan of St John, New Brunswick, was in Germany when the war began. She returned to Canada and enlisted with the CAMC on 4 February 1915 at the age of 33, with a posting to No. 2 Canadian General Hospital at Le Tréport, France. She left for Petrograd in May 1916 and returned to England, posted to the hospital at Shorncliffe.[17] Gertrude Squire of Norwood, Ontario, enlisted in England on 26 January 1915 at the recorded age of 30 (although census records indicate she was almost 33 years old). Her record indicates she had 'prior military experience' in Great Britain, likely as a member of the Queen Alexandra Imperial Military Nursing Service (QAIMNS).[18] The *Canadian Nurse* journal reported her married as Mrs Gibson and living in Regina with a young son in 1927.[19] Mabel Lindsay of Ottawa, Ontario, enlisted at Montreal, Quebec on 13 April 1915 at the age of 40, with prior experience with an American Ambulance at Neuilly, France. She was posted originally to No. 16 Canadian General Hospital.[20]

125

Dorothy Cotton was from Almonte, Ontario, and graduated from the Royal Victoria Hospital (Montreal) in1910. She was appointed as nursing sister in the Canadian Active Militia in October 1914, and to the Canadian Expeditionary Force in January 1915. She went overseas with No. 3 Canadian General Hospital (the McGill University unit) in May, at the age of 29, serving in England and France. In November 1915, Matron-in-Chief Margaret Macdonald selected her as the Canadian representative for a small group of thirty-seven allied forces nurses to staff the newly formed Anglo-Russian Hospital. Following eight months' service, which included a tour to the front with a field unit, Cotton took leave to be with her widowed mother whose two sons (Dorothy's brothers) had been recently killed in France. Her second posting to the Anglo-Russian Hospital was from January to August 1917, after which she returned to England as Acting Matron of the IODE Officers Hospital in London. In August 1918, she became the Matron of Camp Hill Military Hospital at Halifax, Nova Scotia and one year later, in August 1919, she left the military.[21]

There are several accounts of the Anglo-Russian Hospital including Cotton's own publication in the *Canadian Nurse* journal.[22] According to these accounts the hospital effort was driven by Lady Muriel Paget, Honorary Organising Secretary of the Executive Committee who was well-known for her charitable work in both England and Russia, and by Lady Sybil Grey, daughter of Canadian Governor General Earl Grey (1904–11).[23] Michael Harmer, drawing on his surgeon father's letters and diary written from the Anglo-Russian Hospital, referred to these two women as the 'heroines' of the project. Paget and Grey served as co-directors of the hospital with Paget as the 'entrepreneur and organising genius' and Grey as the administrator.[24] Grey's appointment was not without controversy, however, as the *British Journal of Nursing* referred to her as a 'young untrained Lady of Title – backed by social influence' while asserting that 'trained nurses will be in charge of the hospital and their duties will not clash'.[25]

The Anglo-Russian Hospital was clearly promoted as a gift from the Dominions to Russia but its origins were more complex and somewhat controversial. The hospital's status was ambiguous since it was neither an official military hospital nor an official Red Cross hospital, matters that complicated the politics and often left the staff with little medical or nursing work to do. The British Red Cross supported the hospital through a large donation as did the Order of Saint John of Jerusalem in England although both organisations disclaimed 'ownership' of the hospital: 'It was intended to be entirely self-supporting ... the fact that it did not work out that way is no reflection upon those who believed in the ideal.'[26] The chairman of the organising committee was an official of the British Red Cross, the medical and nursing staff was appointed by personal recommendations, and its existence was unsettling to the 'British Colony in Petrograd' which also operated the British Colony Hospital there. Cotton described it as 'a small English hospital here run by Lady Georgina Buchanan [wife of the British ambassador to Russia] and members of the British colony, which opened shortly after war was declared and which we were invited to see over one day'.[27] Anglo-Russian Hospital nurses were asked to help with Red Cross activities such as 'rolling and making of field dressings and bandages' and to 'pack and send off Christmas bags containing sweets, tobacco, books etc. to the soldiers at the front'. Referred to as 'Lady Georgina's personal baby',[28] tensions between the British Colony Hospital and the Anglo-Russian Hospital had to be smoothed over, likely through shared activities such as Cotton described and with considerable diplomacy on all sides.

While the hospital's organisational status was ambiguous, its location was also controversial and based on internal political interests. Dr William Douglas Harmer was Warden of the Medical College and a surgeon at St Bartholomew's Hospital in London when he joined the Anglo-Russian Hospital staff in November 1915. Some 6,000 patients were eventually treated during the years of operation but, as his son wrote, 'My father never talked much about his time in Russia, apart from some personal anecdotes, but his letters and diary leave little doubt that it was a disappointment to him, at any rate in terms of useful surgery and compared with what was happening in Flanders during 1916.'[29] According to Dr Harmer's diary, there were 'several hundred hospitals in Petrograd and over a thousand in Moscow ... more than enough beds to cope with their own casualties from the North-western front ...' He claimed that with 25,000 empty beds in Petrograd, 'we are hardly needed here ... We ought to be nearer the front.'[30] Instead, in his analysis, the hospital had been located in Petrograd because that was 'where the Royal family, the Embassy and the Foreign Office were able to exert their influence', without which the hospital would have withered because Moscow was not interested in British involvement.[31]

Cotton inspected refugee camps in Petrograd and Moscow, and undertook a lengthy trip into central Siberia to visit the Sparsky and Athabasca copper mines on her way to Petrograd at the end of 1915 – apparently as a mandate from the Red Cross since she took pains to document her findings over some twenty pages at the end of her diary. In the report, she compared Petrograd and Moscow, writing that '[I]n Petrograd it seemed to one that as much as possible they were trying to hide the evidences of the war, as the contrast [with Moscow] is great … In [Petrograd] everyone was on the surface gay and going on much as usual, but underneath there was a deep dread of the Germans, and that ultimately the Germans would be in Petrograd.'[32] Later, she commented on the vast number of hospitals set up all over Moscow and the 'refugees pouring in by thousands from Poland and Galicia', claiming there were 800,000 refugees in Moscow alone.[33] Cotton's report painted a grim portrait of the war:

> These poor women and children without their husbands or fathers … Heaps of them had lost their children and crowds of children were orphans belonging to no one. In one morning alone they collected, when I was there, 1000 babies from small girls who were mothering them. Their stories of woe and how they had been treated could only be dragged out of them … [W]hen you see it for yourself it brings forcibly [sic] before one all the horrors of war much more even than seeing the maimed and wounded soldiers. Some of their stories were too terrible to even write about and from what we could make out their stories agreed if you traced up the districts they came from. In some apparently the Commander of the German troops had held his men in check and simply driven them away. In others the Commanders must have been fiends as they had allowed both officers and men to get on with a big drunken orgy. So you can picture for yourself what awful horrors crowds of them had been through.[34]

Her subsequent experiences with the Anglo-Russian Hospital in Petrograd, however, were in stark contrast to the conditions she reported during this inspection trip. Much of the hospital experience involved preparing (and waiting) for patients in a converted palace while taking in visits with royalty, sightseeing and cultural events.

There were four aspects or divisions to the Anglo-Russian

Hospital. The main division was the 200-bed hospital at Petrograd that included an X-ray department and a bacteriological laboratory brought from London, completely staffed by Dominion personnel. The second division was a mobile field hospital unit attached to, and intended to move with, the Russian Guards; it consisted of 42 ambulance and transport carts, staffed by 125 Russian Sanitars (orderlies) and 8 nurses. The third division was to be a smaller surgical hospital unit located in a large barracks at Lutsk under the supervision of a British surgeon. The fourth consisted of a fleet of twenty-two motor ambulances.[35]

While many historical accounts portray military hospitals in drab settings with great hardships to be endured by the staff, the Petrograd hospital was located within the palace of Grand Duke Dimitri Pavlovich, on the corner of Nevsky Prospect and Fontana Canal where 'the ballroom, reception rooms and state apartments made stately wards'.[36] Cotton was placed in charge of the biggest ward, a former ballroom, which she described enthusiastically:

> The walls and ceilings are very elaborate, white plaster, and a boarding has been put up about 5 feet all the way around the sides; otherwise it is left just as it was, a beautiful parquet floor: on one side, huge windows looking into a courtyard, but fortunately on the side that gets all the sun; on the other side, large mirrors; at one end a small alcove, evidently used for the orchestra … It is also to have a couple of large palms, so makes quite a 'show ward' of the place … There are about eight huge gold chandeliers.[37]

This room held seventy beds for sick and wounded soldiers, staffed by three nurses and one member of the Voluntary Aid Detachments (VADs),[38] as well as orderlies about whom she wrote: 'you need several to make up for one real one; they take things so casually, are very willing but slow; they are called "Sanitars" and are men usually from Convalescent hospitals who can work'.[39]

Visibility and publicity were part of a political agenda to reassure the Allies that Anglo-Russian bonds were intact as well as to solicit ongoing public financial support for the endeavour. According to Cotton, the official opening was attended by the Dowager Empress Maria Feodorovna, the Princesses Olga and Tatiana (daughters of Tsar Nicholas II), the Grand Duchess Maria Pavlowa, the Grand Duke Cyril and his wife, as well as other members of the royal family, church dignitaries and 'officers in gorgeous uniforms'.[40] As one historian noted, the hospital opened 'with a fanfare of publicity in the London *Times*' and 'bristled with Lords and Lord Mayors, Field Marshalls and Members of Parliament, to say nothing of the Prime Minister and both Archbishops'.[41] The British Queen Alexandra, who was also the Tsar's aunt, was the hospital's official patroness.

Cotton wrote to her mother about the publicity generated by the opening and blessing of the hospital: 'Splendid photographs were taken and are to appear in the papers, so look for them. I suggested to Lady Sybil that she send a set to the papers in Canada ... I always keep it well to the fore what a handsome gift Canada gave – I don't mean myself, you know.'[42] These photographs were used to raise funds at the Anglo-Russian Exhibition in London (May 1917); a series of twelve photographs were reproduced as postcards and sold in support of the hospital. In yet another political move, since the hospital was supposed to be completely self-supporting, there was a campaign for towns and districts to sponsor a bed or groups of beds within the hospital and committing to raise the funds to fully support these for a year. As added enticement, plaques placed over the beds commemorated individual donors or British towns and cities that had donated funds.[43]

The staff consisted of twenty 'fully-trained and certificated nurses and ten VADs (to act as probationers)' as well as nine physicians and surgeons.[44] Nurses were to wear the uniform of Russian Red Cross sisters, 'except for Miss Dorothy Cotton of the Canadian contingent ... selected by Miss Macdonald, [CAMC] Matron-in-Chief, as the Canadian Sister who should be granted leave to accompany the Mission on the invitation of the Hospital Committee, conveyed through the Matron. She will still be under the Canadian contingent and will wear their uniform.'[45] Whether or not this was a hard-fought battle, given the ambiguous status of the hospital as non-military, Cotton was very pleased with the decision and wrote: 'My uniform is certainly very taking(!) and all the sisters here are terribly interested in it, and call me the "Officer Prince".'[46]

Cotton was aware of the shifting political milieu and referred to the hospital in her writings as having "three distinct phases" characterised by changes in status, patronage and types of patients treated as the 1917 revolutions reached into hospital wards. Clearly patronage and 'prestige' determined when and how the hospital functioned:

> [T]he first [phase] during the Czar's regimé [*sic*], when we had prestige from being under the patronage of the Royal family and had only wounded soldiers as patients; the second during the revolution, with patients of all classes and in all walks of life and of both sexes, garrison soldiers, students, civilians and many scurvy cases. Thirdly, during the Bolshevik régime, when the patients held council to decide if they would allow one another to be operated upon after the M.O.s [Medical Officers] had given their order. This time we had no patronage or prestige from any party.[47]

In January 1918, the hospital closed, owing to unsafe conditions and a state of disorganisation that made it impossible to continue the work. As Lady Paget reported, the hospital had been run by a committee of orderlies since June 1917 (as part of new revolutionary ideology) and many workers simply refused to work any longer.[48] The nurses were left to find their own way back to England, sometimes by circuitous routes for safety. Cotton returned by way of Finland and Sweden while others crossed Siberia to return via North America.

Cotton's three official reports to the CAMC describe nurses' work as being quite similar to work on the Western Front: establishing hospital units in existing buildings, setting up and organising wards, supervising other staff and orderlies, assisting physicians with dressings and surgeons in the operating rooms.[49] She highlighted only a few differences such as the use of a separate 'Bandage Room' in lieu of doing wound irrigations and dressing changes in ward beds, referring to this practice as 'the Continental plan'. The Bandage Room was organised much like an operating room with strict sterile technique followed: 'There were four tables for the patients, small tables beside each for the dressings, instruments, etc., and they were "set up" between each case by one of the dressing room staff.'[50] According to Cotton, this system was even more efficient because VADs changed linens on the ward beds while patients were undergoing their treatments. She seldom mentioned individual patients and when she did, she described them as 'interesting cases'. The majority of her accounts focused on relationships with the royal family and embassy personnel (to whom she carried letters of introduction), relationships between members of the hospital staff, and various trips accompanying Red Cross personnel into prisons and refugee camps.

Cotton felt quite close to Lady Grey and Lady Paget (claiming to be 'real chummy' with her). [51] Both women secured privileged access for her to social events such as Russian ballets and prestigious dinner invitations.[52] After one particular day at the art galleries, a shampoo and several stops for tea, she wrote to her mother: 'Isn't it wonderful for me to have all this. I can assure you I fully appreciate it too … Everything I see I think how Father would love it all or to hear of it from me,'[53] Lady Paget secured her inclusion on trips into central Siberia as well as southern Russia where Cotton recorded observations of the conditions for peasants and refugees. Indeed, it was this close relationship with Lady Paget and her post-war charitable work in Romania that led to an invitation from Queen Marie for Cotton to establish a training school for nurses in post-war Romania in1920.[54]

Cotton's privileged position within the Anglo-Russian Hospital, of which the obvious demonstration was that she was the only one permitted to still wear her distinctive national uniform, heightened her visibility and awareness of her political position. As she wrote to a Montreal friend: 'Being "Canada," I always come in for everything that is going on, and my brass buttons make an awful disturbance. By the way, my nickname is "Sister Buttons". Everyone here is so thrilled with the generous gift from the Canadian government to the Anglo-Russian Hospital. I pretend to think it is nothing, but all the time I am nearly bursting with pride.'[55]

This privileged position must have generated tension with other nursing staff, however. In a letter to her sister, Cotton confessed that English nursing sisters were 'disgusted' that she interacted socially with VADs – that it was perceived as 'unprofessional to associate with V.A.D.s', adding that the English nurses 'are so jealous of them in every way'.[56] VADs were typically of a higher social class than paid trained nurses although within military hospital organisations, VADs fell under the supervision of nursing sisters, which disrupted usual class-based relationships and caused friction on the wards. Considering New Zealand nurses as quite the nicest among the staff, Cotton wrote: 'Most of the others [nursing sisters] are cats and to tell you the truth I never came across a more catty or narrow minded lot of females. But it has not mattered to me. I have had Miss Stevenson [a Red Cross VAD], and there are others of different clay [emphasis in original].'[57]

From its establishment in November until Easter of 1916, Lady Grey noted that the hospital staff were 'marking time' and it was 'high time the hospital opened as a lot of nurses without work are very childish and unreasonable'.[58] She reported that many nurses put in time at the Berlitz School trying to learn the Russian language. Cotton was definitely one of those disenchanted with the posting at Petrograd and seeking a posting to a field hospital unit near the front lines, hopefully in the Caucasus or Dvinsk/Riga areas, writing that rumours of forming such a unit 'will decide the fate of many [nurses] re. staying or leaving after 6 months'. Although nurses were only obligated to commit on a 'month by month' basis after the initial six-month commitment, she admitted that she 'would hate to miss the chance of the field work'.[59] After many delays, the first field hospital got underway, travelling 'for an unknown destination in the direction of Polock, a town south of Dvinsk' where Cotton finally realised her goal of getting to the front in a field unit. She wrote, 'At the beginning the booming of the big guns was distinctively heard, but later on became less frequent. One day about noon, we heard firing, and saw shrapnel busting in the sky just over our heads, apparently firing at an aeroplane of which we saw no signs owing to the cloudy day.'[60]

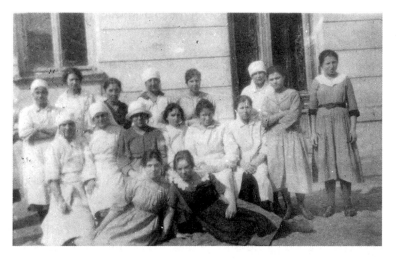

6.1 Nursing personnel of the Anglo Russian Field Hospital, June 1916

On 29 June, there was an incident which must have caused considerable angst and strain on Anglo-Russian relationships. The Anglo-Russian Hospital was highly dependent on the general public for financial support and had been in the news from its inception. Women were to serve behind the lines in safety, according to gendered role expectations; they were not to be injured or killed on front lines. However, as Cotton recorded in her diary:

> It was while the party were [sic] on this trek that Lady Sybil so unfortunately was wounded. They had put in near some camp to rest the horses, and while there went up to a trench to see a company of bomb throwers at practice. The trench or dugout was supposed to be bomb proof, but somehow a tiny piece did come through at that moment Lady Sybil was looking through the smallest opening and the piece of shrapnel hit her in the cheek. They drove her as soon as possible into Maleditchona and from there by special train to Petrograd – where she was X-rayed and operated upon.[61]

Fortunately, the incident was kept quietly out of the media and Lady Grey recovered.

Eyewitness to the revolution

Cotton's front-line experience was cut short, however, by a leave to Canada for several months, following the deaths of her two brothers in France. It was on her return to the Anglo-Russian Hospital at the end of 1916, that hospital staff found themselves in a vantage position as eyewitnesses to the beginnings of the Russian Revolution in Petrograd. At first, Cotton lamented that it was 'hard to know how to look at things, we hear so little', owing to the submarine blockade of Russian ports. Then food and supplies became more expensive while work became 'dreadfully dull'.[62]

As the hospital fell under the influence of shifting governance and ideologies, it gradually lost the ability to function – calling the assumed neutrality of medical services into question. Cotton's main account of events during March 1917, were written to her sister Elsie in a letter with separate entries dated between 4 March and 31 March.[63] All four CAMC nurses had been enjoying a sightseeing day off together when they encountered a regiment of Cossacks in the streets around the hospital on their return. They heard accounts of street rioting during the day from other staff members. The next day, however, as she started out from the hospital, Cotton was on the front steps of the hospital just as a rioting crowd of mounted Cossacks passed through the street in front of her. Over the next several days there were incidents of increased gunfire, street charges with lances drawn, more riots and ever lengthening lines for bread. By 10 March the nurses could no longer walk between the hospital and their billets; instead they travelled to the hospital by motorcars and remained there for meals as well. That afternoon, Cotton wrote:

I was interrupted by one of the Sisters who called me into her ward to look at the Nevsky. We watched the crowds collecting ... Then suddenly everyone ran wildly in all directions, most of them falling flat and crawling along on their stomachs. The soldiers had fired on the people. They had been placed across the Nevsky higher up, and it was quick rifle fire ... Did I tell you before that we had a guard at the front door?

When Cotton went on duty the next day, the infantry was patrolling streets and buildings with machine guns and ammunition

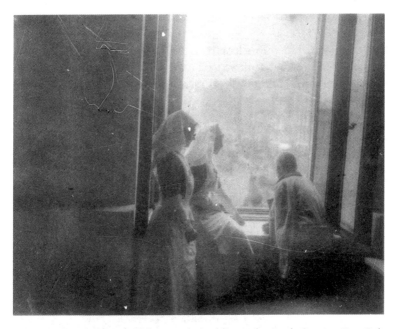

6.2 Two nursing sisters with wounded soldier at the Anglo Russian Hospital in the Dmitri Palace, Petrograd, 1916

wagons. As she wrote, there was 'an uncanny stillness in the air' during the afternoon as soldiers revolted and joined 'the people'. For the next week, the nurses slept at the hospital with an occasional foray out for baths as events became much more 'exciting' and even the hospital came under fire: 'The People came at about 12 o'clock midnight, searched the place, and demanded that we at once hang out a Red Cross flag, so we hurriedly made one up on the machine, made out of an old Santa Claus coat and a sheet. That night we sat up all night. Some lay down, but I wandered around, as I did not want to miss anything.' By 20 March, 'Everyone was armed and the streets were crowded. Motor lorries flying around – everyone's motor was taken – lots of firing from the bridge, both rifle and machine gun. The Police were using the Dowager Empress's Palace directly across from us, so there was heavy firing on it.' On 24 March, 'all Imperial signs and coats-of-arms over the shops or anywhere were taken down and burnt ... A guard with fixed bayonets came and demanded that we take down the Russian flag. Everyone is wearing a red rosette or ribbon. The Red flag is flying from the Winter palace and the Dowager Empress's.'

Cotton concluded this lengthy letter by writing: 'The Revolution has really been wonderful. So well managed for a Revolution, quick, clean & very tidy. Little dirty work. Although we hear new & awful

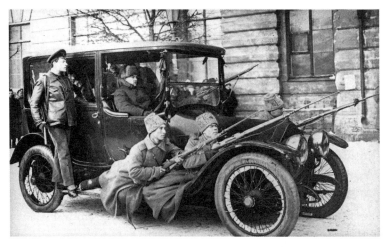

6.3 Group of armed Russian soldiers with automobile, Petrograd, 1917

stories almost every day. I do wish I could write freely, but I feel so much my letters may be censored.' To her mother, she added, 'After all, being here for the revolution has been a wonderful experience.'[64] Later she took her camera to a demonstration march and 'walked with them to the Duma' where: 'We arrived quite a long time before the procession and being Sisters, were allowed in. I was awfully thrilled, I can assure you, and tried to picture the doings there last month.'[65]

Initially valorising the revolutionists, Cotton became quickly disenchanted as events played out within the hospital and the new republic began to take shape. For example, she described how: 'The Sanitars now choose what wards they will work on, and have a committee composed of four of themselves, who rule.' She now referred to the men on her unit as 'so dreadful' and by the end of April 1917 declared that 'the hospital has gone down dreadfully, and I am only hoping that after Lady Muriel's show in London [the Anglo-Russian Exhibition] it [the hospital] will close'.[66] Over time, other experiences dampened Cotton's views of the war and she was quite ready for the hospital to close by fall of 1917. She returned to No. 3 Canadian General Hospital in England and subsequently to Canada where she was demobilised in August 1918.

In 1920 Cotton accepted a two-year civilian assignment to Eastern Europe as the leader of a group of Montreal nurses who were invited to Romania to establish a school for trained nurses at Coltzea Hospital in Bucharest on behalf of the Canadian Nursing Mission. Lady Paget enabled Cotton's connection with Romania through her friendship with Queen Marie who invited the Canadians to come there.[67] By 1921, however, she was once again very discouraged and felt little progress had been made with that project.[68] After working briefly for the Rockefeller Institute in Paris (1921–22), she completed a diploma in Public Health and worked in Saskatchewan as a public health nurse with the Victorian Order of Nurses.[69] Nothing further is known about her post-war life or career.

Symbolic diplomatic gesture

Cotton's descriptions of the Anglo-Russian Hospital experience was a mixture of travelogue, political intrigue, vicarious danger and a sense of witnessing (and recording) history in the making. Russia appeared mysterious to Cotton who referred to Petrograd as 'exotic' on her arrival:

> [W]hen Archangel came in sight it was like nothing we had ever seen before … the rounded and exotic shaped domes of the Russian churches, painted in bright blues, and the glistening of the gilded spires and crosses … We were fortunate enough to see several Laplanders in their picturesque costumes, and teams of reindeer; washerwomen doing their week's laundry in the broken ice about the boats, and a hut and coach built by Peter the Great.[70]

During her second stint at Petrograd, she wrote similarly that 'I always feel here as if I was living in Arabian Nights'.[71] In May 1916, she participated in a sightseeing trip with Drs Harmer and Flavell and her VAD friend, Miss Stevenson, to Moscow where they visited the Palace and Treasury among other sites.

There is no evidence that Cotton was aware of any incompatibility between privilege, social class, and the impoverished conditions that partly precipitated the Russian Revolution and ultimately, disillusioned her. She readily acknowledged the usefulness of her position as a privileged woman and used personal and political connections to her advantage. She capitalised on her professional credentials as a trained nurse from a prestigious Montreal training hospital, her officer's status in the CAMC, and her social relationships (first with Matron-in-Chief Macdonald and then with both Lady Muriel Paget and Lady Sybil Grey) to position herself as the Canadian representative for the Anglo-Russian Hospital mission.

The 1917 Russian Revolution, however, compounded the chaos of war and disrupted the formerly close associations between Russia and England. With the executions of the Tzar and his family, both Cotton and the Anglo-Russian Hospital lost privileged status, ultimately becoming unable to function as an organisation or to assure the safety of the staff. The hospital lost its political and diplomatic mandates, and the work achieved had been neither remarkable nor extensive in terms of the number of wounded cared for at the hospital. But it had served its purpose as a symbolic gesture of support to the Russian government and its army, intended to keep Russia within the Western alliance. It extended caregiving work into the realm of politics and diplomacy, ultimately meeting its demise at the hands of the revolutionists and the ensuing chaos. Military nurses, such as Dorothy

Cotton, enabled the political and diplomatic work of caregiving while capitalising on opportunities to experience Russian culture and forge relationships that would potentially further their careers.

Notes

1 Sir Edward Kemp, *Report of the Ministry: Overseas Military Forces of Canada, 1918* (London, Overseas Military Forces of Canada, 1919), 383.

2 G. W. L. Nicholson, *Canada's Nursing Sisters* (Toronto, A. M. Hakkert, 1975), 90. A newspaper obituary clipping for Dorothy's brother, Captain Charles Penner Cotton, details his death in France in June 1916. It identifies their father as the late General William Henry Cotton, the eldest son as Harry Cotton who died in the South African War (1899–1902), and the youngest son as Captain Ross Penner Cotton who was also killed in France during the same month as Charles. Cotton refers to the event in her diary as the battle of Sanctuary Woods 'where the Canadians had been reported under siege and fighting fiercely'. See R. C. Fetherstonhaugh, 'War Diaries and Letters: Dorothy Cotton', v. 8, Rare Books and Special Collections, McGill University Library, Montreal [hereafter as the Fetherstonhaugh fonds].

3 Dorothy Cotton, 'A word picture of the Anglo-Russian Hospital, Petrograd', *Canadian Nurse* 22, 9 (1926), 486–8. Her diary and some of her letters and photographs [MG 30 E464], have been digitalised by Library and Archives Canada [hereafter as LAC] (accessed 28 May 2011), at www.collections canada.gc.ca/nursing-sisters/025013-2203.01-e.php?isn_nbr=97730&PHP SESSID=6shsukj392trp8auo5f85sekf0 Additional letters and photographs are part of the Fetherstonhaugh fonds. For a British VAD's perspective, see Joyce Wood, 'The revolution outside her window: New light shed on the March 1917 Russian Revolution from the papers of VAD nurse Dorothy N. Seymour', *Proceedings of the South Carolina Historical Association* (2005), 71–86.

4 Cotton, 'A word picture of the Anglo-Russian Hospital', 486.

5 'Gift of Canada', newspaper clipping [newspaper unnamed], 25 November 1915, Fetherstonhaugh fonds; Michael Harmer, *The Forgotten Hospital: An Essay* (West Sussex, Springwood Books, 1982), 17.

6 David Mackenzie, 'Introduction: Myth, memory, and the transformation of Canadian society', in David Mackenzie (ed.), *Canada and the First World War: Essays in Honour of Robert Craig Brown* (Toronto, University of Toronto Press, 2005), 3–14, quotation p. 4.

7 Douglas McCalla, 'The economic impact of the Great War', in Mackenzie (ed.), *Canada and the First World War*, 138.

8 Katie Pickles, *Female Imperialism and National Identity: Imperial Order Daughters of the Empire* (Manchester: Manchester University Press, 2002).

According to Pickles, the IODE was 'first and foremost a patriotic organization, advancing its own particular brand of female imperialism'. It 'celebrated all things British and advanced Canada's destiny as a part of the British Empire'. Quotes from p. 2.

9 Pickles, *Female Imperialism and National Identity*, 5 and 9.

10 Jeffrey S. Reznick, *Healing the Nation: Soldiers and the Culture of Caregiving in Britain during the Great War* (Manchester and New York, Manchester University Press, 2004), 1.

11 John F. Hutchinson, *Champions of Charity: War and the Rise of the Red Cross* (Boulder, CO, Westview Press, 1996).

12 Julia Irwin, 'Nurses without borders: The history of nursing as US international history', *Nursing History Review* 19, 1 (2011), 93–4.

13 Heather Jones, 'International or transnational? Humanitarian action during the First World War', *European Review of History* 16, 5 (2009), 709.

14 Jones, 'International or transnational', 710.

15 Rebecca Gill, 'The rational administration of compassion: The origins of British relief in war', *Le Mouvement social* 227 (2009), 9–26; and 'Networks of concern, boundaries of compassion: British relief in the South African War', *Journal of Imperial and Commonwealth History* 40, 5 (2012), 827–44.

16 Gill, 'Networks of concern, boundaries of compassion', 840–1.

17 'Edith Tilley Hegan', LAC, RG 150, Accession 1992–93/166, Box 4232–40; *Quebec Chronicle*, 27 March 1919, 12; 'Canadian Great War Project' (accessed 31 May 2011), www.canadiangreatwarproject.com/searches/soldierDetailPrint.asp?ID=88600.

18 'Lucy Gertrude Squire', LAC, RG 150, Accession 1992–93/166, Box 9212–51; 'Canadian Great War Project' (accessed 31 May 2011), www.canadiangreatwarproject.com/searches/soldierDetail.asp?ID=8589.

19 'News', *Canadian Nurse* 23, 10 (1927), 547.

20 'Mabel Lindsay', LAC, RG 150, Accession 1992–93/166, Box 5655–40; 'Canadian Great War Project' (accessed 31 May 2011), www.canadiangreatwarproject.com/searches/soldierDetail.asp?ID=93523.

21 'Dorothy Cotton', LAC, RG 150, Accession 1992–93/166, Box 2036–22; Fetherstonhaugh fonds.

22 Harmer, *The Forgotten Hospital*; Anthony Cross, 'Forgotten British places in Petrograd/Leningrad', *Europa Orientalis* 5 (2004), part 1: 135–47 (accessed 30 May 2011), at www.russinitalia.it/europa_orientalis/Cross.pdf; Cotton, 'A word picture of the Anglo-Russian Hospital'; Nicholson, *Canada's Nursing Sisters*, 90–2; 'The Anglo-Russian Hospital', *British Journal of Nursing* (9 October 1915), 293–4; and Herbert F. Waterhouse, W. Douglas Harmer and Charles J. Marshall, 'Notes from the Anglo-Russian Hospitals', *British Medical Journal* 2, 2962 (6 October 1917), 441–5 (accessed 28 May 2011), at www.jstor.org/pss/20308399.

23 Cross, 'Forgotten British places', 137.

24 Harmer, *The Forgotten Hospital*, 5.
25 Harmer, *The Forgotten Hospital*, 20.
26 Harmer, *The Forgotten Hospital*, 10, 23–4.
27 Cotton, '1st Official Russian report – Covering Period November 2, 1915 – January 31, 1916', Fetherstonhaugh fonds.
28 Harmer, *The Forgotten Hospital*, 23–5.
29 Harmer, *The Forgotten Hospital*, 10.
30 Harmer, *The Forgotten Hospital*, 57–8, 76.
31 Harmer, *The Forgotten Hospital*, 151.
32 Cotton diary, 43–4.
33 Cotton diary, 55.
34 Cotton diary, 57–8.
35 Waterhouse *et al.*, 'Notes from the Anglo-Russian Hospitals', 441.
36 Cotton, 'A word picture of the Anglo-Russian Hospital', 487.
37 Cotton, letter to her mother, 25 January 1916, Fetherstonhaugh fonds.
38 For more on VADs, see Cynthia Toman, 'Help us, serve England: First World War military nursing and national identities', *Canadian Bulletin of Medical History* 30, 1 (2013), 156–7; Linda J. Quiney, 'Assistant angels: Canadian Voluntary Aid Detachment nurses in the Great War', *Canadian Bulletin of Medical History* 15, 1 (1998), 189–206, and 'Sharing the halo: Social and professional tensions in the work of World War I Canadian volunteer nurses', *Journal of the Canadian Historical Association* 8 (1998), 105–24; Henriette Donner, 'Under the cross – why VADs performed the filthiest task in the dirtiest war: Red Cross women volunteers, 1914–1918', *Journal of Social History* 30, 3 (Spring 1997), 687–704; Vera Brittain, *Testament of Youth* (London, Virago, 1978 [1933]).
39 Cotton, letter to her mother, 25 January 1916, Fetherstonhaugh fonds.
40 Cotton diary, 26; 'Second official Russian report', Fetherstonhaugh fonds.
41 Cross, 'Forgotten British places', 137.
42 Cotton, letter to her mother, 25 January 1916, Fetherstonhaugh fonds.
43 Cross, 'Forgotten British places', 139; Harmer, *The Forgotten Hospital*, 17.
44 'The Anglo-Russian Hospital', 293.
45 'The Anglo-Russian Hospital', 294; Susan Mann, *Margaret Macdonald: Imperial Daughter* (Montreal, McGill-Queen's University Press, 2005).
46 Cotton, letter to her mother, 24 November 1915, Fetherstonhaugh fonds.
47 Cotton, 'A word picture of the Anglo-Russian Hospital', 488.
48 'Tells how anarchy is sweeping Russia', *New York Times*, 14 May 1918, 11.
49 Cotton, 'Reports to the CAMC', Fetherstonhaugh fonds. For medical perspectives on surgical and medical treatments at the Anglo-Russian Hospital, see Waterhouse *et al.*, 'The Anglo-Russian Hospitals'.
50 Cotton, 'A word picture of the Anglo-Russian Hospital', 488; see also Cotton's diary.

51 Cotton, letters to her sister Mary, 8 December 1915 and 4 March 1921, Fetherstonhaugh fonds.
52 Cotton, letters to her mother, 25 December 1915 and 1 January 1916, Fetherstonhaugh fonds.
53 Cotton, letter to her mother, 24 November 1915, Fetherstonhaugh fonds.
54 Cotton, letter to her sister Mary, 4 March 1921, Fetherstonhaugh fonds.
55 Cotton, letter to Bob [Robert Fetherstonhaugh] from Petrograd, 16 December 1915, Fetherstonhaugh fonds.
56 Cotton, letter to her sister Elsie, 31 March 1917, Fetherstonhaugh fonds.
57 Cotton, letter to her mother, 10 June 1916, Fetherstonhaugh fonds.
58 Lady Sybil Grey in Harmer, *The Forgotten Hospital*, 65.
59 Cotton, letters to her mother, 28 February 1916 and 5 April 1916, Fetherstonhaugh fonds.
60 Cotton diary, 39–40.
61 Cotton diary, 37–8.
62 Cotton, letters to her 'family', 18 February 1917, 2 March 1917 and 27 March 1917, Fetherstonhaugh fonds.
63 Cotton, letter to sister Elsie from Petrograd, 4 March 1917 with entries sub-dated between 9 and 21 March, 1917, Fetherstonhaugh fonds.
64 Cotton, letter to her mother, 27 March 1917, Fetherstonhaugh fonds.
65 Cotton, letter to her mother, 29 April 1917, Fetherstonhaugh fonds.
66 Cotton, letters to her mother, 21 April 1917 and 29 April 1917, Fetherstonhaugh fonds. The Anglo-Russian Exhibition was a fund-raising project organised by Lady Muriel Paget for the ongoing support of the Anglo-Russian Hospital. It was held at the Grafton galleries (London) during May 1917. See Cross, 'Forgotten British places', 139.
67 'Tells how anarchy is sweeping Russia'. Interestingly, five of the eight nurses who went to Romania were former CAMC nursing sisters and two others had wartime service experience in France. See Nicholson, *Canada's Nursing Sisters*, 90–2, and 'The Canadian nursing mission to Rumania [Romania]', *British Journal of Nursing* 30 (October 1920), 248.
68 Cotton, letter to sister Mary, 4 March 1921, Fetherstonhaugh fonds.
69 Brian Douglas Tennyson, *The Canadian Experience of the Great War: A Guide to Memoirs* (Lanham, Maryland: Scarecrow Press, 2013), 103.
70 Cotton, 'A word picture of the Anglo-Russian Hospital', 487.
71 Cotton, letter to her mother, 30 January 1917, Fetherstonhaugh fonds.

7

The impact of the First World War on asylum and voluntary hospital nurses' work and health

Debbie Palmer

In 1918, poor work conditions at the Cornwall Lunatic Asylum resulted in the deaths of six nurses. The high mortality rate, according to the asylum's medical superintendent, was the result of long working hours and the severe shortage of nurses during the First World War.[1] In contrast, voluntary hospital nurses at the South Devon and East Cornwall Hospital, Plymouth saw little deterioration in their mortality and morbidity rates. Increasing numbers of nurses were recruited to care for sick and wounded soldiers between 1914 and 1918 but little is known about how staff shortages and other disadvantages of war affected nurses' work at home. To explore this question, this chapter compare nurses' work in two very different hospitals situated thirty-two miles apart in the south-west of England. It reveals the significant differences and similarities between asylum and voluntary hospital nurses' work at a time of duress. And, finally, it compares levels of nurses' sickness as a barometer of the impact of war. Historians tend to assess mental and physical illness separately so this comparison of hospitals and treatments is an innovative addition to the scholarship.

The Cornwall Lunatic Asylum

The Cornwall Lunatic Asylum (CLA), known locally as St Lawrence's Hospital, opened in 1820 in Bodmin, the county town of Cornwall. Cornwall's economy was based on agriculture and mining with little secondary industry or commerce. The asylum was an important source of employment and, in 1914, seventy female nurses and seventy-five male attendants cared for 1,013 patients (476 male and 537 female). The overwhelming majority were pauper patients, maintained out of the poor rates. There were only fifty-three private patients. Male and female patients were separated and nursed by staff of the same sex. Patients were also divided into categories of chronic; sick and infirm; recent and acute; and epileptic. Classification of mental illness began in the mid-nineteenth century and varied between asylums.[2]

Asylum nurses were traditionally drawn from the working classes.[3] For example, attendant George White had previously worked as an 'outfitter's apprentice' and his sister was a 'servant'.[4] Supervising patients' work on the farm, in the laundry and in workshops took up a major part of attendants' daily activities and manual skills among staff were prized. Jennifer Laws argues that attitudes towards the value of patients' work changed during the war from the late-nineteenth century justification of economic and managerial goals.[5] According to the *Lancet*, in 1914, work was the major therapeutic agent for mental disease: 'there [was] nothing like work, particularly physical exertion, to overcome the "blues" or to distract the mind during great trouble'.[6] The majority of asylum patients, the journal argued, should be put to work and only delusional patients be kept under observation until fit. Those with previous manual occupations, such as carpenters, continued their profession within the asylum and those without any work experience were employed on the farm or making mattresses.[7]

At the outbreak of war, over half of CLA patients (645) were compulsorily employed as a form of rehabilitation and a way of returning patients to the national labour pool.[8] Recovery was often judged by an ability to work particularly during the war when labour was in short supply. When patient Samuel G. applied to be discharged in 1915, he was told that if he worked on the farm for two months his application would be considered.[9] The CLA had a large farm, which was an important financial asset as well as the main source of food during the war.[10] Attendants fulfilled a number of other roles vital to the smooth running of the asylum, as well as its economic viability. Volunteers to the asylum's fire brigade were paid an extra £24 annually, the chapel choir (£6) and organ blowers (£1).[11]

The asylum had both a different legislative framework from that of the SDEC and a distinct culture. Senior nurses at both hospitals played no part in management but CLA matrons did not even give regular reports. Elizabeth Taylor was appointed matron in March 1914 and had a background of general and mental nursing work having trained at the Royal Infirmary Manchester.[12] At the time, the notion that 'the successful asylum nurse must also be a good general nurse' was widely discussed, in part, to increase the number of senior posts open to general nurses.[13] Ideas about the causes of insanity had shifted in the late nineteenth century and, by 1914, were considered to be physiological and 'not as a possession by demons or sheer outburst of temper', therefore making room for the general nurse in the care of the insane. As a result it was argued that asylum nurses' work was similar to general nursing requiring qualities of tact, kindness and self-control.[14]

The CLA was governed by Dr Francis Dudley, a member of the Medico-Psychological Association (MPA) and senior assistant medical officer before his appointment as medical superintendent in June 1914. It is difficult to offer an analysis of asylum nurses' work without mentioning the theory and practice of psychiatry, which had begun to exert some influence since the middle of the nineteenth century.[15] But, as Peter Nolan notes, the early psychiatrists 'were neither scientists nor clinicians; their work was primarily custodial and experimental', often guided by personal whims and pet theories about how asylums should be run and patients treated.[16]

Some MPA members were interested in nurse training as a way of raising psychiatry's status and, in 1894, persuaded the General Medical Council to introduce a certificate in psychological medicine.[17] A *Handbook for the Instruction of Attendants on the Insane* was published in the same year that prioritised personal discipline, order, cleanliness and obedience.[18] Known as *The Red Handbook*, it provided the basis of CLA nurse training in 1918. During the war, nurses learnt through apprenticeship but this system became strained when large numbers of experienced attendants were called up for military duty. Nevertheless, seven nurses passed the MPA preliminary certificate in November 1917 and were awarded £1 for their effort.[19] In 1919, nursing staff 'had to attend nine out of twelve lectures given by the doctor in [their] own time, very often after 13 hours of duty, after 8 pm'. The lecture consisted of the doctor reading from *The Red Handbook* for an hour.[20] According to charge nurse Woods, who worked on the epileptic ward, 'there was no treatment' in this period and 'very few of the staff were capable of taking a pulse or temperature or giving a simple enema'. Instead, work focused on keeping epileptic patients clean, fed and free from injury.[21]

Dudley managed the asylum in conjunction with a lay visiting committee drawn from landowners, clergy, magistrates and Members of Parliament. They set and enforced the regulations governing nursing staff, subject to regular inspection by the Board of Control. The Board, like its predecessor the Lunacy Commission, provided a framework for the provision and administration of institutions designed to confine the lunatic. Commissioners' roles were limited, confined to inspections and public criticism of poor standards.[22] Both the committee and the Board regularly inspected the CLA and their construction of patient care shaped nurses' work.

The Board's and the committee's priorities were the cleanliness of both the environment and the patient. In October 1914, the committee reported that the asylum was 'in good order and well aired … We were very struck with the cleanliness of the patients and especially regards the beds and floors which were scrupulously clean.'[23] The preoccupation with hygiene was based on the miasmic theory of disease, which supported the notion that dirt was the main cause of bad health in mind and body.[24] Dudley subscribed to both the miasmic and the germ theories of disease, which seems contradictory today but was not uncommon in the late nineteenth and early twentieth centuries.[25] As a result of both these understandings, CLA nurses' work, regulated and controlled by Dudley's strict timetable, was dominated by cleaning. In 1914, attendants and nurses spent two of their thirteen hours on duty cleaning the ward and scrubbing and polishing the floor. A further hour and thirty minutes was devoted to washing patients. For example, Attendant Vanderwolfe started work at 7 a.m. when patients were got out of bed, washed and made ready for breakfast at 8 a.m. He then cleaned the ward, scrubbed and polished the floor until 10 a.m. At 7.30 p.m patients were cleaned and put to bed and Vanderwolfe went off duty at 8 p.m.[26] Bathing was a communal, factory-like procedure with nurses allocated to separate tasks.[27]

Dudley, like other psychiatrists of the time, considered taking patients into the open air a treatment for mental illness. According to the germ theory of disease, individuals, rather than smells, were the vectors of disease.[28] Nurses' work involved long periods of patient supervision outside, either walking or sitting in the airing courts. Patients were turned out on the airing courts or sent to work at 10 a.m. and counted back into their ward at 11 a.m. Dinner was served at 12 p.m. and then patients were sent outside again from 2 p.m. till 4.30 p.m. when tea was served. Despite the shortage of staff during the war, patient care continued to revolve around access to the open air and, on a fine day, most patients went out of doors.[29] In June 1915, the visiting committee brought waterproof capes for patients so that they could go outside even in the rain.[30] In May 1916, the asylum's annual summer picnics to Trebetherick beach, Polzeath commenced and continued until the end of July.[31] How many patients went or how they travelled the twenty-eight mile round trip is unclear. Even in 1917, when nurses' work conditions were at their worst, the idea of walking and picnics as treatment continued. For example, on 7 May 1917, twenty men walked the six miles to and from Helman Tor and dinner was sent out to them. The 'experiment of a picnic' was judged a success by the committee and repeated a week later.[32] Dudley's emphasis on the open air meant that patients experienced life outside the asylum walls even when there were few staff. This also meant a change to nurses' routine work but with the added responsibility of preventing patients escaping.

Eight months after the outbreak of war, a rapid increase in the number of patients placed heavy demands on a depleted staff. In March 1915, 226 pauper patients were transferred from Bristol Asylum to make room for wounded soldiers. The CLA had accommodation for 1,000 patients but numbers rose to 1,226.[33] Initially, patients slept on the ward floors while the War Office was petitioned to supply bedsteads. Out of a staff of seventy-two male attendants, twenty-seven had already left for military duty by July 1915, leaving a significant gap in experienced staff. Places were filled by retired attendants, men 'above military age' and 'married men with families' – the latter groups having no previous experience of asylum work.[34] Furthermore, some attendants were elderly. For example, temporary attendant C. Weary was 76 when he was advised to retire because of health problems.[35]

Dudley was initially optimistic about the quality of temporary attendants and told the visiting committee in 1914 that the asylum was 'unusually lucky'. However, by 1915, difficulties recruiting 'suitable substitutes' prompted him to lobby the Parliamentary Recruiting Committee to refrain from calling up any more staff.[36] An initial promise was unfulfilled and the numbers of male attendants called up rose from 34 in 1915, to 43 in 1916, to 49 in 1917.[37] The introduction of temporary attendants brought with it an increase in staff turnover. Prior to 1915, male attendants formed a stable workforce that was prepared to tolerate poor work conditions and ill health in the hope of receiving a pension. However, in 1916, one-fifth resigned or were found to be unsatisfactory.[38]

In an attempt to encourage staff to stay, the visiting committee introduced a war bonus for head attendants, head nurses and married male attendants in May 1915, eight weeks after the arrival of the Bristol patients. The committee explained that the bonus was because of an 'increase in patient numbers and the extra cost of living caused by the war'.[39] Reinforcing the notion of the male breadwinner, head male attendants received significantly more than their female colleagues: married male attendants pay was raised by two guineas a week compared to the two assistant head nurses who only got a £1. Unequal pay continued throughout the war and while all male attendants were given the war bonus in 1916, the majority of female staff had to wait until November 1918.[40]

Nurses' increased workload resulted in an immediate rise in staff sickness, which continued until 1919. Prior to the arrival of the Bristol patients the average sickness rate was two nurses per month.[41] But four weeks after their arrival, in April 1915, levels rose to sixteen female nurses and eleven attendants.[42] They remained high until 1918. In March 1916 ten staff members were on sick leave, rising to eleven in May and to twenty-six in January 1917.[43] Whereas physical injury from violent patients had posed the greatest health risk in the late nineteenth century, the main risk during the war was from infectious diseases. For example, three female nurses contracted diphtheria and three nurses caught scarlet fever in 1915.[44]

Nurses' and attendants' work involved caring for violent patients without the use of force but this goal often proved problematic. Sedative drugs, such as bromides and barbiturates, were considered harmless and non-addictive treatments for mental disorders. Restraint by straitjacket had to be officially sanctioned by Dudley and was officially only used once during the war when a noisy patient was moved to the isolation unit and put into the jacket. Once there he escaped and smashed a window, door and mantelpiece. He was then moved to the 'strong room' and kept in seclusion.[45]

The mid-nineteenth century saw a movement among some psychiatrists to outlaw violent behaviour towards patients, and attendants who treated patients roughly at some asylums risked dismissal.[46] Some CLA nurses were disciplined for physical violence during the First World War including nurse D. who admitted that she hit patient Margaret S. making her nose bleed.[47] But often no action was taken, as in the case of patient David M. who was found to be 'extremely bruised on the buttocks' after attendant M. kicked him.[48] Despite increasing rights for patients to be free from summary violence, the visiting committee was reluctant to prosecute staff, particularly male attendants who were in short supply. According to historian Geertje Boschma, tensions were high on wards for disturbed patients and nurses, who themselves were under strict hierarchical supervision and took out their strain on the patient. Boschma argues that cases of patient abuse usually remained concealed and only came to light when a patient complained to a third party or staff reported on each other because of a disagreement. Abuse, she concludes, was part of complex staff–patient interactions.[49] Whistleblowing was also discouraged: nurse Lobb, forced to retract her complaint to the visiting committee that two nurses had forced a patient to eat, was reprimanded for making allegations she could not substantiate.[50]

A system of strict discipline and rigid timetabling was intended to prevent violent altercations between staff and patients. Dudley never contemplated relaxing discipline as a way of attracting new recruits or encouraging staff to stay. He maintained that the ability to obey orders determined whether a nurse proved satisfactory. In the first two years of the war, nurses Pitts, Penelly, Scutlebury and Kendall were discharged for failing to 'peg the clock' three times in a row on night duty.[51] A system of 'peg clocks' was used to prevent staff sleeping on night duty; each nurse would insert and turn a key every hour and the clock would record the time pegged. Nurse Scutlebury's appeal that she had been unable to peg the clock because she was with 'a troublesome patient' failed because she had not recorded this information at the time in a book situated next to the clock.[52]

Despite the shortage of staff, nurses' work included the supervision of patients' entertainment. The idea of 'moral management', of replacing mechanical restraints with non-physical methods of control, had grown in popularity in the early nineteenth century. In 1916, outdoor summer dances were held and over 350 patients went to Bostock's circus in Bodmin, paid for by the asylum. How a skeleton staff of largely untrained staff achieved this logistical feat is unknown.

As the war progressed, nurses' work conditions deteriorated. Working hours increased and leave was often cancelled. Nursing staff were required to live in the asylum, often sharing bedrooms on the wards but only with staff members of the same sex. Staff used patients' bathrooms and, without any recreation area, also ate their meals on the wards. Nurse Clara Williams joined the CLA on 22 October 1914 and left five months later without permission from the medical superintendent. In a letter to the visiting committee, she explained that she left because 'she did not feel well' and 'had repeatedly asked for three days leave but had been told that she could not be spared'. Throughout her period of employment she had slept in a patient's room, which she described as uncomfortable, without a lock, and giving her no privacy. During a month of night duty in February 1915, according to Williams, matron had persistently interrupted her daytime rest.[53]

The shortage of staff began to affect patient care in 1915 when the Board of Control commented that nine of the patients who died that year had bedsores.[54] Furthermore, the Board interpreted the fact that more patients wet the beds at night as indicative of poor nursing care rather than admit that staffing levels were dangerously low.[55] Nurses' workloads were further burdened by the rapid increase in the incidence of dysentery and diarrhoea among staff and patients following the arrival of the Bristol patients. Opinions about the cause of asylum dysentery were divided. Harold Gettings, medical superintendent of the West Riding Asylum, Wakefield, suggested that it was not simply overcrowding, as others argued, but more a question of isolating the 'carriers'.[56] An isolation unit had opened at the CLA in 1900 but its lack of effectiveness during the war may have been because it only had ten beds and there were thirty-five cases of dysentery among patients in 1917 and 163 cases in 1918. The policy of isolating all cases was resumed in 1919 and immediately produced a dramatic reduction. Only three cases were recorded in 1919, a fact Dudley attributed to the success of segregation 'together with improved diet'.[57] At the same time, nursing staff began formal training and were given 'strict injunctions ... to personal ablutions and cleanliness'.[58]

Nurses' work during the war involved caring for shell-shocked soldiers. The visiting committee initially resisted the Board of Control's requests in 1916 to admit soldiers on the grounds that 'to relegate them to asylums would impose on them the stigma associated with pauperism'. Instead, the committee suggested that soldiers should be housed in large houses, which had no association with asylums or mental hospitals.[59] Despite their objections, the CLA received seven cases in 1917 and eight in 1918. They were treated as private patients and wore distinctive badges according to their service background. There are no details of treatment or nurses' role but elsewhere ideas revolved around bed rest, persuasion, hypnotism and electroconvulsive therapy.[60]

In 1918, nurses' work conditions deteriorated to the extent that their health began to suffer and six nurses died. In his annual report, Dudley explained that:

> It has been an exceptionally trying year for the staff, six more of our attendants and three of the artisans were called up for military service. Below strength in all departments, it had to cope with the increased work due to the abnormal amount of sickness involving extra hours of duty under very depressing circumstances. During the year temporary attendant Matthews, nurses H. Symons, E. Vague and O. Launder died of typhoid fever. Attendant French and nurse E. Cooksly of phthisis and nurse R. Scantlebury of influenza. With one exception they were under 30 years of age.[61]

Part of the problem was a shortage of food. The asylum had introduced food rations in 1916 and again in 1917. The quality of food was poor and bread was often returned to the kitchen uneaten. In response to nurses' complaints, the committee compensated staff with 4 shillings a week.[62] Nurses' anxiety about their risk of illness increased and several resigned or were dismissed by Dudley on the grounds 'that they were not strong enough for the work'.

Tensions among staff increased partly because of the struggle of day-to-day work but also because of difficulties recruiting senior nurses. Matron Taylor left in 1918, after four years in post, to be replaced by Margaret Hiney. Appointing an assistant matron proved more problematic and, in 1917, Dudley embarked on a recruitment campaign visiting general infirmaries in London. One nurse agreed to join the CLA but then found another job, another came and went on the same day.[63] Helen Jones was eventually appointed in August 1918 and became matron in February 1919 when Hiney was dismissed. The pattern of employment among senior staff had changed from the nineteenth century when matrons remained for decades. Periods of employment became much shorter particularly during the latter stages of the war.

Hiney was 33 years old when appointed and had previously worked at St Olave Infirmary, a general hospital attached to Rotherhithe workhouse. She made several immediate changes to long-standing work practices during her first few weeks in post to which junior nurses objected. These included the cost-cutting measure of providing material instead of a ready-made uniform. She also enforced a stricter system of rules, which included moving permanent female night staff on to day duty if they committed a fault at work.[64] Although she made positive changes by increasing nurses' leave to one full day a week, giving nurses two hours' free time every evening and allocating rooms for recreation when not in use by medical locums, these were overlooked.[65] Nurses did not like the change to traditional practices and complained to the visiting committee but without success.

On 21 October 1918, female nurses' resentment about their work conditions came to a head, resulting in a five-day strike.[66] The main complaint was that their relationship with senior nursing staff had broken down. Further grievances included an 80-hour week, lack of a staff bathroom and poor meal facilities, where nurses had to wash the utensils left in the mess room and cook their own food in the twenty minutes allowed for meal breaks.[67] The strike was led by Mrs D. Hawken, a National Asylum Workers' Union (NAWU) member who had been appointed from Prestwich Asylum, the site of previous industrial action by nursing staff. The NAWU was formed in 1910 and its main concerns during the war were to reduce working hours from 80 to 60, and to protect male attendants' jobs and wages.

Hawken had only been in post four days, according to the *Bodmin*

Guardian, when nurses began telling her about their grievances.[68] The rapid recruitment of 62 of the 70 female staff to the NAWU upset matron Hiney, who immediately banned nurses from wearing their union badges on duty reminding them of the rule forbidding the wearing of jewellery. Dudley dismissed Hawken and the other four 'ringleaders' for breaking this rule with one month's notice, without consulting the visiting committee. His refusal to reinstate the five women prompted thirty-nine nurses to strike. There was considerable sympathy for the strikers in Bodmin who joined a rally at the asylum gates, where Hawken gave a scathing exposure of work conditions. By 25 October, the number of nurses on strike had risen to fifty, all of who were dismissed by Dudley for insubordination.[69] Strikers rejected the visiting committee's proposal to allow all but the five leaders to return to work. But when 72 of the 75 male attendants took up NAWU membership in support of their female colleagues, the committee, fearing a male strike, reinstated all the women. Hiney, on the other hand, was given six weeks' sick leave because of 'worry and overwork'[70] and was eventually dismissed because of health problems.[71]

As a result of the strike, the visiting committee revised pay and work conditions. Before the war, male attendants had received £27 per annum rising to £47 after twenty years but this now increased to £58 4s. for all male attendants. Female nurses had been paid from £15 to £28 after fifteen years but this rose to £33. Working hours were reduced from 80 to 63 hours, and overtime introduced. For the first time, a contract of employment was introduced for new staff to sign after a three-month probationary period.[72] Staff were given separate sleeping accommodation away from the wards and a designated wing with dining and recreation rooms.[73] Some nurses still slept on the wards but were provided with separate bathrooms from the patients.[74] Clearly, the war eventually had a positive impact but life was particularly hard for those nursing on the Home Front in asylums. We now explore its influence on voluntary hospital nursing in Devon.

The South Devon and East Cornwall Hospital

The SDEC, a provincial voluntary hospital in Plymouth, Devon, opened in 1840 and at the start of the war employed 50 female nurses to care for 124 patients. Nurses were called up for military service but there is no record of how many went. Because there were no male nurses working at the SDEC, staff shortages were not as acute as at the CLA. But the numbers were high enough to affect the smooth running of the hospital and, in March 1916, chairman Sir Henry Lopes congratulated matron Harriet Hopkins for 'the way she had met the difficulty caused by the serious depletion of the nursing staff'.[75]

Hopkins had been in post for twenty-eight years at the start of the war and was very experienced. Trained at Charing Cross Hospital, London, she had been a member of the general council of the British Nurses' Association (BNA), and the executive committee of the Matrons' Council in the late nineteenth century.[76] These organisations were committed to registration and education and, unsurprisingly, nurse training continued at the SDEC throughout the war.

In July 1916, a shortage of nurses prompted Lopes to apply to the Red Cross Society to supply voluntary aid detachment nurses (VADs). The VAD scheme, originated in 1909, supplied 12,000 VADs to military hospitals and 60,000 to auxiliary hospitals by the end of the war. Some VADs had full hospital training, others more limited nursing experience while the remainder were unqualified.[77] Regular nurses feared competition and were anxious that their superior status should be given formal recognition in the form of registration. Animosity between the two groups of nurses was fuelled by the *British Journal of Nursing's* criticism of the 'hauteur' of the VAD.[78] The promotion of nursing as a way of helping the war effort elevated the occupation's image and temporarily influenced a change in the class background from which nurses were drawn. VADS were often from the upper and middle classes and this was the case at the SDEC.[79] Two VAD probationers had upper-class backgrounds: Kathleen Lopes' father was Sir Henry Lopes and Constance Robartes' father was the Honourable Charles Agar Robartes, owner of the 1000 acre Lanhydrock estate in Cornwall.[80]

Nearly half of the SDEC probationers who entered training during the war paid twenty-six guineas. The remainder did not pay but neither did they receive a salary, which was only introduced in September 1919 prompted by a shortage of recruits.[81] The selection of new recruits was based on whether matron Hopkins considered them suitably 'respectable.' The term not only suggested that the recruit came from a middle-class background but that they understood and exemplified a set of unwritten moral values Hopkins believed necessary to elevate the status of nursing. For example, G. Gray of the Falstaff Inn, Plymouth complained to the *Western Morning News* in 1913 when his daughter's application for nurse training was rejected on the grounds that she 'was a publican's daughter and would have to come to his house in uniform'. Hopkins explained that 'it would not add to the dignity of the institution to have a nurse going into a public house, though it was her home'.[82] Successful applicants came from professional backgrounds, like Kathleen Forster-Morris, whose father was a vicar, and Geraldine Aldons whose father was a senior surgeon. Hopkins, supported by the medical staff, encouraged nurses to aspire to a middle-class lifestyle. The house committee purchased a croquet set for nurses and encouraged them to use the hospital's lawn tennis court by screening it to provide privacy.[83] Nurses had their own sitting room, which was furnished with upholstered easy chairs, a mahogany writing table, chesterfield sofa, bookcase and piano.[84] They also had a library and their own dining room.[85]

Although the number of patient beds increased from 124 to 199 in 1915, mostly to accommodate injured soldiers, not all were occupied with a daily average of thirty empty beds.[86] In September 1914, fifty beds were allocated to the military, rising to sixty beds in October 1915. This caused consternation amongst the medical staff, who successfully complained that they were unable to admit sick civilians while beds allocated to the military remained empty. In response, military beds were reduced to twenty-five.[87] Medical staff also complained that soldiers occupied beds unnecessarily, arguing that they were often fit for discharge and 'convalescent home treatment' shortly after admission. The problem of fit ambulant soldiers, according to the doctors, was that they took up valuable nursing time because nurses had to keep a close eye on them to prevent them escaping to the pub.[88]

Although the soldiers were mostly mobile and required little nursing care, nurses faced considerable demands from a number of heavily dependent civilian patients. In 1916, for example, the average length of patient stay was thirty-five days compared to a national average of twenty-two days.[89] Doctors wanted to reduce the number of long-stay 'chronic and incurable' patients and increase the turnover of surgical cases and gave the shortage of nurses as reason for the change.[90]

Nurses worked an average of sixty hours a week with one whole day and two half-days off. Like CLA nursing staff, SDEC nurses' work was regulated by a strict timetable that again prioritised cleaning the patient and their environment. Nurses were woken at 6.30 am, attended compulsory prayers at 7.20 am, started duty at 7.30 am and finished at 9 pm. They had three half-hour breaks for meals during the day. The first part of their daily routine involved taking all patients' blood pressures and temperatures. The importance of measuring blood pressure was recognised at the end of eighteenth century but had only become part of nurses' work in the early twentieth century with the development of the sphygmomanometer and stethoscope.[91] Any nurse unfortunate enough to break a thermometer was sent to matron's office to pay a fine of one shilling.

Cleaning the environment was very important and nurses spent one hour and thirty minutes daily wet dusting and polishing the lockers, beds and tables, sweeping the wards and cleaning the sluices and the bathrooms. Once cleaning was finished, nurses performed dressings. Helping patients eat lunch was also listed on their timetable. The afternoon's work included another blood pressure round, tidying beds and the admission of visitors for a short period. Patients, who spent most of their day in bed, waited until the end of the day to be blanket bathed. Beds were re-made after tea and any evening treatments given before the laundry was put away.[92]

SDEC nurses enjoyed better living conditions than their CLA counterparts and did not experience problems of overcrowding. All nurses had their own bedrooms in hospital accommodation and shared a bathroom. As a result, nurses' health did not deteriorate to the same extent as at the CLA. Indeed, rates and causes of sickness at the SDEC remained similar to the previous decade. Tonsillitis and skin infections remained the most frequent causes. The SDEC did not admit infectious patients and so nurses faced less risk of occupational ill health than those at the CLA. Nurses made several complaints during the war over minor issues, such as the night nurses' objection to the noise of soldiers playing croquet during the day.[93] All complaints were quickly resolved perhaps prompted by a desire to retain prestigious nurses like the chairmen's daughter.

Staff turnover increased from 1916 onwards. For the first time since the introduction of training in the 1880s, over 50 per cent of probationers left before qualifying. This may be an effect of the war but could also be attributed to a change in the style of nurse management. In 1916, Hopkins retired to be replaced by Alice Dickson, age 33, who had trained and worked as a ward sister at the SDEC.[94] She was much quicker than Hopkins to dismiss nurses as unsuitable suggesting that she had a different set of expectations than her predecessor.

Conclusion

The First World War had a much greater impact on asylum nurses' work in Cornwall than their voluntary hospital counterparts in Devon. The asylum was overcrowded, lost more staff to military service and its population suffered from food rationing. As a result of poor living conditions, nursing staff were unable to control and contain infectious diseases which overwhelmed its isolation policy. The SDEC nursing staff, on the other hand, were under less physical and mental pressure: the nurse-patient ratio was much higher and even though a high proportion of civilian patients required considerable nursing care, a significant number of beds allocated to the military were routinely empty. Whereas CLA staff called up for military service were replaced by untrained novices or elderly retired staff, VADs replaced SDEC nurses, many of whom had previous nursing experience and were educated on the hospital's training programme. The introduction of new styles of nurse management at the end of the war caused tensions between senior and junior nurses in both hospitals but only prompted militant strike action at the CLA.

There were strong similarities between asylum and voluntary hospital nurses' work. Regulated timetables controlled working days, which prioritised cleaning both the environment and the patient. Work was task orientated particularly at the CLA where even bathing patients was separated into tasks. The most significant difference in work patterns was the asylum's emphasis on work and fresh air. Although SDEC patients were, on average, admitted for over a month they were largely confined to bed and nurses' work did not extend to promoting exercise or entertainment. Instead it focused on relatively new technical skills of monitoring the patient's condition. In contrast, asylum nurses spent the majority of their day outside working or walking with their patients. The most surprising revelation is that asylum nurses' work during the war included patient entertainment. This presents an alternative view to the notion that it was a custodial role involving violent restraint.[95] The fact that a skeleton nursing staff enabled 350 patients to go to the circus suggests a more complicated story than previously told. Overall, the First World War had more of an impact on asylum nurses' work on the Home Front and the rising mortality rate of nurses' at the CLA suggests that many were overstretched and overwhelmed by their arduous working lives.

Notes

1 99th Annual Report 1918, 24, HC1/1/3/9.
2 Peter Nolan, *A History of Mental Health Nursing* (London, Chapman & Hall, 1993), 39.
3 Robert Dingwall, Ann Marie Rafferty and Charles Webster, *An Introduction to the Social History of Nursing* (London, Routledge, 1988), 126.
4 1901 Census online, RG13, 2201: www.1901censusonline.com/results. asp?wci=person_results&searchwci=person_search (accessed 17 February 2012).
5 Jennifer Laws, 'Crackpots and basket-cases: a history of therapeutic work and occupation', *History of the Human Sciences* 24, 2 (2011), 65–81.
6 Anonymous, 'Work as a therapeutic agent', *Lancet* (2 May 1914).
7 Anonymous, 'Work as a therapeutic agent'.
8 Charles Thomas Andrews, *A Dark Awakening: A History of St. Lawrence's Hospital, Bodmin* (London, Cox & Wyman, 1978), 217.
9 Cornwall Record Office (CRO), HC1/1/1/16, Cornwall Lunatic Asylum Visiting Committee (CLAVC) Minutes (Mins) (26 July 1915), 220.
10 CRO, HC1/1/1/16, CLAVC Mins, 30 March 1914, 219, 328.
11 CRO, HC1/1/1/16, CLAVC Mins, 26 July 1915, 194.
12 Anonymous, 'Appointments', *British Journal of Nursing* (27 July 1912), 69.
13 Anonymous, 'The mental nurse', *Lancet* (13 May 1911).
14 Anonymous, 'The mental nurse'.
15 Nolan, *A History of Mental Health Nursing*, 10.
16 Nolan, *A History of Mental Health Nursing*, 11.
17 Nolan, *A History of Mental Health Nursing*, 61.
18 Nolan, *A History of Mental Health Nursing*, 64.

19   CRO, CLAVC Mins, HC1/1/1/16, 26 November 1917, 62.

20   Andrews, *A Dark Awakening*, 259.

21   Andrews, *A Dark Awakening*, 259.

22   Jo Melling and Bill Forsythe, *The Politics of Madness: The State, Insanity and Society in England, 1845–1914* (Abingdon, Routledge, 2006).

23   CRO, HC1/1/1/16, CLAVC Mins, 12 October 1914, 294.

24   Nolan, *A History of Mental Health Nursing*, 61.

25   Debbie Palmer, *Who Cared for the Carers? The History of Nurses' Occupational Health* (Manchester, Manchester University Press, 2014).

26   Andrews, *A Dark Awakening*.

27   Andrews, *A Dark Awakening*, 257.

28   Nolan, *A History of Mental Health Nursing*, 39.

29   CRO, HC1/1/1/16, CLAVC Mins, 28 June 1915, 199.

30   CRO, HC1/1/1/16, CLAVC Mins, 28 June 1915, 194.

31   CRO, HC1/1/1/16, CLAVC Mins, 1 May 1916, 34.

32   CRO, HC1/1/1/16, CLAVC Mins, 28 May 1915, 310.

33   CRO, HC1/1/3/9, 96th Annual Report 1915, 74.

34   CRO, HC1/1/3/9, Board of Control Report, July 1915, 26.

35   CRO, HC1/1/1/16, CLAVC Mins, 25 October 1915, 293.

36   CRO, HC1/1/1/16, CLAVC Mins, 25 January 1915.

37   CRO, HC1/1/3/9, 96th Annual Report 1915.

38   CRO, HC1/1/3/9, Board of Control Report, July 1916.

39   CRO, HC1/1/1/16, CLAVC Mins, 31 May 1915.

40   CRO, HC1/1/1/18, CLAVC Mins, 25 November 1918, 316.

41   CRO, HC1/1/3/9, 95th Annual Report 1914.

42   CRO, HC1/1/1/16, CLAVC Mins, 29 March 1915, 101.

43   CRO, HC1/1/1/16, CLAVC Mins.

44   CRO, HC1/1/3/9, 96th Annual Report 1915.

45   CRO, HC1/1/1/17, CLAVC Mins, 27 March 1916, 11.

46   Richard Hunter, 'The rise and fall of mental nursing', *Lancet* 1 (14 January 1956); Nolan, *A History of Mental Health Nursing*, 57.

47   CRO, HC1/1/1/16, CLAVC Mins, 26 October 1914, 391; HC1/1/1/18, CLAVC Mins, 26 March 1918, 146.

48   CRO, HC1/1/1/16, CLAVC Mins, 26 July 1915, 220.

49   Geertje Boschma, *The Rise of Mental Health Nursing: A History of Psychiatric Care in Dutch Asylums 1890–1914* (Amsterdam, Amsterdam University Press, 2003), 122.

50   CRO, HC1/1/1/16, CLAVC Mins, 22 February 1915, 75.

51   CRO, HC1/1/1/15, CLAVC Mins, 27 July; 28 September; 26 October 1914; 26 February 1915.

52   CRO, HC1/1/1/15, CLAVC Mins, 26 February 1914, 394.

53   CRO, HC1/1/1/16, CLAVC Mins, 29 March 1915, 100.

54   CRO, HC1/3/9, 99th Annual Report 1915.

55 CRO, HC1/3/9, 99th Annual Report 1915, 25.
56 Hugh Pennington, 'Don't pick your nose', *London Review of Books* 27, 24 (13 December 2005), 29–31.
57 CRO, HC1/1/3/9, 100th Annual Report 1919, 8.
58 CRO, HC1/1/3/9. Board of Control Report, April 1918, 27.
59 CRO, HC1/1/1/16, CLAVC Mins, 25 September 1916, 135.
60 Ben Shephard, *A War of Nerves: Soldiers and Psychiatrists 1914–1994* (London, Jonathan Cape, 2000).
61 CRO, HC1/1/3/9, 99th Annual Report 1918, 24.
62 CRO, HC1/1/3/9, 98th Annual Report 1917, 7.
63 CRO, HC1/1/1/18, 29 October 1917, 42; 29 July 1918, 232.
64 Anonymous, *NAWU Magazine* (October–December 1918), 6.
65 CRO, HC1/1/1/18, CLAVC Mins, 29 October 1917, 42.
66 Mick Carpenter, *Working for Health The History of the Confederation of Health Service Employees* (London, Lawrence & Wishart, 1988), 71.
67 Anonymous, *NAWU Magazine* (October–December 1918), 6.
68 Anonymous, *Bodmin Guardian* (29 October 1918).
69 CRO, HC1/1/1/18, CLAVC Mins, 26 October 1918, 276.
70 CRO, HC1/1/3/9, 99th Annual Report 1918.
71 CRO, HC1/1/1/18, CLAVC Mins, 27 January 1919, 359.
72 CRO, HC1/1/1/18, CLAVC Mins, 30 December 1918, 335.
73 CRO, HC1/1/1/18, CLAVC Mins, 1 July 1919.
74 CRO, HC1/1/1/18, CLAVC Mins, 26 April 1919.
75 CRO, HC1/1/1/18, CLAVC Mins, 26 April 1919.
76 Anonymous, *Nursing Record and Hospital World* (14 June 1888), 127.
77 Brian Abel-Smith, *A History of the Nursing Profession* (London, Heinemann, 1960), 86.
78 Ann Marie Rafferty, *The Politics of Nursing Knowledge* (London, Routledge, 1996), 77–8.
79 Anne Summers, *Angels and Citizens: British Women as Military Nurses 1854–1914* (London, Routledge, 2000), 278.
80 Plymouth and West Devon Record Office (PWDRO), 1490/24, South Devon and East Cornwall (SDEC) Register of Nurses, 1903–23.
81 PWDRO, 1490/24 SDEC Register of Nurses, 1903–23.
82 Anonymous, 'Licensee's Protest', *Western Morning News* (11 July 1913).
83 PWDRO, 606/1/18, SDEC Hospital house committee minutes, 29 July 1904.
84 PWDRO, 606/1/18, SDEC Hospital house committee minutes, 28 May 1907.
85 PWDRO, 606/1/7, SDEC general hospital committee minutes (Gen Com Mins), 10 June 1902; 15 December 1905; 16 February 1906.
86 PWDRO, 606/1/11, SDEC Gen Com Mins, March 1916, 192.
87 PWDRO, 606/1/11, SDEC Gen Com Mins, 4 May 1916.
88 PWDRO, 606/1/11, SDEC Gen Com Mins, 17 February 1915.

89 PWDRO, 606/1/11, SDEC Gen Com Mins, 15 March 1916, 199.

90 PWDRO, 606/1/11, SDEC Gen Com Mins, 15 March; 27 October 1916.

91 Jeremy Booth, 'A short history of blood pressure measurement', *Proceedings of the Royal Society of Medicine* 70, 11 (November 1977), 793–9.

92 PWDRO, 606/1/11, SDEC nursing committee minutes, 23 July 1914.

93 PWDRO, 606/1/22 SDEC house committee minutes, 19 November 1915.

94 PWDRO, 606/1/22 SDEC house committee minutes, 30 June 1916.

Part III
Technological warfare

8

Blood and guts: Nursing with the International Brigades in the Spanish Civil War, 1936–39

Angela Jackson

Blood and guts: words that could resonate with nurses in any war but have a particularly powerful significance in the case of the war in Spain. 'But Spain is Red', one anti-communist heckler protested at a public meeting in England where a nurse, recently returned from the front, was speaking to raise funds. 'Yes it is', she replied, 'red with blood. The blood is splashed over the streets and the gutters often run with it. For weeks my fingernails were blocked up with clotted blood, and my arms were splashed to the elbows with it.'[1]

Blood permeated the daily life of the nurses who volunteered for Spain.[2] Not only did they often spend their days dealing with the haemorrhaging wounded and slipping on the gory floors of hastily improvised operating theatres, they were also involved in the huge strides being made in the field of blood transfusion. Guts were a prominent feature of life in a variety of ways. In addition to helping the surgeons search through yards of intestines for shrapnel and bullet holes, nurses also played a key role in caring for soldiers during outbreaks of typhoid and dysentery. Inevitably, they frequently suffered from the same illnesses themselves.[3] In another sense, the word 'guts' could also describe the courage shown by these young women. However, it would be an oversimplification to regard them merely as stereotypical heroic figures in the history of 'women worthies'.[4] The faults and frailties that are revealed both wittingly and unwittingly in their own testimonies and in other archival material have allowed a more extensive analysis of that notion than is possible here.[5] Nevertheless, it should be noted that by going to Spain they

165

had willingly volunteered to face all the dangers of carrying out their duties in the midst of a bitter conflict, despite the fact that the war was regarded by many British people in those days as just another 'quarrel in a far away country between people of whom we know nothing'.[6] The challenges they met when serving in Spain were many: the sudden burden of responsibility; the difficult conditions when caring for patients in temporary locations such as tents, old farmhouses and caves; exhaustion and, on top of all that, the emotional trauma of loss, not only of patients who could not be saved but also of brothers, husbands and lovers who died at the front. The way in which the majority dealt with these challenges was, indeed, admirable.

When civil war divided Spain in 1936, qualified nurses from many different countries volunteered to go to help the wounded, working almost exclusively in the areas held by the elected Republican government.[7] Their reasons for doing so varied considerably: some, like the majority of male volunteers in the International Brigades, were motivated by political awareness, believing that by helping the Spanish Republican government they would not only be fighting General Franco and fascism, but would also be helping to prevent another world war. Other nurses went primarily for humanitarian reasons, knowing little of the deep-seated, essentially Spanish causes that had led to war, nor the wider implications of a conflict that quickly took on a more international perspective.[8] From the early days in hospitals organised and run by voluntary groups such as the Spanish Medical Aid Committee in London, many nurses transferred to medical units of the International Brigades, and were soon incorporated in the Spanish Republican Army.[9] In addition to military casualties, including prisoners from Franco's forces, at times they also cared for civilians, usually the victims of bombardments.

Their work in Spain was wide ranging. At the height of battle, a theatre nurse might work for thirty-six hours at a stretch or face a constant stream of almost impossible choices in triage. In the wards, nurses gave intravenous injections by the flickering flames of candles, cigarette lighters or from a wick floating in a dish of oil.[10] During the hot summer days they fought the swarms of flies that plagued their patients. At night they scared away the rats that would creep in to gnaw the wounds of unconscious men. In the bitter deep snows of Teruel, where the only method of heating was to burn alcohol in a bowl, one of their tasks was to find the line of demarcation for amputation on frostbitten limbs. In the lulls between battles, nurses with midwifery training visited the villages to help civilian mothers give birth, though amid the turmoil of the retreats they could find themselves delivering babies by the roadside or in the soot and grime of a disused railway tunnel. Some made radio broadcasts from Spain or wrote articles for newspapers and magazines, appealing for more nurses and funds. All too often, they took on the sad task of recording the last messages of dying soldiers to send to their families at home.

The work of these women can be explored in depth using a variety of sources. Official records from the medical units did not survive the war, though other archival reports and minutes of committee meetings are accessible. Retrospective memoirs and oral testimonies of the volunteer nurses themselves can be contrasted with contemporary sources such as their letters from Spain and published articles. In the case of Patience Darton, for example, it has been possible

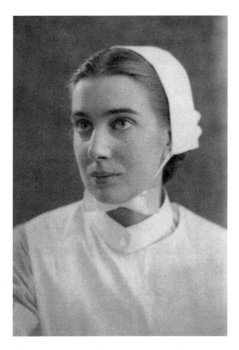

8.1 Patience Darton

to write a full biography, drawing not only on the interviews carried out in her later years, but also on the remarkably vivid letters she wrote as young woman working in the medical units in Spain.[11] In this chapter, such varied sources are used to examine several aspects of nursing experience that were at the forefront of changes taking place at the time. These changes took various forms. Although antibiotics were still unavailable and even sulphanilamide was a rarity, and despite the fact that shortages of food and basic supplies were all too frequent, the chances of survival for patients improved significantly during the course of the war as a result of certain key practical, surgical and medical innovations. Some of these were detailed in contemporary journals by doctors working near the front lines in Republican Spain.[12] Another type of change was to have a notable sociological impact. Many of the qualified volunteer nurses were committed to passing on their expertise to others. As the care of patients in Spain had been traditionally the province of nuns and professional training for nurses was in its infancy, the transmission of nursing skills to the young untrained Spanish girls who came to work in the International Brigade medical units was of vital importance, both in practical and political terms, demonstrating the capabilities of 'modern' women.[13]

This chapter takes as its focus four themes relating to the challenges the nurses faced. 'Mobilisation' examines the challenges of logistics and improvisation; 'The wounded' explores the challenges of surgical nursing; the section on 'Typhoid fever' looks at the challenges posed by epidemics, and the profound challenges to tradition are discussed under the heading of 'Teaching'. This chapter and its conclusion show how nurses' skills impacted not only on those they were trying to help, but also on their own lives.

Mobilisation: the challenges of logistics and improvisation

The aim of treating the wounded as soon as possible after they were injured by transporting the surgeon to the patient had already become common policy during the First World War, but evolved further in Spain, creating extra duties for nurses.[14] As the fronts moved and new battle lines were drawn, nurses carried out much of the hard work entailed in preparing old and frequently unsanitary buildings for use as provisional hospitals. They were also usually responsible for ensuring that all equipment was dismantled and packed safely to be moved elsewhere. Thora Silverthorne, a theatre nurse among the first to volunteer in 1936, spoke of one particularly crucial skill in which the English nurses excelled:

> None of us had been in a war situation. It was quite different working in hospitals, you know where everything is – hospitals in England were arranged, you knew exactly where you were, but we had to improvise everything, improvise instruments often. We'd have to try and make something do and try and keep the theatre as clean, you know, in war conditions. When I think of it now, how we ever coped – young people with no experience of coping under conditions of bombing. If you couldn't do it you improvised as well as you possibly could.[15]

Thanks in part to the huge efforts made by fund-raising committees and generous donations from thousands of ordinary people in countries such as Britain, a number of vehicles were converted for use as mobile operating theatres known as 'auto-chirs', with lighting provided by a motorbike engine, portable operating tables and autoclaves for sterilisation. Lillian Urmston, a nurse from Stalybridge, wrote an article for the *Nursing Mirror* explaining how the auto-chirs were equipped, the journeys she made in convoy sitting on top of a pile of mattresses in the back of an open lorry, and the duties of a nurse on arrival at their destination.[16] Another English nurse and midwife, Patience Darton, an experienced camper with the Girl Guides and a Wolf Cub leader, was able to advise the doctors on the team about some of the equipment that would be needed to set up such a unit during the fighting near the city of Zaragoza. As the wounded had to be housed in tents that offered no protection from attack, they were evacuated to a safer location as soon as possible after treatment.[17] Later on in the war Patience was asked to organise a similar mobile unit with an eight-bed ambulance and the necessary assistants and stretcher-bearers to move as close as possible to the front. Everything was stowed away tightly around the people travelling in the back, while Patience and the doctor sat in the front with the driver. Unfortunately, the ambulance crashed during the long and arduous journey and she was thrown through the windscreen, suffering quite severe facial injuries.

Her courage was put to the test afterwards in the hospital when the

Spanish hospital staff would come in, take one look at her face, burst into tears and go out. The mayor came to visit her and made a marvellous speech to the staff about how she had given her 'all' to Spain. In a terrible temper, but unable to speak properly because of her injuries, she related how she had tried to say, 'I hadn't given my all, my face was nothing like my all – there was lots of me left.'[18] Plastic surgery was in its early days, but luckily, she was eventually sent to Dr Leo Eloesser, one of the leading American surgeons in Spain, who had set up a clinic closer to the French border at Mataró. He was able to restore her features to a great extent, though her nose was never quite the same again.

Moving during the retreats was often a terrifying experience for the nurses. With the battle drawing closer by the minute, everything would have to be packed rapidly for transport to a new location. Frequently, there were not enough vehicles to do this all together, so a system of leap-frogging had to be used. Nurses could be left waiting with some of their patients for the lorries and ambulances to return. 'It was hell', said Lillian Urmston, explaining how at night, it was such 'a horrible feeling' to hear a vehicle arriving because it might belong to the enemy. Atrocity stories abounded of rapes and the killing of patients being perpetrated by the 'Moors', frequently used by Franco as shock troops when advancing. Lillian remembered that although, at last, their own vehicles arrived, her knees would be knocking for hours afterwards and other nurses would be white and vomiting.[19]

Throughout the conflict, for over two and half years, as the fronts moved, so did the nurses. Often they had little idea of where they were, and never knew where they would be going next until the last moment. Hospitals where they worked were bombed, and on the retreats the ambulances were machine-gunned along with the columns of refugees. As in other wars, nursing was often a very dangerous occupation. To contain their fears for the sake of their patients and carry on despite the traumatic sights they witnessed showed enormous strength of character.[20]

The wounded: the challenges of surgical nursing

In interviews and memoirs, nurses often referred with pride to the success of new techniques employed in Spain for the treatment of open wounds and compound fractures. Techniques for the management of these injuries had been pioneered by the Catalan surgeon, Josep Trueta Raspall, thereby greatly reducing the number of amputations required.[21] Patience Darton recalled the details:

> The surgeons worked out a method whereby they did a tremendous 'debridement', they cut away all the bits that might be infected instead of doing the minimum and sewing them up. They used to open up the things, cut away all the dead parts, put them in a plaster and leave them sometimes for two or three months and they would heal up under the plaster. So we didn't get gas gangrene by this method, it was very rapidly found out how to prevent it. You see, the gas gangrene in the First World War was a terrible thing, hundreds died of it in the most dreadful way, the most agonising thing. I saw it later in Spain, but I never saw it from our surgeons and operations.[22]

She did not refer to the problem of the nauseating smell that resulted from having to leave the plaster casts in place for so long. In the convalescent hospitals, nurses would cope with this by caring for the patients whenever possible on open balconies. The almost overwhelming odour was found not to be an indicator of wound infection, which was more reliably diagnosed by a rising temperature and pulse rate, or oedema of the affected limb.[23]

Sadly, although the technique was put into quite widespread use in the areas held by the Republican government, there were still occasions when nurses in the International Brigades had to deal with patients who were already suffering from gas gangrene when they arrived. Patience Darton recalled several such cases; their slow deaths indelibly imprinted on her memory. Whilst working in a disused railway tunnel, she was caring for some Spanish patients who had been picked up from an abandoned hospital during a retreat, some already dying from gas gangrene. 'An absolute nightmare – and they wouldn't die. We filled them up with morphia, there was no treatment.' The fact that they took four days to die despite such massive amounts of morphia is recalled again in another interview ten years later.[24] Her degree of distress had not diminished. The way in which nurses sometimes coped with these levels of intense pain among the wounded was highlighted by Molly Murphy:

> It was a relief to them and to us when death stilled their anguish. We felt it deeply and it is a mistake to think that a nurse becomes immune to the

171

suffering because in such circumstances as these we must work like fury and cannot stand by to weep.[25]

She recalled one colleague exclaiming on finding a patient had died, 'Now I can have his pillow for some other poor devil.' Then, immediately regretting her callous remark, she burst into tears saying, 'Oh Murphy, what is this war doing to us? How could I say such a thing?'[26]

Nurses were closely involved with the work of blood transfusion in Spain, giving their own blood for transfusion as well as administering supplies intravenously. Improvements were made in the technology for the preservation of bottled blood, increasing the scale of its collection and transportation from civilian donors, thereby saving many lives. Early in the war, nurses and other staff in the medical units frequently gave blood by direct arm to arm transfusion. Using this method it was easy to donate rather too much. Patience, for example, 'puffed for a day' afterwards. Her blood had actually not been a good match for the injured man and had made him rather ill. Nevertheless, he and his family were full of gratitude and excitement, thinking that this now made them blood brothers and sisters. Patience recalled that it all seemed 'very dramatic and lovely' for them.[27] The miracle of direct transfusion was also remembered by Nan Green, an administrator in the International Brigade medical units: 'Blood goes from your arm and colour comes to his lips – it was an experience I wouldn't have wanted to miss.'[28] Sometimes, wrote Margaret Powell, when blood was needed urgently, the nurses 'behaved like vampires', waylaying lorry drivers going back and forth to the front, taking a pint of blood in return for a swig of rum.[29]

However, a system of collecting blood from donors in the cities was soon well established, and functioned efficiently for much of the war, although when demand was especially high, direct transfusion could be the only option. After collection in cities such as Barcelona, a rudimentary classification into blood groups was carried out when possible and a citrate anticoagulant added before the supplies were transported to hospitals near the front in lorries adapted for refrigerated storage.[30] Not only did the successful calls for donors increase the availability of preserved supplies for the wounded, but the very act of giving blood encouraged solidarity between civilians and the soldiers

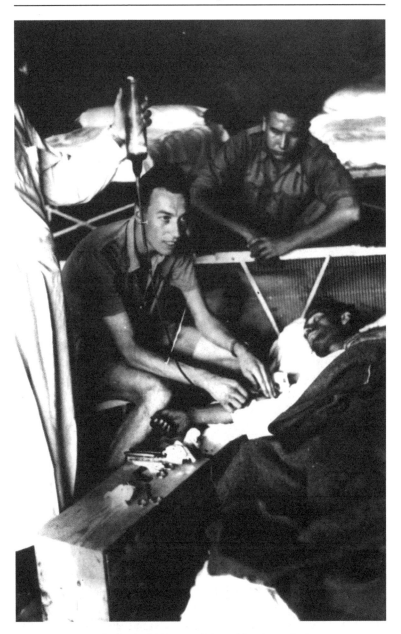

8.2 Dr Reginald Saxton giving a blood transfusion

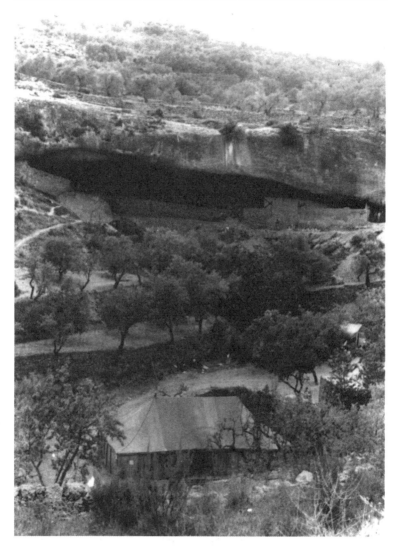

8.3 The cave hospital at La Bisbal de Falset

at the front. What better way to create a sense of national identity than for the non-combatant population to become blood brothers with the soldiers who were fighting and dying for the Republic? The symbolic importance of donating must have been particularly strong in the case of women who could not fight themselves but who must have felt their blood was empowering those who could.[31]

Winifred Bates visited many hospitals and medical units in Spain, checking on the well-being of English-speaking staff. During the Ebro offensive she visited the hospital set up in a cave near the village of La Bisbal de Falset where she had a particularly vivid experience of blood transfusion:

> It is so hard to make a man, and so easy to blast him to death. I shall never forget the Ebro. If one went for a walk away from the cave there was the smell of death. In the beds beside the soldiers were women and children brought in from the villages round about after bombing raids. I do not know if the girls who worked with me were ever aware that under my placid countenance I had a secret sin, the sin of jealousy. Many a time they had been called upon to give their blood to a soldier in a transfusion. I, being a rare and not very useful group, had never been called. It hurt a little, to know that I was not useful. Up in the cave an Englishman was dying. I watched the doctor give him the universal group from the ampoule, and he said, 'If this does not do we'll take you.' I have since seen pictures of elaborate blood transfusions in hospitals with all the performers dressed up in white. In the cave, work was more direct. I sat down on the floor, stuck my legs under the bed and put my arm on the table. It was a simple matter. There was nothing in it, but it eased my vanity and helped my self respect.[32]

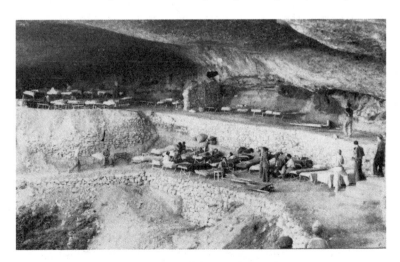

8.4 Interior of the cave hospital

Patience Darton referred to the subject of blood transfusions in the cave to illustrate another point she was anxious to clarify, namely, that of the treatment of enemy wounded. The usual issues surrounding their treatment, exacerbated when supplies were short, were rendered even more complex in this case by Franco's use of Moorish troops. As historic enemies, racial tensions already existed between Spaniards and Moors, and their reputation for extreme cruelty intensified feelings against them. Patience spoke frankly about the problems that had to be overcome when they needed medical attention:

> There was one Moor I remember, a Moorish prisoner we'd taken, a Franco Moor, very badly wounded in the neck. God, how he hated us, he used to give terrible looks to us, he didn't trust us at all, he expected we'd kill him the same as they killed people. But he was admitted amongst the others, and he ought to have had a blood transfusion, and the [Spanish] chaps got together and said they weren't going to give the blood of the women of Spain to the Moor.[33]

Although the Moors were hated, and Franco despised for bringing them to fight in Spain, Patience believed that there was also an awareness of other aspects of the situation amongst the Spaniards and Catalans in the unit. 'They knew quite well', she said, 'that they shouldn't have been fighting the Moors anyway in Morocco. That was also a disgrace. They were very clear about that.' The main purpose of her story becomes clear when she stresses the fact that the men, much to her admiration, overcame their prejudices. She recalled: 'When I looked round, he was getting one – this lot of sheepish faces as he got his blood transfusion.'[34]

Typhoid fever: the challenge of epidemics

Good nursing care often made the difference between life and death, not only for the wounded but also for those with diseases such as typhoid fever. Outbreaks among the troops were not unusual, but impacted far more severely on the foreign soldiers, owing to their lack of natural immunity. Nurses from Britain were more aware than some of the Spanish doctors of recent developments in the treatment of those suffering from the disease. Patience Darton came into conflict with one such doctor soon after she arrived in Spain. She had been sent to Valencia to nurse the Commander of the British Battalion, Tom Wintringham, believed to be gravely ill with typhoid after being wounded. When she arrived, she found her patient 'very wretched', the place 'filthy' and the flies 'awful'. Following the common practice at the time, he had not been given solid food for weeks. Fortunately, while at University College Hospital, Patience had some training and experience of nursing typhoid cases:

> And I remembered quite well then that the old method for nursing typhoid was that you kept them on no food at all, sips of milk and thin bread and butter, nothingness, for six weeks, so they wouldn't perforate because that's what you do with typhoid if you get it badly, your intestines perforate and you get general intestinal poisoning and you die. And this was not considered a good thing. They had looked into it and the little 'Peyer's patches', the bits that get the infection in your intestines, give out in the second week of your infection. If you don't perforate in the second week, you're not going to perforate – that phase is over, and you'd better be fed, because people were taking a long time to recover from typhoid because they were starved. Now I remembered that and I thought 'Oh, well, thank goodness for UCH.'[35]

Patience decided to 'tepid sponge' her patient to make him more comfortable. Just then, the doctor arrived and Patience welcomed him with smiles, but he responded with a furious tirade in Spanish. Eventually, when someone was able to act as interpreter, it transpired that he was firmly convinced that washing the patient was almost sure to be lethal. A form was produced for Patience to sign, to take complete responsibility for the likely death of her charge. She signed her acceptance when perhaps other, more timid young women would not have dared to do so. She also worked out that her patient's temperature fluctuations were due to a wound infection beneath his sutures. She re-opened the wound and drained the abscesses. Her intervention, in combination with good nursing and a diet of light foods, soon resulted in Tom Wintringham's recovery.[36]

During the first year of the war, conditions for the care of soldiers with typhoid patients were at times appalling and suitable food was frequently unavailable. An epidemic on the Aragon front in the spring of 1937 resulted in a mortality rate of almost 20 per cent. By October 1937, a major outbreak of around 1000 cases had a reduced mortality rate of 8 per cent, despite continuing problems with the inadequacy of provisions.[37] This outbreak was described in harrowing terms in the notes of Rosaleen Smythe, who was working as an administrator in the unit:

> – It has been raining for days and days. This prevents attacks. The river is rising hourly; it has reached the door of the hospital, which is only a wooden hut. Operating room and triage are divided from the wards by sheets. My office is in triage.
> – We had orders to pack up and move off, but the floods have prevented the lorries from coming up. For two and a half weeks we have been in a state of package. We have scarcely any food and what there is, is bad … Dr Saxton has to chlorinate the water every morning.
> – The cases are increasing. We have no clean water, no fires, no heating, no lavatories.
> – Existence is a misery. Rain is coming in. Rats run across the floor.
> – We have no milk, eggs or potatoes for the typhoid patients … I cannot say enough about the splendid way Ada Hodson, Patience Darton and Lillian Urmston are working. How Ada makes us laugh when she tries to drink the peculiar liquid which is neither tea, coffee nor cocoa, but a mixture of all. In the evenings, by the light of a few candles we put on a gramophone. The records we have are Beethoven's Fifth Symphony, one movement of Schubert's Unfinished and one Haydn. We play them over and over again to the drip, drip of the incessant rain. We put on extra pullovers to go to bed in, we have given our blankets to the patients.
> – A bitter cold wind and a frost has set in. Those poor *chicas* (Spanish girls) have to clean the few bed pans in the icy river water.[38]

This same epidemic was remembered vividly by one of the doctors, Reginald Saxton, when he was writing a glowing reference for Patience Darton just before the start of the Second World War. Part of his letter refers to her work on the ward of around forty cases of typhoid fever. It clearly demonstrates his belief in the value of skilled nursing care for the survival of typhoid patients:

> I worked with Nurse Darton as my Ward Sister on many occasions in Spain, and never had a more efficient or justifiably self-confident nurse. In particular I recall a typhoid epidemic in October and November 1937, when, with a severe shortage of food, clothing, heating and lighting, utterly inadequate sanitary accommodation, completely untrained assistant nurses and overcrowded and uncomfortable staff quarters with a minimum of furniture and privacy, Miss Darton ran a typhoid ward with great

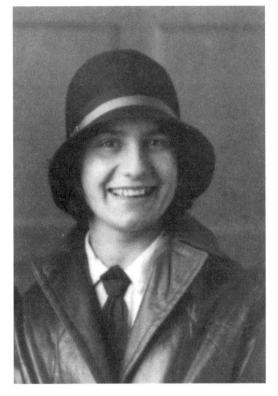

8.5 Penny Phelps

efficiency. I could only give the patients a minimum of attention as I was Superintendent of the hospital as well as Medical Officer for that ward, but I had complete confidence, justified by results, in leaving the major part of the treatment in her hands.[39]

Penny Phelps, who had trained as a nurse to escape her impoverished background in London's East End, was one of the few with experience of working in a fever hospital before she volunteered for Spain. Because of this, she was sent to deal with an epidemic of scarlet fever in the Italian 'Garibaldi' Battalion of the International Brigades. Their own doctor had fallen ill too. When she arrived, she found a ward packed full of sick men, one of whom she realised had typhoid:

I went in and it – stench – and there was pots of urine, you know, all over-flowing with urine, bits of bread and crusts all over, no pillows, people in clothes and on clothes, and it was terrible, and the windows were closed. And I thought, 'God, what am I in for?' And then I looked as I walked by and I thought, 'God, that man's ill.' And I went up, and I thought, 'God, he's almost moribund.' And talk about lice, you could imagine that they'd be running off with people.[40]

In addition to attending to those who were ill, Penny organised staff for a programme of thorough disinfection, fumigation and inoculation against typhoid for the entire battalion of 600 men. This certainly turned out to be a challenge for a rather 'green' young nurse. The soldiers were unaccustomed to vaccinations and tried to avoid having them. She had to threaten to report them and told them that, if they contracted typhoid, the battalion would become a liability to the Republic, not an asset. The ordinary soldiers then submitted to the needle, but the officers still believed it was not necessary. She was very resourceful, hiding a tray of vaccines in the Officers' Mess before their arrival. When they were eating, she went in and locked the door. They tried to escape like naughty school-boys, but eventually, with the help of the political commissar, she convinced them of the need to have the TAB vaccine, for the good of 'the cause'.[41]

Penny Phelps was one of the nurses who contracted typhoid herself and was sent home to convalesce in Britain for a while before returning to Spain bearing a consignment of desperately needed medical instruments. With a high risk of contaminated water sup-plies, vaccines still not in general use and anti-typhoid far from completely effective, it was not surprising that nurses too sometimes succumbed to the disease. When they did, they were inclined to feel guilty, not only because they felt they were being a nuisance and were unable to carry on caring for their patients, but also because during their nursing training they had been taught that, 'If we got typhoid it was our own fault for being careless.'[42] As the war went on, specially designated hospitals were set up in the Republic for typhoid patients. The town of Valls, for example, had a hospital for infectious cases where local archives record that at least one of the Spanish nurses also died from typhoid.[43] The disease took its toll not only on soldiers but also among those who cared for them.

Teaching: the challenge to tradition

Many of the British nurses were enthusiastic about training the Spanish women who volunteered to work in the hospitals and were well aware of the social and political implications of what they were doing but, as Patience Darton explained, this was not true in every case. Before she joined the International Brigade medical services, Patience was among several British nurses working in a provisional hospital at Poleñino. There, she found herself in open disagreement with some of the other nurses on a professional level as a result of their attitudes to Spanish girls who were working in the hospital:

> And there were seven of us (British nurses) by the time I got there, all trained, and we weren't training Spanish girls who wanted to come in and help – which was a very brave thing to do because it wasn't the thing for a good Spanish girl of any sort, to go and work in a hospital with men, it wasn't at all proper. And we were letting them do the skivvying, which was a thing I disagreed with profoundly. I thought we should train them. I mean, this was our chance to train them to do the things we could do.[44]

Subsequently, Patience worked with other qualified nurses in Spain who recognised the importance of training local women volunteers, and shared her commitment to do so.[45] For some of the Spanish women who had been brought up within the constraints of strict Catholic traditions, coming into contact with these professional foreign nurses could be an eye-opening experience, as Patience Darton recalled:

> And to them it was an enormous thing – we were modern women that they hadn't ever come across, you see. We didn't mind talking to men, we didn't mind throwing our weight around either, which we did a good deal, because you know what nurses are! And without thinking much about it, you see, but a Spanish woman couldn't have done that, and she couldn't have nursed a stranger – she couldn't have touched a strange man, let alone washed him or looked after him. For them it was a tremendous thing they were doing, to accept it, you see. The Spanish men didn't like it particularly.[46]

Medical volunteers who had come to Spain from the USA also soon became aware of the importance of passing on their skills to others. Celia Seborer, a trained clinical laboratory technician working in Murcia, wrote about the classes in basic nursing skills that were taking place there every afternoon to train Spanish girls. However, she recognised that more still could be done, commenting: 'Probably the most vital part of our work and one that till now we have underestimated and neglected is our work with the Spanish girls and women here in the hospital.'[47] The American nurse, Ruth Waller, broadcast from Madrid about the nursing school in the hospital where she worked, describing in detail what was being taught in the classes. Some students had progressed to a second, more advanced course, though as she pointed out, this was still very elementary and not to be compared with the three-year course of instruction given in America. Nevertheless, she was pleased to report that 'the girls are learning enough of the fundamentals to make of them competent and responsible nurses' aids'. She was particularly pleased with the continuing enthusiastic attitude of the students:

> The novelty of the class has surely worn off for the older pupils, but I know that it is not a chore for them; it is the major interest of their day. You could easily understand why this is if you could see them at their usual work; on their knees scrubbing the cold marble of the long halls with colder water. The school is for these Spanish girls an assurance that life can hold something more for them than the scrubbing brush and pail. We, at home, are apt to take such an assurance as everyone's birthright. However, in Spain it is a new idea – the new idea that we are all working to see realised in the coming life of this people.[48]

Unlike many girls in Spain who, until the days of the Republic, were not even taught to read, Aurora Fernández was relatively well educated and had been studying English when the civil war began. She quickly volunteered to work in the medical units:

> All the English nurses taught us, the volunteer nurses, how to work, but in such a considerate way, they never showed any 'superiority' towards us. They usually said, 'Could you come and help me?' That was the introduction to do 'together' something ... I must stress the non-obtrusive way in which this was done in order not to hurt anybody's feelings. They did not say 'I am going to tell you how to do this,' but rather, 'Come, let us get this ready.[49]

This method was not only 'very soothing' but, in the eyes of Aurora Fernández, 'of high political significance in those days'. There can be no doubt of the importance of this contact with qualified nurses for some of these young Spanish women. The life of Aurora Fernandez was changed completely. After working for much of the war with British nurses, on Franco's victory she left Spain for exile in France, but was eventually helped by her friends in the medical units to go to London.

Conclusion

It is difficult to assess the work of qualified nurses in Spain during the civil war in precise terms. There were no targets set, no budgets met, and the carefully kept records of the patients in individual hospitals have not survived.[50] However, the significance of their contribution can be evaluated in other ways. The knowledge they had gained in Spain soon proved useful once again for the treatment of casualties in the Second World War. Among the many examples of how this occurred is an illustrated series of fascinating articles by Lillian Urmston in the *Nursing Mirror* in 1939, covering many aspects of her work at the front, giving information about procedures, treatments and individual cases.[51] Another example can be found in the minutes of the Spanish Medical Aid Committee in January 1939, recording that a letter had been received from 'Nurse Darton, returned from Spain, asking whether we could assist her to obtain a non-resident post under the London County Council [LCC]'.[52] She was interviewed by the LCC and offered work lecturing nurses on the organisation of hospital services under war conditions and surgical nursing in wartime. She spent three months teaching the hundreds of LCC nurses the new techniques and practices she had learned in Spain.[53] The immense responsibilities of qualified nurses in Spain had included not only giving intravenous injections and general anaesthetics, but also the complex tasks of triage and dealing with dressings for severe wounds. In Spain, their work had frequently overlapped with that of doctors or their Spanish assistants, the 'practicantes'.[54] Many nurses must have felt their duties to be mundane and limited when they returned to work in their home countries.[55]

Recognition of the work done by British nurses in the Spanish Republic during the civil war was complicated by the fact that the government was defeated in 1939 and the dictatorship of Francisco Franco lasted for almost forty years. Nevertheless, the Republican government in exile made one British nurse, Margaret Powell, a Dame of the Order of Loyalty to the Spanish Republic in recognition of her 'valiant action as a nurse' and her 'self sacrifice and devotion to our wounded and to our war victims'.[56] The names of certain individual nurses appear on plaques in memory of local volunteers in the International Brigades. However, appreciation of their role during the war is demonstrated most clearly by the reception they were given whenever they returned to Spain after Franco's death in 1975. One example can be noted in particular. For many years, Patience Darton did not go back to Spain on trips to the battlefields with the other International Brigaders. This was not only because there were 'too many ghosts' for her there, but also because she was well aware of the emotional nature of the welcome other nurses had been given on their return. 'The Spaniards', she said, 'always made such a 'terrible fuss' of the nurses. 'One does get much more attention, and it was they who did all the fighting – the chaps – much worse for them.'[57]

However, Patience Darton did eventually go back to Spain. She died in Madrid on her first return visit in 1996 while attending a 'Homage' to the International Brigades.[58] When asked in an interview in her later years if she had any regrets, she admitted there were things in her life she wished she had done differently. But, like the majority of British nurses who went to Spain, she never regretted having volunteered:

> Only when I think of Spain, yes! I believe it was a wonderful thing to be able to feel so united. We – the International Brigaders – were so fortunate. We were so lucky that the Spaniards let us go to their country. We were so fortunate to be able to be with people who were committed to such a just cause, people who were really fighting against fascism.[59]

Notes

1 Penny Phelps, report of speech at Welwyn Garden City, 6 May 1937. See also her memoirs, Penny Fyvel, *English Penny* (Devon, Arthur H. Stockwell Ltd, 1992). For more on Penny Phelps and other British nurses in Spain see Angela Jackson, *British Women and the Spanish Civil War* (London and New York, Routledge/Cañada Blanch Studies on Contemporary Spain, 2002; rev. pb. edn, Barcelona, Warren & Pell Publishing/Cañada Blanch Studies on Contemporary Spain, 2009).

2 Nursing was a profession almost exclusively taken up by women rather than men at the time of the war in Spain. There were very few female doctors. Only one British nurse, Priscilla Scott-Ellis, is known to have worked in the Nationalist hospitals with Franco's forces. See Priscilla Scott-Ellis (ed. Raymond Carr), *The Chances of Death: A Diary of the Spanish Civil War* (Norwich, Michael Russell, 1995); Paul Preston, 'All for Love', in *Doves of War: Four Women of Spain* (London, HarperCollins, 2002); Jackson, *British Women and the SCW*.

3 Penny Phelps was seriously wounded by shrapnel when the hospital in which she was working was bombed. She was repatriated for several abdominal operations but was never able to have children. Many nurses were badly affected by their poor diet in Spain and suffered repeatedly from dysentery. See Jackson, *British Women and the SCW*.

4 'The history of women worthies' is a term that has been used by historians such as Natalie Davis and Gerder Lerner to describe a type of 'compensatory history' found in certain studies of notable women.

5 See for example honest admissions by Nan Green in her memoir, *A Chronicle of Small Beer: The Memoirs of Nan Green* (Nottingham, Trent Editions, 2005) and Angela Jackson's biography of Patience Darton, *For us it was Heaven: The Passion, Grief and Fortitude of Patience Darton from the Spanish Civil War to Mao's China* (Brighton, Sussex Academic Press, 2012).

6 Neville Chamberlain, radio broadcast, 27 September 1938.

7 Due to the lack of surviving official records and the variety of organisations that sent out volunteer nurses from different countries, it is not possible to calculate the exact numbers who served in Republican Spain. Research for this chapter is based on the work of English-speaking nurses. At least 170 English-speaking women volunteers have been documented as being involved with the work of the medical services, but the total might be considerably higher. Jim Fyrth and Sally Alexander (eds), *Women's Voices from the Spanish Civil War* (London, Lawrence & Wishart, 1991), 29, fn. 1.

8 For more on the motivation of British women see Jackson, *British Women and the SCW*, chapter 2. In addition to the military aid sent to Franco by Hitler and Mussolini, the non-intervention pact promoted by Britain and France was to have a devastating effect on chances of victory for the democratically elected Republican government.

9 For example, the Spanish Medical Aid Committee (SMAC) had its headquarters in London and around 200 branches all over the UK. It raised funds to send out several groups of medical personnel, ambulances and equipment, and set up provisional hospitals, including one of the first, at Grañen.

10 See, for example, Margaret Powell, 'Nurses there work in wards lit by cigarette lighters', *Daily Worker*, 7 January 1938.

11 Jackson, *For us it was Heaven*.

12 See for example R. S. Saxton, *The Lancet*, 'The Madrid Transfusion Institute', 4 September 1937 and 'Medicine in Republican Spain', 24 September 1938; Paul Preston, 'Two doctors and one cause: Len Crome and Reginald Saxton in the International Brigades', *International Journal of Iberian Studies* 19, 1 (2006), 5–24.

13 Standards of hygiene and asepsis were low at that time in Spain, and there was no tradition of nursing training comparable to that in Britain. When the Second Republic was established in 1931, nursing schools were set up in some regions of Spain. The Catalan government began an ambitious project for training nurses, the first school opening in Barcelona in 1933, but in general, numbers of trained nurses were still minimal and nursing care of the patients was carried out by other family members or by nuns. See Roser Valls (Coordinator), *Infermeres catalanes a la Guerra Civil espanyola* (Barcelona, University of Barcelona, 2008).

14 For more on the organisational structure of the medical services in Republican Spain see Nicholas Coni, *Medicine and Warfare: Spain, 1936–1939* (London, Routledge/Cañada Blanch Studies on Contemporary Spain, 2008), chapter 7, and Linda Palfreeman, *¡Salud! British Volunteers in the Republican Medical Service during the Spanish Civil War, 1936–1939* (Brighton, Sussex Academic Press, 2012), chapter 6.

15 Thora Craig, née Silverthorne, Imperial War Museum Sound Archive (IWM) 13770.

16 Lillian Urmston, 'English Nurse in Spain', *Nursing Mirror* (27 May 1939), 293; Palfreeman, *¡Salud!*, 114–5.

17 Patience Edney née Darton (PE), interview with Angela Jackson (AJ), 18 March 1994.

18 PE, IWM 8398. For more on this episode see Jackson, *For us it was Heaven*, 81–3.

19 Lillian Buckoke, née Urmston (LB), Tameside Local Studies Library, Stalybridge, 203.

20 For more on the subject of 'containment' and how nurses coped with the experience of war, see Christine E. Hallett, *Containing Trauma: Nursing work in the First World War* (Manchester, Manchester University Press, 2009).

21 Coni, *Medicine and Warfare*, 49–57 and the autobiography of J. Trueta, *Surgeon in War and Peace* (London, Gollancz, 1980).

22 PE, IWM 8398.

23 Coni, *Medicine and Warfare*, 52.

24 PE, IWM 8398 and AJ, 18 March 1994.

25 Molly Murphy, *Molly Murphy: Suffragette and Socialist* (Salford, Institute of Social Research, University of Salford, 1998), 144.

26 Murphy, *Molly Murphy*, 144.

27 PE, AJ, 18 March 1994.

28 Nan Green, IWM 13799.

29 Margaret Powell, unpublished memoir, 1980, courtesy of her daughter, Ruth Muller.

30 Barcelona had more than 14,000 listed donors in 1938, a figure which had doubled by the end of the war according to Coni. For a brief account of medical advances during the war see his article, 'Medicine and the Spanish Civil War', *Journal of the Royal Society of Medicine* 95 (2002), and for more information on blood transfusions during the civil war see chapter 5 of his book, *Medicine and Warfare*.

31 For more on the subject of women 'milicianas' who fought at the front in the early months of the war, see Mary Nash, *Defying Male Civilization: Women in the Spanish Civil War* (Denver, Arden Press, 1995).

32 Winifred Bates, 'A woman's work in wartime', unpublished memoir, International Brigade Archive, Marx Memorial Library (MML), London.

33 PE, IWM 8398.

34 PE, IWM 8398.

35 PE, AJ, 8 March 1996. Patience Darton would probably also have been aware that rehydration was of key importance in typhoid cases, usually with intravenous or occasionally, with intramuscular or subcutaneous saline infusions.

36 For more on Patience in Valencia see Jackson, *For us it was Heaven*, chapter 4.

37 Reginald Saxton, *The Lancet* (1938).

38 Rosaleen Smythe, *SMAC Bulletin*, May 1938, MML, and in Fyrth, *Women's Voices*, 83.

39 Reginald Saxton, reference for Patience Darton, Brighton, 16 August 1939, courtesy of her son, Bob Edney.

40 Penny Feiwel, née Phelps, AJ, 22 February 1996.

41 TAB – typhoid-paratyphoid A and B vaccine: a suspension of killed typhoid and paratyphoid A and B bacilli.

42 Joan Purser, IWM 13795.

43 The Rafael Campalans School, today known as Mare de Déu de la Candela, was the location of this hospital for infectious cases. See Juan Roberto Zepeda Iturrieta and Jordi Pérez Molino, 'L'Hospital de Sang de Valls', *Quaderns de Vilaniu 51* (Valls: Institut d'Estudis Vallencs, May 2007).

44 PE, IWM 8398.

45 See for example, Lillian Urmston, 'Training nurses in the battle line', *Nursing Mirror*, 24 June 1939, 435–6; Louise Jones, 'The monastery at Uclés', in Fyrth, *Women's Voices*, 93.

46 PE, AJ, 18 March 1994.

47 Celia Seborer, 11 July 1937, in Fyrth, *Women's Voices*, 161.

48 Ruth Waller, Madrid Radio Broadcast, 10 January 1938, MML.

49 Unpublished short memoir, Aurora Edenhofer (née Fernández), Prague, January 1983, MML. Other Spanish girls who came into contact with British

nurses and wished to emulate them included Josefa from Seville, *SMAC Bulletin* (October 1937), 4, MML, and Lola, LB, Tameside, 203.

50 Nan Green and Rosaleen Smythe were among the British women who carried out the vital work of record keeping, important at the most basic level in order to inform families when a patient died. Green, *A Chronicle of Small Beer*.

51 Lillian Urmston, *Nursing Mirror*, 1939: 13 May, 231, 234; 20 May, 273–4; 27 May, 293; 3 June, 335–6; 10 June, 368–9; 17 June, 403–4; 24 June, 435–6.

52 SMAC minutes, 4 January 1939, Modern Records Centre, University of Warwick.

53 Patience Darton, Curriculum vitae, 1931–41.

54 For more on the Spanish male 'practicantes', the doctors' assistants with up to two years' training, see Coni, *Medicine and Warfare*.

55 For more on the lives of British nurses after their return home see Jackson, *British Women and the SCW*, chapter 6, and *For us it was Heaven*, chapters 11–17.

56 Colin Williams, Bill Alexander and John Gorman, *Memorials of the Spanish Civil War* (Stroud, Alan Sutton Publishing, 1996), and Jackson, *British Women and the SCW*, chapter 6.

57 PE, IWM 8398.

58 For more on this subject and the symbolic significance of the death of Patience Edney, see Jackson, *For us it was Heaven*, chapters 16–17.

59 Patience Edney in Petra Lataster-Czisch, '*Eigentlich rede ich nicht gern über mich*' *(Lebenserinnegungen von Frauen aus dem Spanischen Bürgerkrieg 1936–1939)* (Leizpzig and Weimar, Gustav Kiepenheurer Verlag, 1990), 9–105.

9

'Those maggots – they did a wonderful job': The nurses' role in wound management in civilian hospitals during the Second World War

David Justham

The wound care practices of nurses that persisted into the Second World War period were reminiscent of the nineteenth-century sanitarian movement's quest for cleanliness. It is the contention of this chapter that civilian nursing in the UK just before and during the Second World War was governed by a series of highly routinised practices affecting the totality of nursing work including wound care. Taken as a whole, these practices provided a coordinated approach aimed at keeping the care environment clean, the patient clean and wounds clean.

Oral histories provide the primary source of evidence for this chapter.[1] In the 1980s Jocalyn Lawler found very few first-hand historical accounts of the practice of nursing.[2] Since then, using the techniques of oral history, historians of nursing have started to explore the largely hidden work of nurses.[3] Most oral history interviewees in this study trained prior to, and during, the Second World War. Some of their practices appeared so archaic that it seemed as though they had been in place since a time just before germ theory, when the predominant theory of disease causation was due to miasma.[4] Apart from the intrinsic value of understanding the clinical work of nurses in this period, the data may give insights into approaches to care that may be needed in a post-antibiotic era.[5]

During the period when germ theories were evolving, nurses

adapted their understanding of disease yet maintained a strong emphasis on environmental cleanliness.[6] Time delays appear to have existed between evolution of theory and its practical application.[7] Thus, Alison Bashford found evidence that nursing textbooks continued well into the twentieth century with sanitarian concepts that had emerged decades earlier.[8] The surgical management of wounds by the medical profession had been debated and developed from Lister's use of carbolic acid as an antiseptic.[9] The First World War had seen further developments by the medical profession in the management of battlefield casualties, yet between 12 and 15 per cent of wounded soldiers died from infections.[10] Germ theory was acknowledged but, at times, nurses failed to capitalise on it, as seen in the preparation of dressings. Moreover, maggot infested wounds found during wartime raised anxiety and created difficulty in terms of defining what was unclean.

Into this milieu of transition must be added the cultural dimension of UK nursing that was grounded in routinised care practices learnt via an apprenticeship system. Obedience to superiors was paramount. The system was slow to adapt, and was associated with recruitment and retention difficulties, giving rise to a number of reports in the late 1930s and early 1940s.[11] The influences of wartime compound the challenges of exploring the history of the clinical work of civilian hospital ward-based nurses. There are many accounts of the wartime experiences of nurses, with several collected accounts of the experiences of British military nurses during the Second World War.[12] These accounts generally contain a minimum of clinical details. The memories of wartime nurses focus on the journeys to the battlefields, troop movements, and the horrific nature of many battle injuries. The challenges of setting up and working within casualty clearing stations and field hospitals are reported with a minimum of detail. There are some descriptions of the multiple trauma and gross disfiguration that can follow bomb blast injuries, shrapnel wounds or close combat. The ways that nurses delivered care in civilian hospitals has been largely overlooked by historians of wartime nursing.[13]

This chapter outlines the memories of nurses in relation to wound care in civilian hospitals collected to examine nursing work before the availability of antibiotics. Participants commented on the redressing of both surgical and traumatic wounds, yet details of specific wounds were not recalled during the interviews. Some respondents remembered aspects of wound management during surgical procedures in the operating theatre. Analysis of the interview data is organised under a series of themes which address wartime challenges, the dressing round, the preparation of equipment and materials for wound dressing, and the management of wound infection. These themes serve to illustrate the routinisation of nursing work within a sanitarian perspective.

Wartime challenges

British civilian nursing services experienced recruitment difficulties during the war. A number of government and other reports had been commissioned to examine these difficulties from the early 1930s.[14] The intense routines for nursing care, particularly the rigorous ward cleaning routines, were identified as contributing factors.[15] Wartime compounded the recruitment difficulties. Qualified nurses volunteered for service with the military nursing services thus draining civilian hospitals of a substantial proportion of their qualified and skilled workforce.[16] Penny Starns refers to a Control of Engagement Order being extended in 1943 to restrict the recruitment of nurses into the armed forces.[17] Recruitment into the military nursing services from a number of branches of nursing work was controlled so that civilian nurses were retained in certain branches, including paediatrics and mental health nursing.

In order to increase the number of nurses in general hospitals, restrictions on married state registered nurses were lifted. Carol Clark returned to hospital work during the war because of staffing shortages.[18] It was also a time when materials were in short supply. Alice Allen recalled that 'all the wounds were sutured with black thread because there weren't any sutures as they were all gone to the troops'.[19] Both Edith Evans and Jane Jones reported that tagged gamgee swabs, used to mop the operating field during surgery, were recycled.[20] These gamgee swabs were counted in at the end of an operation to make sure none were left in the patient, washed and re-sterilised in readiness for re-use. The reported shortages did not alter wartime wound care practices, even though there were substantial changes to the patients for whom they cared.

British battlefield casualties were treated in both casualty clearing stations and field hospitals before evacuation back to Britain. Many civilian hospitals received wounded personnel from the battlefronts, whether allied troops or prisoners of war (PoWs). Phyllis Porter recalled how wartime casualties, some with horrific injuries, arrived at hospital at night by train.[21] Day staff used to have to get up to help receive casualties, and then could go back to bed to be up again a few hours later for the day shift. Admitting casualties 'en bloc' at night would minimise disruption to daytime routines, but were they were received under blackout conditions. Porter remembered a patient with a high temperature that caused him to hallucinate. One night he 'opened the blackout with lights full on – soon brought somebody down to the ward to see what was happening'.[22] Despite these challenges nursing continued to use routines of working that pre-dated the war.

The dressing round

Cleaning duties were always timed to take place before wound care. All participants in this study reported rigorous daily environmental cleaning routines often in association with ward domestic staff. Such routines had a lasting effect on the work of first-year probationers. Often demoralising, cleaning was also recognised as important in the battle against the risk of infection. Janet Wilks, who started nursing in November 1935 expressed how, as a new probationer, she hated the menial jobs, of which cleaning was the most tiresome and disheartening.[23] She then recounted how a ward sister helped her understand that meticulous cleaning regimes were essential to minimise infection risks.[24] Wilks's comments refer to a time before sulphonamides drugs and antibiotics were available and when streptococcal and staphylococcal infections could prove fatal. The Medical Research Council (MRC) recommended that ward dressing rounds were 'preceded by a quiet interval of at least one hour' when no dust raising activity took place.[25] The emphasis on a quiet period preceding the round to allow dust to settle assumed a ward routine that required environmental cleaning took place as one of the first tasks of the morning, to which Susan Shaw, Violet Vickers and Wendy Woods all attest.[26] The importance of the cleaning routine is illustrated in Allen's recollection, as a junior staff nurse, of an incident when the ward maid did not arrive on duty and 'you couldn't start the dressings 'til one and a half hours after the damp dusting was finished'.[27] So, to enable the dressing round to take place, she undertook the damp dusting. Dust was considered a potential wound contaminant.[28] Allen's very clear memory illustrates that cleaning by damp dusting followed by a quiet period was important in the overall routine of wound management.

All the participants reported that hospital acquired infection in wounds was a rare event. The sanitarian strategy for cleanliness used by nurses took precedence over the germ theory approach of reducing the presence of pathogenic organisms. Edith Evans recalled that 'dirty dressings were removed – never left' on any patient.[29] A soiled dressing was dirty, but not necessarily harbouring infection.

The organisation of the dressing round was the responsibility of either the sister or staff nurse. Thus Clark reported that the dressing round wound be undertaken by the same person each time so changes in the conditions of wounds were noticed.[30] Vickers remembered that the staff nurse, with a probationer to serve as an assistant, would redress wounds.[31] Harris added that there might be a role reversal with the staff nurse allowing the probationer to undertake the redressing of the wound.[32] Both Allen and Woods reported that a list of dressings was prepared by the sister or staff nurse with the cleanest at the top and dirtiest at the bottom.[33] The implication was that the person undertaking the redressing of wounds would progress from clean to dirty wounds. This would be possible at a time when work patterns were based on task allocation, and working hours meant a presence by the staff for at least six days in each week. Evans, who trained at the Manchester Royal Infirmary between 1936 and 1939, recalled that the ward sister always went to theatre so she knew what had happened and could redress the wounds or direct others.[34] This was perhaps a luxury not afforded at other hospitals. Her account identified that the sister took responsibility in theatre for the swabs rather than the scrub nurse who was solely responsible for the instruments. In this interpretation, the sister would have a clear vision of the surgical field and would, therefore, know what had happened to the patient's wound during the surgery. She remembered that the sister, together with a junior member of staff, redressed clean wounds. The staff nurse was allocated to replace the dirty dressings using a different trolley.

This is in stark contrast to Porter's account. Trained at Nottingham's General Hospital between 1939 and 1942, Porter reported that the person undertaking the dressing round would go from one patient to another around the ward, irrespective of whether the wound was clean or dirty. She continued: 'I can remember going round and thinking it shouldn't be this way.'[35] However, she accepted this process and did not challenge her superiors. This illustrates both the subservience of juniors to seniors, and the fact that senior nurses were maintaining traditional nursing practices. Similarly, Nancy Newton reported that the dressing trolley was taken from bedside to bedside, without cleaning and irrespective of the state of each wound, and only taken back to the clinical room to get extra materials if the nurse ran out of items.[36] Allen remembered that clean stitched wounds were redressed first, 'Then you went on – you didn't strip your trolley down between each dressing.'[37]

Preparation of the dressing trolley was thus reported to require the equipment and dressing materials for several patients. Allen reported that: 'You had on the trolley a pile of dissecting forceps and a pile of sinus forceps and a pile of probes and then all the drums of dressings and things but you kept them covered with the linen towel and took out what you needed.'[38] Clark's memory was that the clean items on the top shelf of the trolley were not replaced between patients. The dirty dressings and forceps which had been placed in receivers on the lower shelf 'were removed before you went onto the next bed ... you'd a lot of walking about when I think about it'.[39] Likewise, Woods recalled that the person undertaking the dressings would 'Go from bed to bed. There was no setting up of trolley each time. A runner [another staff member] was used to replenish instruments.'[40] In contrast, Thelma Taylor's memory was of the necessity to return back to the clinical room between dress-ings for the trolley to be stripped down, cleaned and restocked. She added that for 'minor wounds you might go from bed to bed'.[41] The MRC guidance allowed for the dressing trolley to be taken from bedside to bedside provided that separate instruments, dressing packs and gallipots for wound cleaning solutions were available for each patient.[42]

Participants were generally vague about the precise detail in setting a dressing trolley, although guidance can be found in nursing texts.[43] The trolley would be prepared in the clinical room and then taken to the bedside. Wound redressing took place at the bedside, a practice remembered by Reed.[44] The MRC made recommendations as to the layout of items on a dressing trolley.[45] They also recommended sterilised pre-prepared wound dressing packs, a luxury which one respondent, Florence Farmer, experienced. A new pack would be opened for each patient minimising the risk of cross-infection.[46] However, these were not generally available. In contrast, the drum system retained the risk of contamination of remaining dressings within the drum once it has been opened.[47] This was not a problem in a sanitarian vision where the contents of the drum were considered clean.

Woods recalled cleaning the trolley with spirit before putting the items on it.[48] A basic principle recalled by many respondents was that sterile items for the dressing were kept on the top shelf, and un-sterile items and receivers for dirty items kept on the lower shelf. The top shelf might be covered with a sterile towel. Sterilised equipment was placed on the trolley using Cheatle's forceps.[49] The trolley could carry three drums containing dressing materials, one with cotton-wool balls, one for gauze swabs, and one for dressing towels.[50] Another feature of the MRC recommended trolley layout was provision of space for a sulphonamide insufflator or castor.[51] Sulphonamide in powder form was sometimes blown into a wound to prevent infection developing or to help treat localised infection.

The accounts show different approaches to the organisation of the dressing round. Yet all approaches had the common feature of being routinised and grounded in links to maintaining cleanliness derived from sanitarian nursing.

Preparation of equipment

Instruments and gallipots were prepared on the ward by immersion in boiling water. Two of the participants reported the length of time for immersing instruments. Jones reported that all instruments were boiled for at least five minutes and in some cases up to twenty minutes.[52] Woods mentioned that instruments were boiled for 'three minutes or so'.[53] While Woods started her training after the end of the Second World War, it is of interest to note that the boiling time she reported was quite short. Nursing textbooks from the period show a reducing amount of time recommended for boiling instruments. Both Ashdown and Pearce recommended twenty minutes.[54] When Riddell published her account it was fifteen minutes though she did advocate the subsequent placing in Lysol for twenty minutes before use.[55] Boiling times had further reduced within Houghton's text to ten minutes.[56] The MRC suggested that two minutes was sufficient time for boiling instruments.[57] It is reasonable to suggest that the MRC boiling time guidance followed advice from their expert committee of bacteriologists given in the light of improved understanding of the survival characteristics of micro-organisms. The longer boiling times in nursing texts illustrate a cautionary approach to germ theory. However, these processes must have been extremely onerous for nursing staff.

Instruments were cleaned and sterilised on the ward and sometimes placed in Lysol after use. Nursing texts put the cleaning process before sterilising. This suggests a pre-eminence of cleaning over sterilisation.[58] Jones remembered soaking sharp instruments in pure Lysol followed by rinsing in sterile water before use.[59] The use of disinfection by soaking rather than sterilisation by boiling was due to the belief that boiling blunted sharp instruments. Ashdown advised that sharp instruments should be boiled for five minutes then immersed in alcohol until required or, alternatively, that they 'may be sterilised without boiling by placing in pure carbolic for one minute'.[60] The MRC noted that wherever possible instruments should not be disinfected by immersion because of the subsequent need to rinse with sterile water and then dry the instrument.[61] The sanitarian quest for cleanliness pre-dated the concept of asepsis.[62] Both approaches pursued absolute cleanliness, albeit sanitarians wanted to remove dirt, germ theorists wanted to disinfect. The evidence reported here shows that there was some variation in the sterilisation processes for instruments, both in terms of a reducing amount of time that instruments were boiled, and that, in some hospitals, instruments would be cleaned and disinfected in Lysol rather than sterilised by boiling. The evidence reveals that nurses held the responsibility for ensuring that the equipment used was clean and fit for purpose.

Preparation of dressings

All participants, except Farmer, reported that nursing staff prepared dressings for autoclaving (an autoclave being a vessel used for sterilising objects, usually by steam at high pressure). Both Clark and Jones reported that dressings, made of plain gauze that came in six-yard lengths were cut to the size required.[63] Jones also recalled that nurses made the cotton-wool balls before packing them into drums.[64] Barbara Bennett mentioned that drums were packed 'each evening to go down to the sterilising department' though there was no more precise information as to whether this activity was undertaken in the early part of the evening or later.[65] Allen was more specific, recalling that drums were packed during visiting hours.[66] Both Shaw and Woods reported that drums or tins were packed on night duty with cotton-wool balls for swabbing and pieces of gauze for dressings.[67] The accounts generally indicate that the preparation of the drums for autoclaving was undertaken in the evening or at night. Woods added that these drums were put outside the ward entrance daily to be taken by the porter to the autoclave. The autoclaved dressings were returned to the ward in the morning prior to the dressing round.

Consistent accounts of dressing preparation can be found in archival sources.[68] One such account added that patients could be involved in preparing dressings.[69] Riddell describes the preparation of dressings and swabs but cautions that the nurse needs to prepare them as hygienically as possible.[70] Providing patients with a useful task could jeopardise the quest for hygienic preparation of dressings, however well-intentioned the occupational therapy benefit. Gauze was also available ready cut in 6 inch by 4 inch pieces, each having several layers, partially sterilised and packed in sealed paper, or as pieces in sealed tins and completely sterilised.[71] None of the respondents referred to these options.

Woods suggested that the packing of the drum was done in reverse order to the anticipated requirements for the dressing round the following day.[72] This resulted in the dressings required for first patient having their wound dressed being at the top of the drum. The last patient included in the dressing round would have their dressings placed at the bottom of the drum. This account demonstrated that the dressing round was a well-organised event, and prior thought was given as to the dressing requirements. It is unknown how unanticipated demands for additional dressing materials were dealt with. No other respondent suggested this level of sophistication in the packing of dressings into the drums.

The accounts suggested there was little change to preparing dressings throughout the study period. Dry wound dressings and swabs were usually prepared by staff. The materials were placed in a drum which was normally sent away from the ward for autoclaving during the night. The drums of autoclaved dressings and swabs were returned to the ward in readiness for the dressing round. The evidence suggests that preparing dressings was normally a task to be completed by staff working at night, though in some instances this would happen during visiting times. In addition to wound dressings, staff would prepare cotton wool balls, used for cleaning wounds, from large rolls of cotton wool. Kate King's memory was of the need to be careful with the amount of cotton wool used because of it being in short supply.[73] The MRC provided guidance on the technique for packing the sterilising drums, emphasising the need not to pack materials tightly into the drums. It was important that the superheated steam used in the autoclave could penetrate and circulate through the dressing materials for at least 20 minutes. Additional time was needed to allow initial heating and final cooling of the contents before removal from the autoclave.[74] Only one participant remembered using pre-prepared wound dressing packs.[75] The evidence shows that nurses were responsible for the preparation of dressing materials for use in the wards. Nurses could plan the amount of dressings required, ensuring minimum waste during wartime shortages.

Procedure for redressing wounds

Only a few of the respondents could recall any detail. Evans made the important point that 'You followed procedure – couldn't do otherwise.'[76] The discipline instilled during training was such that the procedure became automatic so as to be one of unconscious competence.[77] The discipline imposed on probationers was quite severe and to step outside of expected procedure was a disciplinary matter.[78]

A non-touch technique, using forceps to hold and manipulate dressings, was the method of choice. Many respondents reported this method. Both King and Reed described the use of a non-touch technique in which forceps were used to manipulate cleaning swabs and dressings.[79] Woods described the removal of dirty dressing with forceps.[80] Used forceps were discarded into container on the bottom shelf of the dressing trolley. As Newton recalled: 'Sterilised instruments were in tray on the top shelf of the trolley, and once used were placed in kidney dish on the lower shelf of the trolley.'[81] Waste materials, such as used swabs and dirty dressings would be disposed of in a receptacle for this purpose. In some texts the receiving bin would be placed at the side of the dressing trolley whereas others would have it attached to the trolley or placed on the lower shelf.[82]

Masks were worn by some staff undertaking wound dressings, though this was not a frequent recollection. King's memory was that these cotton masks were not disposable, and needed to be laundered after use. Sometimes rubber gloves were worn to handle dressings. The gloves were not disposable, and needed to be washed, mended if necessary (using patches made from irreparable gloves), powdered inside and placed in pairs in drums for autoclaving between dressing rounds.[83]

Hand hygiene was also important. Porter recalled that Lysol was used to wash hands. It was a strong solution and would burn if it was not washed off the skin.[84] Carbolic was used on wounds. Taylor remembered that Lysol and carbolic were used a lot, and Vickers reported that Lysol 'used to be around an awful lot'.[85] Lysol was a preparation made from cresol, and used as an antiseptic and disinfectant. It was used as a hand-wash in a 1 or 2 per cent strength in water.[86] Bennett expressed the view that there were not as many infections prior to penicillin since people developed strong immune systems.[87] With the attention to detail regarding environmental and hand hygiene respondents could not recall instances of hospital acquired infections. The general opinion was that patients entered hospitals with infections and did not acquire them in the ward setting.

Wound infections

The Second World War saw great change in the medical management of wound infections. During the late 1930s the impact of sulphonamide drugs heralded a change in the management of infectious disease. However, the sulphonamides had limited effect against staphylococci, the bacterial species most commonly implicated in wound infections.[88] Significant improvements were not seen in the reduction of wound infections until the introduction of penicillin in the latter stages of the war.[89] Prior to this, and in an attempt to minimise acquired wound infections, the MRC made recommendations in 1941 concerning the management of wound dressings in ward environments.[90] This memorandum sought to standardise wound dressing procedures across the country. The authors of the memorandum reported that an increasing incidence of wound infection was due to 'defects of aseptic technique' within hospital wards.[91] There was no nurse representation on the committee responsible for the memorandum, though nurses were acknowledged for supplying evidence and advice.

The feared complication of wound infection was septicaemia, which could be fatal in upwards of 50 per cent of cases.[92] The patient with septicaemia would require careful nursing by a nurse with prior experience of such cases.[93] Sulphonamides were reported to have some success in helping to manage septicaemia.[94] It was generally accepted that battlefield wounds had a greater incidence of wound infection.[95] For example, wounds could be contaminated by bullets, debris from bomb blasts, or exposure to soil. Between 12 and 15 per cent of the wounded of the First World War died from infections.[96] It was a common observation, and welcomed fact, that wounds with maggots in them had a good prognosis. Allen, working in London, recalled that infected wounds from the battlefield might be 'all maggoty but the wounds were clean … those maggots did a wonderful job'.[97] Porter considered maggots were accidental but beneficial, and remembered a civilian TB patient being nursed outside in the open air whose undressed skin wound had become infected.[98] Maggots developed in the wound and cleaned it completely. Taylor remembered one soldier with an infected compound fracture. When the plaster of Paris cast, applied in the field hospital, was removed it was found that maggots had 'eaten the pus away'.[99] The maggots fed on dead tissue and the infected material within the wound.

Yet larval therapy was not a positive wound management strategy within UK civilian hospitals. Maggots were thought repulsive despite their undoubted value in clearing wound infection.[100] The repulsion arose from the association of maggots with dirt and putrefaction. Dirt, being unwanted matter, was the target of sanitarians.[101] Environmental dirt in the ward was removed by nurses through daily and rigorous cleaning routines. Mechanical means or irrigation was used to remove dirt, including foreign material, from wounds. Before the availability of the sulphonamides and antibiotics, infected wounds were cleaned by various methods of irrigation, application of antiseptic lotions, fomentations, and poultices.[102] Deliberately leaving maggots in wounds was thought incredible by nurses and challenged their sanitarian principles.[103] Drugs that had some effect on wound infection arrived saving nurses the dilemma of dealing with 'dirty' maggots.

The sulphonamides and antibiotics had a considerable impact on the management of patients with infections. The sulphonamide family of drugs had been available for some years prior to the outbreak of the Second World War.[104] They were primarily used in the management of infectious disease, particularly pneumonia. Many respondents recalled the impact these drugs had. Referring to caring for patients with pneumonia Harris reported: 'You nursed them to the "crisis" and then it was touch and go whether they came through the crisis or they succumbed. Then of course all the interest went out of that in 1938 with M and B 693 [a sulphapyridine].' The difference made was tremendous, 'they were up and walking around very soon once they got on that'.[105] Likewise, Newton was quick to emphasise the labour-saving benefits of the new drugs. She said: 'You weren't having to give cooling washes and things like that. They took away a lot of the heavy nursing.'[106] Bennett's account indicated that the sulphonamides continued in regular use after the introduction of penicillin. When she was in the armed forces in 1943 she developed a carbuncle on her right cheek and was told: 'We won't give you penicillin. It's too painful and you've got to have all these injections. You'd better have some sulphonamides.' She was prescribed sulphonamide tablets. She found these to be 'horrible. They were big things which you had a job to swallow first and foremost … awful stuff.'[107]

The treatment of streptococcus pyogenes septicaemia, which could arise from an infected wound, was revolutionised by sulphanilamide,[108] The sulphonamides could be taken orally or by injection. Queen Elizabeth Hospital in Birmingham adopted the method of treating infected wounds with sulphonamide as a cream spread onto lint.[109] There is evidence that these drugs were welcomed by nursing staff, and they that had some impact on managing the infection risk in wounds. However, the sulpha drugs were not without their side effects which could be quite debilitating, and they were not deemed suitable for everyone.[110]

The Second World War was the last war conducted before the introduction of antibiotics (supply chains and financial considerations not withstanding). Penicillin, a broad-spectrum antibiotic, was produced in sufficient quantities towards the latter part of the war (1943 onwards) when it was made widely available to troops and PoWs. It was effective against staphylococcal infections, and Spink reported a fall in mortality rate for staphylococcal bacteraemia from 80 per cent to 35 per cent following penicillin's introduction.[111] However, it was not available to civilians until after the war. With injured troops and some PoWs being cared for in civilian hospitals, care staff knew that PoWs were receiving more advanced treatment than that available to the civilian population. Giving penicillin created a moral dilemma for Allen who reported that: 'There was none for the civilians … the POWs didn't want it because they thought we were killing them … And, I am ashamed to say … you would leave a little tiny bit' in the bottom of the vial.[112] All the small amounts would be collected together to get a dose which was then given to a desperately ill civilian. Allen continued that, 'it seemed wrong somehow that they shouldn't have any at all'.[113]

Lloyd recalled that penicillin made an incredible difference. As she said: 'There didn't seem to be side effects.'[114] Penicillin could be a painful injection but the incredible difference seen in the management of infection would outweigh the recollection that some patients may have had side effects. A similar, and perhaps more powerful, comment was that penicillin 'revolutionised everything' in nursing.[115] With specific regard to the management of wounds, Shaw mentioned that penicillin was something to be thankful for 'as it made treating infected wounds so much easier'.[116] Published accounts reflect this sense of amazement at a drug which changed the management of infected wounds. McBryde reported that miracles were occurring every day in surgical wards: 'This yellow powder with the musty smell revolutionised the treatment of wounds.'[117] Prentis recalled that arrival of antibiotics 'shifted the balance of power from nursing as we knew it to a quick jab with a needle and it was all over'.[118]

Penicillin was not easy to work with despite the euphoria. Allen remembered needing to be very careful with penicillin, 'We always swabbed the tops [of vials] very carefully' before adding water to dissolve the powder.[119] Vickers remembered that penicillin was just coming in during her training. 'I can see myself going round with a little trolley with Ward Sister and I used to have to draw it up because she couldn't see very well', she recalled, adding that the syringes she used needed to be boiled between each use.[120] Though Porter never had to mix penicillin, she remembered its use in the early days being 'often milky (not clear), given with a large needle'.[121] Taylor gave a reason for large needles: 'Penicillin by injection was painful – that beeswax stuff was hellish … almost solid, had to warm it to soften it, not too hot by the time you got it to the patient, but you were ages getting it in.'[122] It was usual for trained staff to give penicillin injections. Jones remembered that penicillin was given as an 'intramuscular injection of 10 cc, large needles, three hourly. It was very painful if you weren't very careful, and only qualified staff could give it.'[123] Elsewhere, a three hourly regime of 5 cc intramuscular penicillin injections was used because the penicillin was short lasting and a 'rather' dilute drug.[124] The frequency resulted in dread and hate by patients despite its beneficial effects. Taylor recalled two deaths from penicillin intravenous infusions 'they became oedematous and red. Not sure of the reasons for it.'[125] Penicillin might have had a powerful impact on treating wound infection by shortening the duration of the infection but there was no evidence that it changed the routine of the dressing round.

Conclusions

The participants for this study reported that the preparation of dressings, instruments and wound dressing trolleys was more or less as described by the published texts. Care practices were routinised and driven by senior nurses who valued traditional care practices delivered by an obedient, compliant workforce. The wound redressing round would follow at some point after the morning cleaning routines had been completed. Minor variations existed in relation to sterilisation of instruments on the wards, and some variations were evident in the organisation of dressing rounds. Most participants reported a non-touch technique for the process of wound dressing. Hand hygiene was rigorously practised. The greatest variation was in the organisation of the dressing round with some evidence suggesting that clean wounds were not always redressed before infected (or dirty) wounds. Such practices would increase the risk of cross-infection. Nevertheless, there was universal denial of the existence of many hospital acquired wound infections.

Prior to the availability of penicillin, in particular, septicaemia as a complication of wound infection would require skilled nursing care. The accounts reported a relationship between environmental cleaning and wound redressing, the rationale for which is grounded in sanitarian concepts. This does not mean that nurses in this period were ignorant of germ theory, but that the sanitarians' approach to a clean environment, which had been in place for many decades, worked well. There was no recollection of cross-infection. Yet dirty wounds infected with maggots became clean. Despite doing a 'wonderful job', the maggots were cleaned out of the wound, rather than left in place. Practical nurses did not have a powerful enough voice to enable them to argue for innovation, nor did they have formal membership on the MRC committee that produced the memorandum that directly impinged on their work in wound management.[126]

The arrival of sulphonamides and antibiotics were vectors of revolutionary changes in nursing, not least as a means of treating wound infections and their complications. Nurses no longer had to give close personal care to the patient with septicaemia for weeks. Adoption of the MRC's recommendation for pre-prepared dressing packs would remove nurses' need to prepare dressing materials themselves. On several fronts, nursing workloads were reduced, and the principles of sanitarian nursing that had been in place for a hundred years were threatened by developments grounded in germ theory.

Notes

1 The primary sources are a group of 19 interviews, collected by the author during 2008–10. These former nurses trained in UK hospitals during the

1930s and 1940s. Pseudonyms are used to preserve their confidentiality. Sound recordings are located at the United Kingdom Centre for the History of Nursing and Midwifery (UKCHNM).

2 Jocalyn Lawler, *Behind the Screens: Nursing, Somology, and the Problem of the Body* (Melbourne, Churchill Livingstone, 1991).

3 See, for example, V. R. Yow, *Recording Oral History: A Practical Guide for Social Scientists* (Thousand Oaks, Sage Publications, 1994); Paul Thompson, *The Voice of the Past* (Oxford, Oxford University Press, 3rd edn, 2000); and Lynn Abrams, *Oral History Theory* (London, Routledge, 2010).

4 Margaret Pelling, 'The meaning of contagion: Reproduction, medicine and metaphor', in Alison Bashford and Claire Hooker (eds), *Contagion: Historical and Cultural Studies* (London, Routledge, 2001), 15–38; Margaret R. Currie, *Fever Hospitals and Fever Nurses: A British Social History of Fever Nursing: A National Service* (London, Routledge, 2005), 3–4.

5 G. A. J. Ayliffe and M. P. English, *Hospital Infection: From Miasmas to MRSA* (Cambridge, Cambridge University Press, 2003), 231–2.

6 Michael Worboys, *Spreading Germs: Disease Theories and Medical Practice in Britain, 1865–1900* (Cambridge, Cambridge University Press, 2006); and Pelling, 'The meaning of contagion', 16.

7 David Wootton, *Bad Medicine: Doctors Doing Harm Since Hippocrates* (Oxford, Oxford University Press, 2007), 17.

8 Alison Bashford, *Purity and Pollution: Gender, Embodiment and Victorian Medicine* (Houndmills, Macmillan Press Ltd, 1998), 132–3.

9 Worboys, *Spreading Germs*, 80–107.

10 Peter Neushul, 'Fighting research: Army participation in the clinical testing and mass production of penicillin during the Second World War', in Roger Cooter, Mark Harrison and Steven Sturdy (eds), *War, Medicine and Modernity* (Stroud, Sutton Publishing 1999), 204.

11 Chris Hart, *Behind the Mask: Nurses, Their Unions and Nursing Policy* (London, Baillière Tindall, 1994).

12 See, for example, Eric Taylor, *Front-Line Nurse: British Nurses in Second World War* (London, Robert Hale, 1997); Eric Taylor, *Combat Nurse* (London, Robert Hale, 1999); Eric Taylor, *Wartime Nurse: 100 years from the Crimea to Korea 1854–1954* (London, Robert Hale, 2001); and Nicola Tyrer, *Sisters in Arms: British Army Nurses Tell Their Story* (London, Weidenfield & Nicolson, 2008).

13 See, for example, Brenda McBryde, *A Nurse's War* (London, Chatto & Windus, 1979); Brenda McBryde, *Quiet Heroines: Nurses of the Second World War* (Saffron Walden, Cakebread Publications, 1989); Joan Markham, *The Lamp was Dimmed: The Story of a Nurse's Training* (London, Robert Hale, 1975); Janet Wilks, *Carbolic and Leeches* (Ilfracombe, Hyperion Books, 1991); and E. Merson, 'Nursing in wartime', *International History of Nursing Journal* 3, 4 (1998), 43–6.

14 For summary accounts see Brian Abel-Smith, *A History of the Nursing Profession* (London, Heinemann Educational, 1960); and Hart, *Behind the Mask*, 66–7.

15 Sheila M. Bevington, *Nursing Life and Discipline: A Study Based on Over Five Hundred Interviews* (London, H. K. Lewis and Co. Ltd, 1943).

16 Penny Starns, *March of the Matrons: Military Influence on the Civilian Nursing Profession, 1939–1969* (Peterborough, DSM, 2000), 28.

17 Starns, *March of the Matrons*, 36.

18 Carol Clark, interviewed by David Justham at Abergele on 16 July 2008. Began State Registered Nurse (SRN) training in Manchester in 1934. Recording held at UK Centre for the History of Nursing and Midwifery (hereafter UKCHNM), University of Manchester.

19 Alice Allen, interviewed by David Justham at Sheffield on 14 July 2008. Began SRN training in London in 1942. Recording held at UKCHNM, University of Manchester.

20 Edith Evans, interviewed by David Justham at Lymm on 18 July 2008. Began SRN training in Manchester in 1936; and Jane Jones, interviewed by David Justham at Preston on 6 August 2008. Began SRN training in Manchester in 1944. Recordings held at UKCHNM, University of Manchester.

21 Phyllis Porter, interviewed by David Justham at Nottingham on 24 May 2010. Began SRN training in Nottingham in 1939. Recording held at UKCHNM, University of Manchester.

22 Porter, interviewed on 24 May 2010.

23 Wilks, *Carbolic and Leeches*, 24–5.

24 Wilks, *Carbolic and Leeches*, 27.

25 Medical Research Council (MRC) War Wounds Committee and Committee of London Sector Pathologists, *The Prevention of 'Hospital Infection' of Wounds*, MRC War Memorandum No. 6 (London, His Majesty's Stationery Office, 1941), 15.

26 Susan Shaw, interviewed by David Justham on at Nottingham 18 May 2010. Began SRN training in Nottingham in 1943; Violet Vickers, interviewed by David Justham at Nottingham on 24 May 2010. Began SRN training in Nottingham in 1947; Wendy Woods, interviewed by David Justham at Nottingham on 1 June 2010. Began SRN training in Nottingham in 1950. Recordings held at UKCHNM, University of Manchester.

27 Allen, interviewed on 14 July 2008.

28 M. S. Riddell, *First Year Nursing Manual* (London, Faber & Faber Ltd, 5th edn, 1939), 14.

29 Evans, interviewed on 18 July 2008.

30 Clark, interviewed on 16 July 2008.

31 Vickers, interviewed on 24 May 2010.

32 Hilary Harris, interviewed by David Justham at Clitheroe on 6 August 2008. Began SRN training in Manchester in 1934. Recording held at UKCHNM, University of Manchester.

33 Allen, interviewed on 14 July 2008, and Woods, interviewed on 1 June 2010.

34 Evans, interviewed on 18 July 2008.

35 Porter, interviewed on 24 May 2010.

36 Nancy Newton, interviewed by David Justham at Sturton on 19 December 2008. Began SRN training in London in the early 1940s. Recording held at UKCHNM, University of Manchester.

37 Allen, interviewed on 14 July 2008.

38 Allen, interviewed on 14 July 2008.

39 Clark, interviewed on 16 July 2008.

40 Woods, interviewed on 1 June 2010.

41 Thelma Taylor, interviewed by David Justham at Nottingham on 24 May 2010. Began SRN training in Nottingham in 1943. Recording held at UKCHNM, University of Manchester.

42 MRC, *The Prevention of 'Hospital Infection' of Wounds*, 17.

43 See, for example, A. M. Ashdown, *A Complete System of Nursing* (London, J. M. Dent & Sons Ltd, 1928), 377; Riddell, *First Year Nursing Manual*; M. Houghton, *Aids to Tray and Trolley Setting* (London, Baillière Tindall and Cox, 2nd edn, 1942).

44 Rita Reed, interviewed by David Justham at Nottingham on 18 May 2010. Began SRN training in Nottingham in 1943. Recording held at UKCHNM, University of Manchester.

45 MRC, *The Prevention of 'Hospital Infection' of Wounds*, 17–19.

46 Florence Farmer, interviewed by David Justham at Preston on 4 August 2008. Began SRN training in Manchester in 1936. Recording held at UKCHNM, University of Manchester.

47 For a description of the drum system see, for example, W. T. G. Pugh, *Practical Nursing including Hygiene and Dietetics* (Edinburgh, William Blackwood and Sons, 13th edn, 1940), 175; and Riddell, *First Year Nursing Manual*, 119.

48 Woods, interviewed on 1 June 2010.

49 Graham Thurgood, *Transcript of interview HX2 recorded* on 25 July 2001. Data extracted 19 July 2010. Transcript held at Huddersfield, University of Huddersfield Archives; Houghton, *Aids to Tray and Trolley Setting*, 138–43.

50 From a comment by Woods, interviewed on 1 June 2010, and could refer to a later innovation.

51 MRC, *The Prevention of 'Hospital Infection' of Wounds*, 17.

52 Jones, interviewed on 6 August 2008.

53 Woods, interviewed on 1 June 2010.

54 Ashdown, *A Complete System of Nursing*, 41; and E. Pearce, *Medical and Nursing Dictionary* (London, Faber & Faber Ltd, 6th edn, 1933), 574.

55 Riddell, *First Year Nursing Manual*, 119.
56 Houghton, *Aids to Tray and Trolley Setting*, 3.
57 MRC, *The Prevention of 'Hospital Infection' of Wounds*, 10.
58 Ashdown, *A Complete System of Nursing*, 41; Houghton, *Aids to Tray and Trolley Setting*, 3.
59 Jones, interviewed on 6 August 2008.
60 Ashdown, *A Complete System of Nursing*, 42.
61 MRC, *The Prevention of 'Hospital Infection' of Wounds*, 10.
62 Lynn McDonald, *Florence Nightingale: The Nightingale School* (Waterloo, Wilfrid Laurier University Press, 2009), 13–21.
63 Clark, interviewed on 16 July 2008; Jones, interviewed on 6 August 2008.
64 Jones, interviewed on 6 August 2008.
65 Barbara Bennett, interviewed by David Justham at Dyserth on 15 July 2008. Began SRN training in Manchester in 1938. Recording held at UKCHNM, University of Manchester.
66 Allen, interviewed on 14 July 2008.
67 Shaw, interviewed on 18 May 2010 and Woods, interviewed on 1 June 2010.
68 Thurgood, *Transcript of interview HX2* recorded on 25 July 2001; and G. Thurgood, *Transcript of interview HX5* recorded on 8 August 2001. Data extracted 19 July 2010. Transcript held at Huddersfield, University of Huddersfield Archives.
69 Thurgood, *Transcript of interview HX5 recorded on 8 August 2001*.
70 Riddell, *First Year Nursing Manual*, 123.
71 Scott, *The New People's Physician*, vol. 2, 650.
72 Woods, interviewed on 1 June 2010.
73 Kate King, interviewed by David Justham at Heswall on 7 August 2008. Began SRN training in Manchester in 1939. Recording held at UKCHNM, University of Manchester.
74 MRC, *The Prevention of 'Hospital Infection' of Wounds*, 22–3.
75 Florence Farmer, interviewed by David Justham at Preston on 4 August 2008. Began SRN training in Manchester in 1936. Recording held at UKCHNM, University of Manchester.
76 Evans, interviewed by David Justham at Lymm on 18 July 2008.
77 See, for example, P. Benner, *Novice to Expert: Excellence and Power in Clinical Nursing Practice* (Menlo Park, CA, Addison-Wesley, 1984); S. A. Smith, 'Nurse Competence: A Concept Analysis', *International Journal of Nursing Knowledge* 23, 3 (2012) 172–82.
78 See, for example, Ashdown, *A Complete System of Nursing*, 1; Riddell, *First Year Nursing Manual*, 10; and J. D. Britten, *Practical Notes on Nursing Procedures* (Edinburgh: E. & S. Livingstone Ltd, 1957), 9–10.
79 King, interviewed on 7 August 2008, and Reed, interviewed on 18 May 2010.
80 Woods, interviewed on 1 June 2010.

81 Newton, interviewed on 19 December 2008.
82 See, for example, MRC, *The Prevention of 'Hospital Infection' of Wounds*, 18; Houghton *Aids to Tray and Trolley Setting*, 138–42.
83 Louise Lloyd, interviewed by David Justham at Grantham on 12 August 2008. Began SRN training in Leicester in 1940; and Shaw, interviewed on 18 May 2010. Recordings held at UKCHNM, University of Manchester.
84 Porter, interviewed on 24 May 2010.
85 Taylor, interviewed on 24 May 2010; Vickers, interviewed on 24 May 2010.
86 Pearce, *Medical and Nursing Dictionary*, 379.
87 Bennett, interviewed on 15 July 2008.
88 See, for example, W. T. G. Pugh, *Practical Nursing including Hygiene and Dietetics*; J. A. Ryle and S. D. Elliott, 'Septicaemia and bacteriaemia', in H. Rolleston (ed.), *The British Encyclopaedia of Medical Practice* (London, Butterworth and Co., 1939), vol. 11, 76–89; W. G. Sears, *Medicine for Nurses* (London, Edward Arnold, 4th edn, 1940), 426–7.
89 Neushul, 'Fighting research', 204.
90 MRC, *The Prevention of 'Hospital Infection' of Wounds*.
91 MRC, *The Prevention of 'Hospital Infection' of Wounds*, 4.
92 Ryle and Elliott, 'Septicaemia and bacteriaemia', 85.
93 [The Lord] Horder and A. E. Gow, 'Bacterial diseases', in F. W. Price (ed.), *A Textbook of the Practice of Medicine* (London, Oxford University Press, 5th edn, 1937), 30.
94 See, for example, Ryle and Elliott, 'Septicaemia and bacteriaemia', 85 and 87; Horder and Gow, 'Bacterial diseases', 30; Pugh, *Practical Nursing*, 507.
95 MRC, *The Prevention of 'Hospital Infection' of Wounds*, 4.
96 Neushul, 'Fighting research', 204.
97 Allen, interviewed on 14 July 2008.
98 Porter, interviewed on 24 May 2010.
99 Taylor, interviewed on 24 May 2010.
100 N. M. Matheson, 'Accidental and surgical wounds', in H. Bailey (ed.), *Pye's Surgical Handicraft: A Manual Of Surgical Manipulations, Minor Surgery, and other Matters Connected with the Work of House Surgeons and of Surgical Dressers*, 11th edn (Bristol, John Wright and Sons Ltd, 1939), 67.
101 Mary Douglas, *Purity and Danger: An Analysis of Concepts of Pollution and Taboo* (London, Routledge Classics, 2002), 44.
102 See, for example, Ashdown, *A Complete System of Nursing*; Horder and Gow, 'Bacterial diseases', 25–38; Pugh, *Practical Nursing*; Matheson, 'Accidental and surgical wounds'.
103 See for example, Barbara Mortimer, *Sisters: Memories from the Courageous Nurses of World War Two* (London, Hutchinson), 88–9.
104 Sulphonamide is a generic term for a range of sulphur containing drugs of which the sulphanilamide group was the first to be identified, exemplified by Prontosil, and the sulphapyridine group of which M and B 693 is the

most well known. For further information, see, for example, M. Hitch, *Aids to Medicine for Nurses*, 2nd edn (London, Baillière, Tindall and Cox, 1943), 362–3; and W. G. Sears, *Medicine for Nurses* (London, Edward Arnold & Co., 1944), 426–31.

105 Harris, interviewed on 6 August 2008.
106 Newton, interviewed on 19 December 2008.
107 Bennett, interviewed on 15 July 2008.
108 Ryle and Elliott, 'Septicaemia and bacteriaemia', 87.
109 C. Clifford (ed.), *QE Nurse 1938–1957* (Studley, Brewin Books, 1997), 77.
110 See, for example, M. E. Florey (ed.), *Antibiotic and Sulphonamide Treatment: A Short Guide for Practitioners* (London, Oxford University Press, 1959), 38–45; W. W. Spink, *Infectious Diseases: Prevention and Treatment in the Nineteenth and Twentieth Centuries* (Folkestone, Wm Dawson, 1978), 86.
111 Spink, *Infectious Diseases: Prevention and Treatment in the Nineteenth and Twentieth Centuries*, 283.
112 Allen, interviewed on 14 July 2008.
113 Allen, interviewed on 14 July 2008.
114 Lloyd, interviewed on 12 August 2008.
115 Thurgood, *Transcript of interview HX5 recorded on 8 August 2001.*
116 Shaw, interviewed on 18 May 2010.
117 McBryde, *Quiet Heroines: Nurses of the Second World War*, 135.
118 Evelyn Prentis, *A Nurse in Time* (London, Hutchinson & Co., 1977), 179.
119 Allen, interviewed on 14 July 2008.
120 Vickers, interviewed on 24 May 2010.
121 Porter, interviewed on 24 May 2010.
122 Taylor, interviewed on 24 May 2010.
123 Jones, interviewed on 6 August 2008.
124 Clifford (ed.), *QE Nurse 1938–1957*, 77.
125 Taylor, interviewed on 24 May 2010.
126 MRC, *The Prevention of 'Hospital Infection' of Wounds.*

10

'The nurse stoops down ... for me': Nursing the liberated persons at Bergen-Belsen

Jane Brooks

On 15 April 1945, the British medical and nursing teams, under Lieutenant-Colonel J. A. D. Johnston, Royal Army Medical Corps (RAMC) and Senior Sister B. L. Higginbotham, Queen Alexandra's Imperial Military Nursing Service (QAs), arrived at Bergen-Belsen concentration camp.[1] Six days later when Sister Myrtle Beardwell arrived with the British Red Cross relief teams, she was immediately summoned to a meeting:

> Col Johnson [*sic*] C/O of the CCS [casualty clearing station], took the charter at this meeting. He started by saying that he did not think that women ought to be there – however, we soon prevailed on him to let us remain. 'But,' he said, 'only on condition that you do not go into the horror camp'. His idea, briefly was this. To convert as many barrack buildings into a hospital as possible ... We were to start admitting from the camp the next day.[2]

Much has been written about the involvement of the soldiers, medical students and RAMC personnel in the liberation of Bergen-Belsen but very little about the female registered and volunteer nurses, and how they managed to care for the inmates despite the lack of trained personnel, equipment, medication and appropriate food.[3] The purpose of the chapter is to explore the work of the many different types of nurse involved in the care of the liberated inmates. These included the British Army sisters (QAs), Red Cross registered nurses and volunteer relief workers, German registered nurses and internee nurses, both registered and volunteer and, finally, the 97 medical students from the London teaching hospitals. This chapter examines the

211

work of the nurses through the trajectory of inmates from their initial evacuation from Camp I to the 'human laundry', where they were de-loused and sprayed with DDT by German nurses, to their admission to the ever-expanding hospital in which the majority of the female nurses were employed. The nursing work in the hospital is then exam-ined in more detail, focusing on the various aspects of clinical and psychological nursing work, including the care of diarrhoea, feeding and clothing patients and psychological rehabilitative care.

Many of the sources used in this chapter are personal testimonies, of which four are from registered nurses (RNs), two from volunteer relief workers and several from medical officers, RAMC orderlies and the medical students. There are also a number of both published and unpublished letters from RNs and relief workers. Whilst there are also a few personal testimonies from inmates, there are none from the volunteer untrained internee nurse, or the German trained nurses. It was hoped that the diary of Hanna Levy-Haas would provide some evidence for the work of the untrained internee nurses. However, although Hanna did work caring for the children, during her time at Belsen, this was generally in the capacity as a teacher. Moreover, she had been sent to Theresienstadt with several thousand other Jews at some point between 6 and 11 April, so was not in Belsen at the time of the liberation.[4] In order to comprehend the extent of the work that the nurses were engaged in, the chapter commences with a brief con-sideration of the history of Belsen.

Bergen-Belsen: background to the camp[5]

In her memoir of the Second World War, Brenda McBryde (QA) maintained that although the medical teams went into Belsen in order to 'salvage what they could', 'deliverance came too late for the thousands of men, women and children who had already perished in the gas chamber'.[6] However, she was wrong about this, there were no gas chambers at Belsen; it had not been created as an extermina-tion camp like Auschwitz, but as a transfer camp for influential Jews who could be bartered with the British and Americans.[7] With the end of the Third Reich inevitable, the camp soon became a dumping ground for prisoners from other camps. Anita Lasker-Wallfisch, who had survived Auschwitz, the death march to Belsen and then Belsen itself, described being loaded onto cattle-trucks and rumours circulating that they 'were going to a convalescent camp, and that it was called Bergen-Belsen'. 'Nobody', she continued, 'had ever heard of it.'[8]

On her arrival, Lasker-Wallfisch maintained there were not the bodies piled high, as they were when the British arrived, but as the thousands of prisoners arrived from the death marches, the conditions deteriorated rapidly and 'bodies became so commonplace that one just simply ignored them'.[9] When, in early February 1945, Dr Fritz Leo arrived with eight other doctors and 3,000 people, believing it really was a hospital camp, designed to improve the health of potential slave workers, he was dismayed:

> In the pouring rain our long column drew out of the station on to the long road, and in the rain we stood for a long time, waiting in front of the poverty-stricken, tumble down [sic] wooden huts which were to be our new home.[10]

Belsen was divided into two camps. Camp I was a hutted encampment housing approximately 22,000 women and 18, 000 men. About 90 per cent of the inmates were of Jewish origin, with an average age of 28.[11] Typhus and starvation were endemic, as was TB, dysentery and fever.[12] Many had gastro-intestinal infections, erysipelas and scurvy. Camp II comprised a series of brick buildings and houses with approximately 27,000 inhabitants of a variety of nationalities. Enteric, TB and erysipelas were present, but no typhus and they appeared better fed.[13]

Between 1 to 31 March, 17,000 persons died in Belsen. From 1 to 15 April, the day of liberation, a further 18,000 died. Dr Hadassa Bimko (later Bimko-Rosensaft), a Polish Jew who not only survived Belsen, but also cared for the other inmates throughout her incarceration, recalled that the 'hell of Belsen was at its worst about three weeks before liberation'.[14] Nearly 50,000 died in this camp in the course of two months, not from the gas chambers, but from hunger, disease and probably despair.[15] What is perhaps even more tragic is that between about 12,000 and 14,000 died after liberation.[16] It is the purpose of this chapter to consider the work of the nurses and not to discuss the wider issues related to governmental and army organisational issues. Nevertheless, it seems pertinent to consider the failures which led to these thousands of deaths and examine how the work of the nurses affected these deaths either directly or indirectly.

Evacuating Camp I

According to Johnston, when he arrived, the dead were 'all over the camp and in piles outside the blocks of huts which house the worst of the sick … Approximately 3,000 naked and emaciated corpses in various states of decomposition are lying about this camp'.[17] Private Fisher's first impression of Belsen, when he arrived on 17 April, was of starving people, the gibbet and thousands of pairs of burnt shoes. It was he stated, 'too unbelievable to believe'.[18] Molly Silva Jones, a British Red Cross registered nurse who arrived with Beardwell on 21 April, wrote in her diary, 'shame – remorse, yes, because even in 1934 we had heard of these camps and not realised, not wanted to realise that such things could happen'.[19] Despite the stultifying horror, they realised that the crucial task was to evacuate all 'fit' inmates, away from those with typhus and into the hospital, which was being created in Camp II, the barracks of the former Panzer Training School. However, this in itself was an impossible undertaking since, according to Johnston, about 80 per cent of inmates required hospitalisation. It was, therefore, necessary to create a 'Belsen "Standard of Fitness", i.e. [sic] An individual who was capable of collecting his [sic] own food and maintaining himself'.[20] According to Beardwell, it was a doctor from one of the CCSs, 'who in my estimation had the most gruesome and difficult job of all [and] was to be responsible for deciding which patients were to come to the hospital'.[21] Major Dick Williams, one of the first officers to enter Belsen, commented upon the difficulties of this task, as it was often virtually impossible to decide who was closer to life and who closer to death.[22]

It soon became clear that it was not possible to evacuate all the patients who required it most, as the leaders of each hut would always choose their own compatriots to be moved first.[23] This meant that the inmates of Camp I needed to be cared for in that camp and not in a hospital. This would be difficult with the most experienced nurses, however, and for reasons which are not made explicit in any documentation, women were forbidden from entering Camp I. M. C. Carey, the British Red Cross correspondent described in the

Red Cross Quarterly, 'No women are normally allowed to work in or even visit the concentration camp proper, which is separate and quite distinct from Camp II, the original Army Barracks area.'[24] Silva Jones stated that they were met at the gates by British soldiers, some of whom determined that they should enter the camp in order to believe what they had heard, but other soldiers were much more conservative in their approach to women, arguing that they should not go in, 'no woman should be allowed there'.[25]

Nevertheless, Johnston himself took Beardwell and Silva Jones to see Camp I. According to Beardwell:

> As we were trained nurses he thought we could stand seeing the horrors better than those people who had had no hospital experience. So, on this never-to-be-forgotten day, he took us in his car up to the camp ... The smell was terrible ... The majority of the living inmates looked more like animals than human beings. They were clad in filthy rags and were crawling and grovelling in the earth for bits of food.[26]

Jean McFarlane, a Red Cross relief worker, recalled how on the 23 April she persuaded Lieutenant-Colonel Gonin to take her, even though she was not a registered nurse.[27] Nevertheless, although several of the women did enter Camp I, which according to McFarlane, 'was from no morbid desire ..., but it seemed that the picture would be incomplete without', they still were not allowed to care for the inmates there.[28] Instead, 97 medical students from the London teaching hospitals were brought in to support the care by internee nurses and doctors. Although there would not have been enough female nurses, trained or otherwise to care for the inmates in Camp I, this does still appear to be an odd decision on the part of the military. First, it seems almost barbaric that whilst it was not considered appropriate to allow qualified, experienced female nurses to care for the inmates – the majority of whom were women and children, in Camp I, it was considered appropriate to allow young unqualified men, who had not seen any of the horrors of active service abroad.[29] An article in the *Nursing Mirror* in May 1945, decried the decision to use medical students instead of trained nurses to care for the inmates, asking what 'would Florence Nightingale have done – our founder and ideal – she who "gate-crashed" the Crimea? She would have raised her voice and called for a hundred – two hundred nurses.'[30]

Nevertheless, the presence of medical students appears to have been popular among the inmates. Their 'devoted work' enabled many to be 'nursed back to health'.[31]

Second, it is not clear how the British expected inmates who had been imprisoned, sometimes for years, to be able to carry out nursing work. Jean McFarlane does offer high praise to one trained internee nurse, 'if ever a woman deserved a VC she did', but does not provide her name.[32] The lack of suitability of most of the internees was further exacerbated as many of them were not trained nurses, but had volunteered for nursing work in the camp, possibly in order to receive extra food rations. W. R. F. Collis argued that any effort made by the internee doctors and nurses should be remembered as most of them 'were sick and weak themselves, but, forgetting their tired and wasted bodies, they have worked and fought beside our medical personnel to their utmost power'.[33] In April 1945 Johnston wrote that the internee doctors and nurses were 'apathetic, ignorant'.[34] By June 1945 he wrote that, whilst it was fully appreciated, the internee staff would struggle to assist, owing to their poor state of mental and physical health. However, it was soon realised 'that these people had no interest in anyone other than themselves, and the patients suffered in consequence'.[35] The tone of this somewhat pejorative language to describe the internee doctors and nurses is rather difficult to decipher. Does it reflect criticisms of their inability to function according to their professional calling, or does it reflect a more sinister trope related to inherent anti-Semitism? Certainly, there were concerns from Jewish members of the liberation teams that once the initial horror of what the inmates had experienced was over, the anti-Semitic tendencies of the British would resume.[36] It is possible that the tone was a combination of the two.

Despite the gendered decision as to what was or was not appropriate for women to see, with the arrival of the 97 medical students, the ability to sort out the living from the dead and those who would survive from those who could not, started to be possible. Those who were lucky enough to be chosen were taken to the hospital, which was the responsibility of the army nursing sisters. Once there they were to be cared for by the British Red Cross detachment, but first they were taken to the human laundry.[37]

The human laundry

In his description of the evacuation of inmates from Camp I to the human laundry Carey maintained that the stretcher bearers 'had a queerly sinister appearance, as they went steadily about their grim task', that of sorting through the inmates who had been marked for evacuation by the medical officers. The stretcher bearer then 'stripped off the stinking rags of the patients, rolled them in blankets and carried them out to the waiting ambulances'.[38] The 'human laundry' was located in the stables where 'tables are set in a row down one side, each with its oil stove underneath to counteract shock, and stretchers are brought in at the "contaminated" door at one end, and laid on the floor on the opposite side'.[39] The patients were 'washed ... all over with soap and water and then clipped their hair short and they [the patients] were sprayed with D.D.T'.[40] According to Joan Rudman, a physiotherapist with the 9th British General Hospital, when she visited the area, she saw '50 naked women, so emaciated, you could have cut yourself on their ribs being scrubbed down by German girls just as if they were a lot of cattle'.[41] Carey described the 'poor emaciated creatures feebly trying to wash themselves, but most of them are quite incapable of such an effort and lie there inert'.[42]

The use of language to depict the inmates as less than human was prevalent across many of the personal testimonies of nurses and others. Later in her letter, Rudman comments on the many deaths among the babies, who are 'born all the time', but, she continues, 'although we fight to save them, God knows why, I can't think they'll ever be any good'.[43] McFarlane calls them 'animals' and Sister Elizabeth Biggs (QA) maintained that 'Even now after six weeks of good food they still eat like pigs'.[44] What is not clear is if this dehumanisation affected the care provided by the nurses and relief workers, or if the dehumanising language simply depicted the most obvious comparisons, when the behaviour of the inmates was considered. It is arguable that it was this dehumanising process that enabled the Allied forces to push the corpses, 'to the edge of the pit' and then throw 'them into the huge open wound which was to be the common grave'.[45] Significantly, it was Leslie Hardman, the British rabbi with the liberation force, who requested that more respect be afforded the dead.[46]

Johnston had made early requests for nurses, given the inability of the internees to help in any useful way. In early May he wrote, 'we require (a) The entire staff of 9 (Brit) Gen Hosp incl [sic] C.O., matrons and admin officers'.[47] On 10 May, after the full complement of the 9th British General Hospital had arrived, he wrote again of the need for more staff, 'the greatest problem continued to be the paucity of British supervisory personnel'.[48] However, by this point he also appears to have realised that more workers were required. 'Present requirement (a) A further 75 doctors and 625 nurses (German or other nationalities)'.[49]

The decision to conscript German nationals to care for the Jewish survivors seems to the modern reader to lack any level understanding or appreciation of the psychological needs of the inmates. That this decision was made by medical staff and accepted by the registered nurses is perhaps surprising. However, many of the German nurses were registered nurses from a nearby military hospital and it may be that the decision was based on the need for trained nursing expertise.[50] Muriel Doherty, the Australian Matron who arrived with the United Nations Relief and Rehabilitation Administration (UNRRA) remarked upon the immense fear of the inmates, many of whom were aware of the 'showers' and 'baths' at extermination camps such as Auschwitz.[51] However, as Germany and Britain were still at war, the choices were limited. Silva Jones acknowledged in her diary in her consideration of the nursing in the hospital on 27 April 1945:

> Approximately to every 600 patients there were two Trained Sisters, one English and one Swiss. Close supervision was impossible during the day and there was none at night … It was at this stage that the decision was made to employ German Doctors and Nurses, psychological [sic] a detrimental move but a practical necessity.[52]

The German nurses arrived on 4 May, and according to Sister Muriel Blackman of the British Red Cross, 'Reception as expected – not good.'[53] Others were not so measured in their description of the reception that the German nurses received, describing how they were attacked by the inmates on various occasions.[54] Although some expressed surprise at the lack of animosity shown to the German nurses, the actual attitude of the inmates appears to have been fear, at least initially.[55] Bimko-Rosensaft and her husband Josef Rosensaft both acknowledged that the inmates were shocked when faced with German doctors and nurses in uniform, but as Rosensaft stated, 'we had no choice'.[56] Much of the data suggest that the German nurses were arrogant when they first arrived; it may be that their patriotism, whether or not they were Nazis themselves, made working for the British difficult.[57] However, according to Carey 'eventually the good instincts of their vocation triumphed, as they slowly began to realise the depths of the tragedy which they were being compelled to witness, and their professional training has produced in them, under supervision, efficient workers'.[58] Joanne Reilly argues that they did eventually earn the respect of the British.[59] Blackman admitted, 'they are good nurses and they will help, so I will have them'.[60] Once the inmates had been through the human laundry, they were taken by ambulance to the hospital itself.

Creating the hospital

Silva Jones described how next to the camp were Wehrmacht barracks, which were divided into squares, each square consisted of four buildings. It was these that were converted into a hospital by the British troops and Red Cross. Each building could hold about 160 patients and had a canteen that could hold a further 70. On 21 April, six registered nurses and four Red Cross relief workers reported to the hospital, including Sisters Beardwell, Blackman, Bennett, Robertson, Smith and Cruess along with Misses Brown, Parkinson and Webster. They went to Square 1 to start nursing the first 600 patients who had been admitted the previous day. Silva Jones maintained that there 'were no sheets, no pillows, very few B.P.s [bedpans] (augmented by dog bowls), no washing bowls, few towels, not enough cups'.[61] Beardwell recalled that 500 'beds' were created, which were actually only 'mattresses of straw – there were no luxuries like sheets, pillowcases, and quite an inadequate number of blankets'.[62] According to Annig Pfirter, a registered nurse with the Red Cross:

> Every evening the nurses rushed to meet the lorries returning with supplies to try to obtain a few sheets, blankets, under-clothing, crockery etc. for their patients' use. It can hardly be imagined what it is like to be in charge of sick persons – three quarters of whom were typhoid patients – without any proper equipment or essential medical supplies.[63]

As the days progressed the nurses were able to take over more squares and admit more survivors. Silva Jones maintained that, 'there is no praise too high for those who came to work in the hospital area never having worked in a hospital before. It was difficult enough for the Trained nurses.'[64] Sister Kathleen Elvidge QA Reserve, maintained that 'of all the difficulties, the chief one is that of languages. The majority of patients have some Jewish origin, but are from all countries under the sun. Russia, Poland, Hungary, Czechoslovakia, Belgium, Holland, France & only about four of them have smattering of English.'[65] These language difficulties made it especially difficult for the Red Cross sisters who were required to register the patients. By 19 May 1945, 14,000 beds had been created in the hospital, but not without significant sacrifice and difficulties. The chronic lack of equipment was never completely overcome and the staffing levels remained a fraction of what was required:

> What we had therefore was buildings, 8 nurses, about 300 RAMC chaps, a regt. of LAA [Light Anti-Aircraft] at least 20,000 sick suffering from all the most virulent diseases known to man all of whom required urgent hospital treatment and 30,000 men, women and children who might die if there were not doctors ... What we had not got was nurses, doctors, beds, bedding, clothes, drugs, dressings, thermometers, bedpans or any of the essentials of medical treatment and worst of all no common language.[66]

It is arguable that this lack of equipment was partly to blame for the continued deaths post liberation. However, to what extent this failure to save lives can be directed at the nurses is not clear. According to Rudman, the British registered nurses did not actually do any nursing, but supervised the Red Cross workers, internee and German nurses.[67] Whether she was criticising the registered nurses, or merely stating fact cannot be known, given their lack of numbers, it was probably not possible for the British nurses to do anything more than supervise. In failing to undertake much of the actual nursing they may have missed an opportunity to provide a positive example.[68] The nurses were clearly stymied on some levels by gendered notions of propriety, most especially their forced absence from caring for the victims in Camp I, but also their dismissal from meetings with their medical officer colleagues.[69] However, there is nothing in the nurses' testimonies to suggest they argued against such treatment, or that they presented any knowledge about feeding the starving that they may have learnt from the many articles in nursing press during the war.[70] The question of how far nurse can justify action and inaction by claiming obedience was explored in the work on the involvement of nurse in Nazi atrocities by Hilde Steppe.[71] Nevertheless, it is clear from personal testimonies of nurses during the war that in extreme circumstances there was a general acceptance of the abandonment of the rules of rank.[72] Their inaction does, therefore, suggest some level of culpability. However, given the lack of Allied knowledge about the concentration camps, it had not been possible to train either the doctors or nurses for such a task.[73] Furthermore, despite previous research there remained a great deal of ignorance by even the trained personnel over how the starving should be managed and much of the actual work was done by volunteers.[74]

McFarlane noted that, 'in England and on paper, the set-up for Relief Sections and Hospitals seemed all right, but in the field it was found that all hands at one time or another had to get down to scrubbing and cleaning, hewing wood and drawing water'.[75] Mrs Paton, a British Red Cross relief worker, described the situation to the *Red Cross Quarterly*, 'We do all kinds of work. At first we were needed to organise the hospitals, which hold 150 beds each: I can assure you it was not easy, but all most interesting.'[76] Ben Shephard maintains that only four of the cohort of Red Cross relief workers were trained nurses, and yet all those recruited to nurse were required to help the registered nurses and doctors of the 32 CCS in the hospital.[77] It had been expected that the sisters from the 32 CCS would prepare 500 beds per day and admit 'fresh people from the camp daily at first' into them. Then each day the Red Cross registered nurses and volunteer relief workers would take over the '500 they had admitted the day before'.[78]

While the registered nurses appear to have been able to manage the work, the strain on Red Cross relief workers was palpable. In a letter on 17 May 1945, to Miss Effie Barker the Deputy Commissioner of the British Red Cross Commission stated, 'HEARD [one of the Red Cross workers] – Silva Jones feels that she has had about enough. I suggest we tell her that we want her here to help Barbier, which is in fact true, and she will not feel too badly about being taken away.'[79] Beardwell's analysis of the hospital staffing situation was stark, 'In each block were 160 patients, and what could one British Red Cross person do amongst that number? There were some Doctors and girls with some nursing experience amongst the inmates, and these were the first to be released from the camp.'[80]

The problems with the internee nurses, which quickly became apparent in Camp I, did not abate once they were occupied in the hospital, although it is not clear from the data if these were trained nurses or volunteers. Blackman described how a Polish nurse refused food to a Hungarian patient, and when that patient complained, the Polish nurse slapped her, 'Arranged for the removal of the Polish nurse from these rooms.'[81] Private Page, an RAMC orderly complained that of the eight young women sent to nurse, only a few of whom knew what they were meant to be doing and all the rest were in fact too ill to assist.[82]

Nursing care in the hospital

In her memoir, Pfirter suggested that everything that she had learnt as a nurse, needed to be renegotiated:

> Life in the hospital-centre was quite different from anything we have ever experienced. It seemed to us sometimes that we were living on another planet; we had in fact to forget all our habits, our ideas as to tidiness, cleanliness, moral considerations and human dignity in order to try to comprehend our patients' psychological and mental state.[83]

However, I would argue that her nurse training had probably enabled her and other registered nurses to manage both the patients and those they supervised. The immediate nursing problems involved the most fundamental aspects of nursing work; that is the problems of diarrhoea and starvation. Norna Alexandra, a Red Cross volunteer nurse who arrived at Belsen with the 29th British General Hospital in late May 1945, maintained, 'so I don't say "crude nursing" but it was just trying to keep them alive, but a lot of them could really almost, could never recover at all, they were just sort of down to skeletons with starvation'.[84] William Davies, from the US Typhus Commission maintained that about 25 per cent of those with dysentery in the 'hospitals' died and that the death rates of those left in the hutted areas from dysentery, were 'considered "higher"'.[85] As the British nurses were barred from working at night, because of fears of attack,[86] too often they started their day by removing those who had died the night before.[87]

For those who would live, the situation remained hazardous, as Beardwell's analysis of the problems once again brought into stark relief: 'We had nothing to work with, and nursing proper was impossible. All the patients had dysentery and were too weak to use the dog dishes which were our only form of bedpans, consequently the stench was fearful.'[88] Roberts and Potter maintained that of the 500 admitted to the hospital blocks each day, about 80 per cent had diarrhoea and there were only two bedpans per block.[89] Page claimed that 'consequently it takes the nurses 90 per cent of their time to give and remove bedpans and the urinal-and-faeces buckets originally intended to contain food'.[90] This situation was made worse by the inmates' profound loss of human dignity. Having lived in barracks without any lavatories, those who could manage 'crawled outside [to open their bowels], but hundreds couldn't', and defecated where they lay.[91] The long-term impact of this meant that even once in the hospital, 'Some would roll out of bed to stool on the floor.'[92] Silva Jones' assessment of the situation was that they just did not understand that if they called someone would come to help, so they both urinated and defecated on the floor or where they lay. Pfirter recalled a woman who 'regularly soiled her bed and all round as soon as she had been washed and clean sheets put on the bed, and took great pleasure in doing so. When lying quietly in her dirt she was quite well behaved. On the other hand she was one of the first to make a pair of slippers out of a piece of her blanket to avoid soiling her feet when walking about the room.'[93] The extent of diarrhoea was probably exacerbated by the internee doctors, who, Silva Jones continued, did not consider that patients with diarrhoea should be fed milk or even water, and wanted to give them strong coffee only.[94]

In an article to *The Lancet* in September 1945, Lieutenant-Colonel F. M. Lipscombe (RAMC) argued that, 'better results [with feeding the starving] might be obtained with a larger staff of skilled nurses'.[95] Rowan MacAuslan argues, that 'by modern acceptable standards, at least 10–20 times the initial number of medical personnel available would be regarded as the bare minimum necessary to ensure even a reasonable chance of survival for the existing survivors of Belsen'.[96] Given the level of starvation and the vital importance of feeding work, this lack of experienced nurses ultimately led to unnecessary deaths. As there were three different diets for the patients depending on their level of starvation, feeding regimes were complex.[97] However, there were not even enough nurses to ensure that adequate fluids could be encouraged:

> Then came the job of trying to feed them, some were so starved and emaciated that they had lost all power of swallowing at all, they were fed with tea spoons, and as fast as we put the soup in it dribbled out of the corners of their mouths, this went on for days and days, a few of them were eventually able to swallow, but the majority of them died. Others were so greedy for food that they just choked themselves, it was nothing to come on duty in the morning to find 20–30 of your patients dead.[98]

The profound lack of nourishment that the inmates had suffered, led to an all-encompassing motivation for food which did not abate quickly.[99] This meant that those patients who were fit enough to get food for themselves required constant supervision to prevent them from stealing and hiding food and eating too much for their starving bodies, 'One day a nurse raising a patient's pillow was surprised to find two live chickens; another day, half a calf was found under a bed.'[100] Several of Silva Jones' patients managed to obtain more food than prescribed. After eating the food, the patient would 'vomit or experience acute abdominal pain and on more than one occasion died'.[101]

The nursing aspect of feeding was not only essential for physical recovery, but also, it appears for the psychological recovery of the patients:

> One day a woman aged about 35 was eating her soup in a mechanical fashion; she let fall her spoon, the nurse picked it up, wiped it and gave it back to her. The poor thing did not seem to understand this very natural gesture and started at the nurse with astonishment. A moment later, when she thought that nobody was looking, she threw her spoon on the floor; again the nurse picked it up, wiped it and gave it back to her. Her face lit up and she said, as if in a daze: 'The nurse stoops down … for me.'[102]

This recognition of the patients' humanity by the nurses was an essential part of their relearning of their place in the world as people. The nursing and medical teams soon realised that this psychological rehabilitation took on several aspects. Once the acute physical status of the inmates abated and their rehabilitation was in progress, the problem of suitable clothing became apparent. Collection parties were therefore sent out into the surrounding villages to acquire clothes for the inmates.[103] Under the auspices of Miss Daniels of the British Red Cross, a clothing distribution point, which became known as 'Harrods', was established.[104] The improvement in the psychological state of inmates was also noted when they left 'Harrods' with a new set of clothes, 'when the patients started getting a little better, the sister in charge would say, "oh they can get ready and go down to Harrods"... and the joy on their faces'.[105]

Nevertheless, as with most aspects of the care of the survivors, clothing distribution was not simple or without its hazards. Beardwell went so far as to state that, '"Harrods" was one of the most difficult places to run.' There were only a finite number of clothes and all the patients wanted more, therefore 'each one had to be looked over before leaving the store. Nearly all tried to smuggle more clothes'.[106] Some could not acquire a habit of wearing normal clothes and continued to either wear prison garb, or go about naked.[107] Sister BB wrote to the *Nursing Mirror* of some who thought they were fully dressed once they were given 'vests and underpants'.[108] However, for those who were recovered enough to appreciate their 'new finery', 'their social personalities would return'.[109] Perhaps the clearest and maybe most bizarre example of this social rehabilitation occurred with a shipment of lipstick. According to Gonin the lipstick arrived shortly after the British Red Cross and was considered so ridiculous a consignment, as the need for all the necessities was desperate:

> I wish so much that I could discover who did it, it was the action of genius, sheer unadulterated brilliance ... I believe nothing did more for those internees than the lipstick. Women lay in bed with no sheets and no nightie but with scarlet lips ... At last someone had done something to make them individuals again.[110]

Conclusion

When the British nursing and medical teams arrived at Bergen-Belsen, they were faced with the complete devastation of thousands of people and they had only the most limited resources with which to deal with that devastation. Once in the camp, despite the

225

army and British government's anxieties of placing women in such horror, trained nurses and relief workers from Britain supervised and engaged in clinical nursing with the most physically and psychologically ill people imaginable. Furthermore, the British nurses supervised internee nurses and volunteers and German registered nurses. The internee nurses whose physical health and moral standards been destroyed by the experience of the concentration camps, found the work almost impossible and were soon relieved of their duties and replaced by German registered nurses. This latter group of nurses is particularly interesting as their recruitment understandably caused great fear among the survivors. However, I would argue that their trained nurse status meant that their skills were vital, even if their nationality was of concern. The limited resources and perhaps lack of consideration regarding the needs of the inmates by the nurses and their medical colleagues meant that many thousands of inmates died in spite of liberation. Nevertheless, this chapter has demonstrated that the work of the female nurses and relief workers of all nationalities was able to restore life and humanity into many survivors of Bergen-Belsen.

Notes

1 There is some discrepancy over Higginbotham's involvement at this early date. According to Brenda McBryde, *Quiet Heroines: Nurses of the Second World War* (London, Chatto & Windus, 1985), 182, Sister Higginbotham was the senior sister with the 32 Casualty Clearing Station (CCS), which arrived at Belsen on 18 April 1945. However, Higginbotham's 'Pass' for Belsen Concentration Camp is dated 5 May 1945. Army Medical Services Museum, Aldershot, Royal Army Medical Corps (RAMC), M80 Belsen.

2 Myrtle Beardwell, *Aftermath* (Ilfracombe, Arthur H Stockwell Ltd, c.1953), 38.

3 Jo Reilly, 'Cleaner, carer and occasional dance partner?: Writing women back into the liberation of Bergen-Belsen', in Jo Reilly, David Cesarani, Tony Kushner and Colin Richmond (eds), *Belsen in History and Memory* (London, Frank Cass, 1997), 157. For further discussions on the presence of nurses during the liberation of Bergen-Belsen, see, Ian Hay, *One Hundred Years of Army Nursing: The Story of the British Army Nursing Services from the Time of Florence Nightingale to the Present Day* (London, Cassell & Company, 1953); Jean Bowden, *Grey Touched with Scarlet: The War*

Experiences of the Army Nursing Sisters (London, Robert Hale Ltd, 1959); Juliet Piggott, *Queen Alexandra's Royal Army Nursing Corps* (London, Lee Cooper Ltd, 1975); Penny Starns, *Nurses at War: Women on the Frontline, 1939–45* (Stroud, Sutton Publishing, 2000).

4 Hanna Levy-Hass, *Diary of Bergen-Belsen, 1944–1945* (Chicago, Haymarket Books, 2009).

5 For full and detailed discussions of Bergen-Belsen Concentration Camp, see, Reilly, Cesarani, Kushner and Richmond (eds), *Belsen in History and Memory*; Ben Flanagan and Donald Bloxham (eds), *Remembering Belsen: Eyewitnesses Record the Liberation* (London, Vallentine Mitchell, 2005); Ben Shephard, *After Daybreak: The Liberation of Belsen, 1945* (London, Pimlico, 2005); Donald Suzanne Bardgett and David Cesarani (eds), *Belsen 1945, New Historical Perspectives* (London, Vallentine Mitchell, 2006); Leslie Hardman and Cecily Goodman, *The Survivors: The Story of the Belsen Remnant* (Middlesex, Vallentine Mitchell, 2009); Mark Celinscak, 'At war's end: Allied forces at Bergen-Belsen' (unpublished PhD thesis, Toronto, York University, 2012).

6 Brenda McBryde, *A Nurse's War* (Saffron Walden, Cakebread Publications, 1993), 161.

7 Shephard, *After Daybreak*, 30; Hannah Craven, 'Horror in our time: Images of the concentration camps in the British media, 1945', *Historical Journal of Film, Radio and Television* 21, 3 (2001), 205–53; Ellen Ben-Sefer, 'Surviving survival: Nursing care at Bergen-Belsen 1945', *Australian Journal of Advanced Nursing* 26, 3 (2009), 101–10; P. L. Mollison (Captain RAMC), 'Observations of cases of starvation at Belsen', *British Medical Journal* (5 January 1946), 4.

8 Anita Lasker-Wallfisch, 'A survivor's memories of liberation', *Holocaust Studies: A Journal of Culture and History* 12 (2006), 1–2, 23.

9 Lasker-Wallfisch, 'A survivor's memories of liberation', 24.

10 Fritz Leo, 'The concentration camp for sick people at Bergen-Belsen', Imperial War Museum, London, 01/16/1.

11 Annig Pfirter, 'Memories of a Red Cross mission', 8, sent to Glynn Hughes in 1960, Wellcome, RAMC 1218/2/18.

12 Shephard, *After Daybreak*, 31.

13 WRF Collis, 'Belsen camp: A preliminary report', *British Medical Journal* (9 June 1945), 814.

14 Hadassa Bimko-Rosensaft, 'The children of Belsen', in *Belsen* (no editors acknowledged) (Tel Aviv, Irgun Sheerit Hapleita Me'haezor Habriti, 1957), 104.

15 Anonymous, Extract from *Die Welt* (15 April 1946) Imperial War Museum, London, 01/19/1.

16 Ben Shephard, 'The medical relief effort at Belsen', in Reilly, Cesarani, Kushner and Richmond (eds), *Belsen in History and Memory*, 32; C. E.

Vella, 'Belsen: Medical aspects of a World War II concentration camp. Paper I', *Journal of the Royal Army Medical Corps* (8 July 1984), 34–59. AMS, RAMC/CF/4/5/BEL/13.

17 James Johnston (Lieutenant-Colonel RAMC) Medical Appreciation – Belsen Concentration Camp (18 April 1945), Imperial War Museum, London, 99/86/1.

18 E. Fisher (Private), 'A soldier's diary of Belsen' (17 April 1945), Army Medical Services Museum, Aldershot, RAMC M 80: Belsen. Glyn-Hughes file.

19 Molly Silva Jones, 'From a diary written in Belsen', 2, Imperial War Museum, London, 99/86/1.

20 James Johnston, 'Medical progress report, no. 3: Belsen concentration camp' (10 May 1945), Imperial War Museum, London, 99/86/1.

21 Beardwell, *Aftermath*.

22 Dick Williams (Major) 'The first day in the camp', *Holocaust Studies: A Journal of Culture and History* 12, 1–2 (2006), 27–30.

23 James Johnston, 'Medical progress report, no. 2: Belsen concentration camp' (10 May 1945), Imperial War Museum, London, 99/86/1.

24 M. C. Carey (Red Cross Correspondent for N W Europe) 'Overseas: Progress at Belsen camp', *The Red Cross Quarterly* (July 1945).

25 Silva Jones, 'From a diary written in Belsen'.

26 Beardwell, *Aftermath*, 40.

27 Jean McFarlane, 'Talk to CDA' (March 1949), 11, Imperial War Museum, London, 99/86/1.

28 Jean McFarlane, 'Diary', 19 April–14 May 1945, 7–8. Imperial War Museum, London, 99/86/1.

29 Mark Harrison, *Medicine and Victory: British Military Medicine in the Second World War* (Oxford, Oxford University Press, 2004), 267.

30 Anonymous, 'Letters: Help for horror camps', *Nursing Mirror* (12 May 1945), 82.

31 Boaz Cohen, '"And I was only a child": Children's testimonies, Bergen-Belsen 1945', *Holocaust Studies: A Journal of Culture and History* 12, 1–2 (2006), 155.

32 McFarlane, 'Diary', 19 April–14 May 1945, 8.

33 Collis, 'Belsen camp: A preliminary report', 816.

34 James Johnston, 'Medical progress report: Belsen concentration camp' (April 1945), Imperial War Museum, London, 99/86/1.

35 James Johnston, 'Administrative Report – Belsen Concentration Camp', Imperial War Museum, London, 99/86/1, 3.

36 Jane Leverson, Bergen-Belsen concentration camp (6 May 1945), cited in Johannes-Dieter Steinert, 'British relief teams in Belsen concentration camp: Emergency relief and the perception of survivors', in Bardgett and Cesarani (eds), *Belsen 1945*, 69; Hardman and Goodman, *The Survivors*, 54.

37 Flanagan and Bloxham, *Remembering Belsen*, 22.
38 Carey, 'Overseas: Progress at Belsen camp'.
39 Carey, 'Overseas: Progress at Belsen camp'.
40 Michael Hargrave, 'Diary'. Imperial War Museum, London, 76/74/1.
41 Joan Rudman, MS letter dated, 14 June 1945, 4. Imperial War Museum, London, 94/5/1.
42 Carey, 'Overseas: Progress at Belsen camp'.
43 Rudman, MS letter dated, 14 June 1945, 7.
44 Biggs, MS letter dated 14 June 1945, 1.
45 Hardman and Goodman, *The Survivors*, 16.
46 Hardman and Goodman, *The Survivors*, 16.
47 Johnston, 'Medical progress report no. 2', 2.
48 Johnston, 'Medical progress report no. 3', 1.
49 Johnston, 'Medical progress report no. 3', 1.
50 Mervyn Gonin, 'The RAMC at Belsen concentration camp', 4, Imperial War Museum, London, 85/38/1.
51 Judith Cornell and Lynette R. Russell (eds), *Letters from Belsen 1945: An Australian Nurse's Experiences with the Survivors of War, Muriel Knox Doherty* (St Leonards, NSW, Allen & Unwin, 2000), 54.
52 Silva Jones, 'From a diary written in Belsen', 10.
53 Muriel Blackman, 'Diary', April to December 1945, Imperial War Museum, London, 01/19/1, entry for 4 May 1945.
54 Shephard, *After Daybreak*, 113.
55 Elizabeth Biggs (Queen Alexandra's Imperial Military Nursing Service), MS letter dated 14 June 1945, Imperial War Museum, London, 09/66/1.
56 Bimko-Rosensaft, 'The children of Belsen', 106; and Rosensaft, 'Our Belsen', in *Belsen* (no eds), 26.
57 For a more detailed account of German nursing and nurses under National Socialism, please see Christoph Schweikardt, '"You gained honor for your profession as a brown nurse": The career of a National Socialist nurse mirrored by her letters home', *Nursing History Review* 12 (2004), 121–38; Christoph Schweikardt, 'The National Socialist sisterhood: an instrument of National Socialist health policy', *Nursing Inquiry* 16, 2 (2009), 103–10.
58 Carey, 'Overseas: Progress at Belsen camp'.
59 Reilly, 'Cleaner, carer and occasional dance partner?', 153.
60 Blackman, 'Diary', entry for 17 May 1945.
61 Silva Jones, 'From a diary written in Belsen', 3.
62 Beardwell, *Aftermath*, 38.
63 Pfirter, *Memories of a Red Cross Mission*, 6. It is unclear why Pfirter refers to typhoid patients, when in fact it was typhus from which most patients suffered. The two diseases had been differentiated in the nineteenth century and it may have been expected that a registered nurse would know that they were different.

64 Silva Jones, 'From a diary written in Belsen', 5.
65 Kathleen J. Elvidge (Queen Alexandra's Imperial Military Nursing Service/ Reserve, MS letter dated 26 May 1945, 3. Imperial War Museum, London, 1029.
66 Gonin, 'The RAMC at Belsen', 4.
67 Rudman, MS letter dated 14 June 1945, 5.
68 William A. Davies, 'Typhus at Belsen: I. Control of the typhus epidemic', *American Journal of Hygiene* 46, 1 (July 1947), 78.
69 Gonin, 'The RAMC at Belsen', 5.
70 See for example, Mme Jansens, 'For European relief. 5. – Belgium, the Buffer state', *Nursing Times* (15 January 1944), 40–42; Madame Cathala, 'For European relief. 15. – France of to-day', *Nursing Times* (22 April 1944), 284; J. R. Marrack, 'For European relief. 8. – feeding a hungry Europe', *Nursing Times* (19 February 1944), 182; N. M. Goodman, 'The health of Europe', *Nursing Times* (27 November 1943), 879.
71 Hilde Steppe, 'The war and nursing in Germany', *International History of Nursing Journal* 1, 4 (1996), 61–9.
72 Anon. nursing sister (no date) *December 1939–October 1943, Tobruk No. 62 General Hospital.* Dame Katharine Jones uncatalogued collection: AMS.
73 FM Lipscombe (Lieutenant-Colonel, RAMC), 'Medical aspects', 13 June 1945. I. W. M. McFarlane PP 99/86/1, 9.
74 Anonymous, 'Diarrhoea'. RAMC 792/3/5, 2.
75 McFarlane, 'Talk to CDA', 3.
76 Paton (Mrs), 'From Belsen Camp', Extract from a letter of 2 May 1945 to the County Secretary, Isle of Wight, from Mrs Paton, I.W./100, Team TS/113/ WO, British Red Cross Commission Civilian Relief, BLA, *The Red Cross: Quarterly Review* (July 1945).
77 Shephard, 'The medical relief effort at Belsen', 39.
78 Beardwell, *Aftermath*, 39.
79 K. Magnew (Deputy Commissioner), MS letter dated, 17 May 1945, Imperial War Museum, London, 01/16/1.
80 Beardwell, *Aftermath*, 40.
81 Blackman, 'Diary', entry for 27 April 1945.
82 Fisher, 'A soldier's diary of Belsen', 6.
83 Pfirter, 'Memories of a Red Cross mission', 6.
84 Norna Alexander, 'Red Cross nurse'. Imperial War Museum, London, oral history 15441.
85 William A. Davies, 'Typhus at Belsen: I. Control of the typhus epidemic', *American Journal of Hygiene* 46, 1 (July 1947), 68.
86 Paul Kemp, 'The British Army and the liberation of Bergen-Belsen, April 1945', in Reilly, Cesarani, Kushner and Richmond (eds) *Belsen in History and Memory*, 144.

87 Hilda Roberts and Petronella Potter, 'Belsen camp', *British Medical Journal* (21 July 1945), 100; Beardwell, *Aftermath*, 43.

88 Beardwell, *Aftermath*, 4; F. M. Lipscombe (Lieutenant-Colonel, RAMC), 'Medical aspects of Belsen concentration camp', *The Lancet* (8 September 1945), 313.

89 Roberts & Potter, 'Belsen camp'.

90 Page, 'A soldier's diary of Belsen', 6.

91 Rudman, MS letter dated 14 June 1945, 3.

92 Beardwell, *Aftermath*, 43; and Gonin, 'The RAMC at Belsen', 5.

93 Pfirter, 'Memories of a Red Cross Mission', 8.

94 Silva Jones, 'From a diary written in Belsen', 4.

95 Lipscombe, 'Medical aspects', 314.

96 Rowan MacAuslan, 'Some aspects of the medical relief of Belsen concentration camp April–May 1945' (unpublished masters' thesis, University of London, 2012).

97 Rudman, MS letter dated, 14 June 1945, 5. For a detailed analysis of the nurse feeding work on the liberation of Belsen, see, Jane Brooks, '"Uninterested in anything except food": The work of nurses feeding the liberated inmates of Bergen-Belsen', *Journal of Clinical Nursing* 21 (2012), 2958–65.

98 Biggs, MS letter dated 14 June 1945, 1.

99 Biggs, MS letter dated 14 June 1945, 1.

100 Pfirter, 'Memories of a Red Cross Mission', 11.

101 Silva Jones, 'From a diary written in Belsen', 4; Pfirter, 'Memories of a Red Cross mission', 6.

102 Pfirter, 'Memories of a Red Cross mission', 9–10.

103 Biggs, MS letter dated 14 June 1945, 1.

104 Silva Jones, 'From a diary written in Belsen', 7; Johannes-Dieter Steinert, 'The British teams in Belsen concentration camp: Emergency relief and the perception of survivors', *Holocaust Studies: A Journal of Culture and History* 12, 1–2 (2006), 73.

105 Alexander, Oral history.

106 Beardwell, *Aftermath*, 54.

107 Steinert, 'Emergency relief and the perceptions of the survivors', 73.

108 BB, Nursing Sister, 'Nursing in Belsen Camp', *Nursing Mirror* (14 July 1945), 204.

109 Shephard, *After Daybreak*, 118.

110 Gonin, 'The RAMC at Belsen', 11.

11

The Norwegian Mobile Army Surgical Hospital: Nursing at the front

Jan-Thore Lockertsen, Ashild Fause, Christine E. Hallett and Jane Brooks

'Why I did go to Korea? I guess it was the same reason that I left my home and travelled 1,000 kilometres to train as a nurse. I was young and adventurous.'[1] The Korean War is 'the forgotten war', the war 'in between' the Second World War and the Vietnam War. Margot Isaksen was one of the 111 nurses who served as a ward nurse or theatre nurse at The Norwegian Mobile Army Surgical Hospital (NORMASH) in the period during which it was operative (July 1951–October 1954).

The Korean War started on 25 June 1950, when Communist North Korea invaded the Republic of South Korea. Armistice was declared 27 July 1953. NORMASH was operative from 18 July 1951 to 18 October 1954. During this period, over 90,000 patients were received and treated, 14,755 as inpatients. Of these, 12,201 were treated before the armistice and 2,554 between the armistice and the closing down of the hospital. More than 9,600 operations were performed.[2] NORMASH was a Norwegian unit and a part of the United Nations Army that, following a resolution in the UN Security Council, offered military support to the Republic of South Korea.[3] Tactically it was a part of the 8th US Army and was equipped as an ordinary US MASH.[4] Alongside the British Commonwealth, it served the US First Corps.[5]

The end of the Second World War saw the birth of the Mobile Army Surgical Hospital. The idea behind MASH was to utilise a mobile surgical hospital that could move quickly and operate close to the combat zone. As a unit, MASH was fully equipped with vehicles and tentage, and it could operate and move by itself in coordination with the movements of the front line.[6] The Korean War was the first war during which this idea was tested.[7] The evacuation line in Korea was from a battalion aid station, to MASH, to the evacuation hospital and then on to the general hospital.[8] But given the lack of sufficient evacuation hospitals, MASHs soon evolved from 60-bed surgical hospitals to 200-bed hospitals that also functioned as evacuation hospitals. This situation lasted until 1952, when most MASHs returned to 60-bed hospitals.[9]

NORMASH was one of six MASHs that were active during the Korean War; the other five were all from the USA. The mortality in the Korean War was 2.5 per cent. NORMASH had a mortality of 1.2 per cent overall.[10] During one period in 1952, Norwegian figures suggest that the mortality rate was as low as 0.6 per cent.[11]

When assembling NORMASH in Japan before departure to Korea, the Norwegian nurses were aware of the shortage of nurses in the USA, which had a subsequent effect on the staffing in US MASHs. It is claimed that this shortage had led to nurses needing to work longer hours and under increasing pressure when on duty.[12] Norwegians observed that the work was much more fragmented than they were used to in Norway. Individuals who were not trained as nurses did nursing work, something that the Norwegians believed to be a result of the shortage of nurses. They observed that non-nurses performed dressings on patients, and that there was a team administering medication such as penicillin and streptomycin.[13] US MASHs used both nurses and technicians as assistants for physicians during operations.[14] It has been claimed that the use of surgical technicians in the US MASHs had a significant influence on the subsequent introduction of surgical technicians to civilian hospitals in the USA.[15] This did not happen in the NORMASH, which used fully trained operating room nurses wherever possible, or registered nurses where necessary, for instrumentation during operations.

This chapter argues that the use of highly trained nurses for both theatre work and ward work in the NORMASH had a significant impact on the success of the hospital (including its low mortality rate). Specialist nurses were employed in operating theatre work, whilst fully trained nurses cared for patients in the wards. These nurses exercised a significant amount of autonomy in their care and treatment of patients. Like US nurses, they were obliged to rely on untrained assistants for support. However, assistants were not used for instrumentation in the NORMASH. The chapter explores the nursing done by trained theatre nurses and registered nurses. It also considers how they educated and trained orderlies and 'The Boys' as auxiliary helpers for defined tasks.[16]

Approaches used

The Korean War is 'the forgotten war'. For this reason primary data are scarce. Brunk says: 'In spite of the popularity of military nursing as a topic for scholarly inquiry, no studies exist that explicate the role of nursing during the Korean conflict (1950–1953).'[17] The study presented here uses oral history methodology alongside archive research and contemporary journal sources. Significant and illuminating data were obtained from oral history interviews with four nurses who worked in the NORMASH. It is believed that these are the only four nurses still living. Oral history is an effective way of collecting testimonies from eyewitnesses.[18] Their stories, told in open interviews nearly 60 years after serving, along with photographs and other materials, give a picture of perioperative nursing at NORMASH.

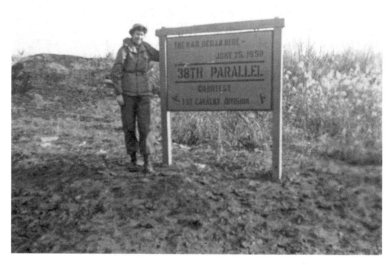

11.1 Gerd Semb, reproduced by kind permission of Gerd Semb

Captain Gerd Semb served with the first contingent at NORMASH. Semb trained as a nurse in Trondheim during the Second World War. In 1944 she fled to Sweden and joined up with the Norwegian Constabulary Force, which was trained in preparation for the liberation of Norway from German occupation. In February 1945 she went with a Norwegian field hospital to Kirkenes, a small town close to the Russian border. The Soviet Red Army had liberated Kirkenes in October 1944. German forces were retreating from Northern Norway, using a scorched earth tactic, and the Norwegian field hospital was established in the destroyed landscape. After the war she stayed in the army, working as a ward nurse; and she was a nurse with The British Army of The Rhine (BAOR) as a part of the occupation force in Germany after the war in Europe.[19] Semb continued working as a nurse with the army until 1967. Like Gerd Semb, First Lieutenant Kari Roll Kleppstad was an army nurse before Korea. She had served with BAOR, and continued to serve with the army after NORMASH. Kleppstad also served in a refugee camp in Austria in 1958. She participated in many military manoeuvres in Norway, only eventually leaving the army to care for an elderly parent. Inga Årdalsbakke was not a theatre nurse, but worked in the operation theatre at NORMASH. After Korea she worked as a nurse both in England and the USA. Like many other veterans of NORMASH she went back to South Korea, where she worked as Head Nurse at the National Medical Centre and CNMC (from 9 August 1959 to 22 October 1960).[20] Margot Isaksen had no military background before NORMASH, but worked as a theatre nurse. Isaksen was only allowed to have one mission in Korea. She was replaced because the Head Nurse of the army, Ruth Andresen, wanted as many nurses as possible to have combat experience.

The oral histories were complemented by additional archival evidence and published sources, including official reports about NORMASH produced on behalf of the Norwegian Army, and books and memoirs written by veteran soldiers. Although these were not nurses, their close observations of the nurses give value to their writings. Their writings both confirm and amplify the oral histories. Soldiers such as Olav Sandvik and Herman Anker educated themselves as veterinarians and orthopaedic surgeons after the Korean War. Their written memories about their duties in the operation theatre confirm official reports about nurses' duties as educators and supervisors.[21]

Establishing NORMASH

The United Nations (UN) wanted Norway to participate with armed forces, but this was not possible. The army was rebuilding after the Second World War and needed all its personnel to secure Norway and to fulfil its obligations to England by providing one brigade to BAOR.[22] Although the Norwegian government wanted to give aid to the civilian population of South Korea through the Norwegian Red Cross, the UN had a greater need for a military hospital and demanded a MASH rather than civilian aid. The burden on the US MASHs had increased, and there was a lack of general and medically trained personnel.[23] Norway did not have a MASH, but did possess a field hospital, Tungt feltsykehus (TFSH), which was not sufficiently mobile and therefore unsuitable for use in Korea. An existing plan for a TFSH was put aside, and a MASH was bought from the USA instead.[24]

The staff of NORMASH were not able to draw upon any prior experiences or written accounts for this type of work – everything was a first-time experience. NORMASH was initially assembled in Japan with 60 beds, before being transferred to Korea where further development and staff training took place. An ambulance platoon was also assigned for duty at NORMASH.[25] NORMASH was planned with fourteen physicians in every contingent. Because there was a shortage of surgeons in Norway, however, NORMASH was not able to recruit the required number.[26] Some surgeons visited US MASHs to learn from their experiences from one year in the combat zone.[27] Peter Lexow served as a physician in the first contingent. He maintained that war surgery was learned at first hand, and with feedback from the evacuation hospital such as 'never do …' and 'always do …'[28] Contacts when educated nurses came to NORMASH for visiting and learning are only recorded late in the assignment and after ceasefire.[29]

From Japan the NORMASH unit was shipped by boat to Pusan in Korea. After disembarking in Pusan the first contingent went by train and lorries to Uijongbu. The journey took them through a war-scorched landscape in which they were faced with fighting armies four times.[30] After reaching Uijongbu NORMASH was established in an idyllic garden, 'The Orchard'. NORMASH was hence stationed between fifteen and thirty kilometres from the front line, and was in fact the MASH closest to the front line.[31]

The war theatre in Korea developed from a blitzkrieg that swept most of the country four times, to a trench war along the 38th parallel. When NORMASH was established, the UN army had complete dominance in the air, enabling a good logistic chain. Supplies to the front and evacuation of patients could be carried out safely. NORMASH received all its material and medical supplies from US depots. All medical technical supplies were stored in wooden boxes marked with numbers so that essential equipment could be identified in cases of emergency.[32]

Korea had at that time not only been totally destroyed; it was also plagued by infections such as typhus, typhoid, pox and tuberculosis.[33] Experience from previous wars had shown that the greatest losses were caused by infections. Personnel were therefore vaccinated before service in Korea. This, along with good personal hygiene, had a beneficial effect, and hardly any contagious disease was recorded among the Norwegian personnel.[34] This was particularly noteworthy given that human waste was used as fertiliser in Korea; hence Koreans, both soldiers and civilians, who underwent surgery at NORMASH had ascaris (intestinal worms).[35] To avoid ascaris among themselves, the Norwegian personnel did not eat local food or vegetables; instead everything came from US sources. Nurses describe the food as good but boring and very 'American', most particularly, they complained of too much bacon.[36]

Recruitment of nurses

There were eighteen nurses in every contingent. Seven positions were theatre nurses and six were ward nurses or deacons (male nurses with an ecclesiastical education in addition to social welfare and nursing). Deacons served with the first four contingents but were not assigned as commissioned officers like the theatre nurses and registered nurses. Two nurses were X-ray nurses and one was a laboratory nurse. In addition, there was one matron and one head nurse for the operation theatre. Both ward nurses and theatre nurses were supposed to be recruited from among those who had served with BAOR.

However, the demand for experienced nurses always exceeded the supply, and it was never possible to fill all the specialist positions in X-ray and theatres with specialist nurses.[37] Very few of the seven contingents had more than a handful of personnel with both medical and military training.[38]

Training was provided for those in the first contingent who lacked military training, when they arrived in Japan. This was basic and consisted largely of learning how to salute, as well as military dress code. All nurses were dressed in uniforms from the US Army. Already, from the first contingent they learned that they were now under US supreme command and that Norwegian officers had limited authority.[39] Disciplinary rules were adopted from US Army regulations, and discipline among the nurses was described as high.[40] Semb stated

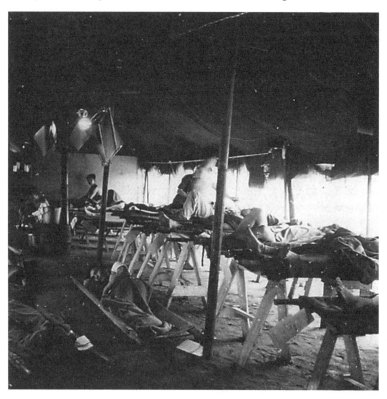

11.2 NORMASH ward, reproduced by kind permission of Ragnhild Strand

that the use of US field uniforms, ranks, food and rules made them feel that everything was Americanised.[41] The nurses maintained that walking around saluting and addressing each other as Lieutenant or Captain felt peculiar.[42] In fact, no one in the first contingent was commissioned as an officer. The Norwegian Red Cross operated the first contingent of NORMASH. The Ministry of Foreign Affairs administrated it, and the staff were denied Norwegian military rank by the Minister of Foreign Affairs. Upon arrival in Japan, the staff changed from Norwegian uniforms with Red Cross distinctions and ranks, to US Army uniforms and ranks. When Norway realised that NORMASH in fact operated as a military unit in Korea in August 1951, the administration was transferred to The Ministry of Defence, and members of staff were given military ranks.[43]

Education of nurses

Until 1974, registered nurses had to work two years as apprentices in operation theatres in order to become specialist nurses. However, there was no additional curriculum for theatre nurses, and they continued to use the same textbooks as other registered nurses. The main differences were the two years of training and the daily experience of working in an operation theatre.[44] From 1948 Norway had a uniform three-year education for nurses. This secured a standard level for all nurses.[45] Every school had long practice periods for students in operation theatres. During practice, students assisted theatre nurses with daily tasks. All operating theatres depended on a supply of well-maintained surgical instruments and a supply of sterilised dressings, gowns and linen for use. Single-use equipment was not commonly in use in Norway until nearly twenty years after the Korean War. Packing and sterilisation was therefore an important topic in Norwegian textbooks and a key aspect of the students' training whilst in the operating theatre.[46]

In the 1950s, theatre nursing had developed into two functions. One nurse had the responsibility for establishing a sterile field, draping patients in sterile linen and assisting the physician during surgery with instrumentation and haemostasis. The other nurse circulated and was responsible for positioning patients for surgery. This nurse also served the physician and scrub nurse in the sterile field if they required additional surgical instruments. Students mainly followed the circulating nurse. Operation theatre training has been criticised for using students as unpaid janitors. However, the practice gave every student nurse an education in sterilising and handling sterile goods. It also gave them a fundamental knowledge of theatre nursing.[47]

Norway got the first medical anaesthetist, Otto Marius Mollestad, in 1947.[48] Previously, providing anaesthesia was the surgeon's responsibility, but a theatre nurse under guidance from the surgeon very often carried out the task. After the Second World War, a course in anaesthesiology was mandatory for theatre nurses who specialised in anaesthesia. Intubation and the use of anaesthetic machines were reserved for theatre nurses with this additional course. Anaesthesia with ether on mask was still commonly in use. Student nurses still had the use of ether anaesthesia in their curriculum and training in dripping ether on a mask.[49] Through education and personal experience, the theatre nurses and registered nurses had become well prepared for working with, and supplementing, each other in the MASH units. Gerd Semb, for instance, had several times acted as a theatre nurse and also given ether anaesthesia as a nurse during the last war winter in Europe.[50]

Baptism by fire

During the first forty days, NORMASH received 1,048 patients – twenty-three of them civilians. Everything came to the hospital, including patients with appendicitis, victims of traffic accidents and those with somatic illnesses.[51] A total of 184 surgical interventions were conducted, of which only sixteen were combat wounds. A grenade that landed on a lorry during an evacuation of civilians was the baptism by fire, at which point forty-one Koreans and soldiers from Canada and Australia were sent to NORMASH. The critically wounded were transported by helicopter, and those less critical were moved by ambulances. Once they arrived at NORMASH all patients were 'triaged', and with four surgical teams operating four operation tables all staff members could retire to bed twelve hours later.[52]

The next test came in October 1951 after moving closer to the front, to Tongduchon. The staff at NORMASH understood that something

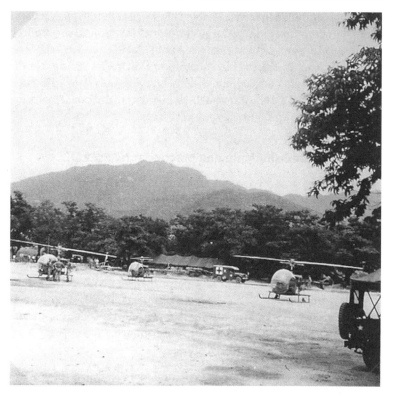

11.3 Evacuation by helicopter, reproduced by kind permission of
Ragnhild Strand

was about to happen. While soldiers were moved to the front, NORMASH was ordered to complete an inventory of the equipment and to ensure that the blood bank was filled. The October offensive started with midnight shelling. The staff could hear the thunder from the artillery. Then the infantry attacked, and soon helicopters, ambulances and jeeps with stretchers arrived at the field hospital.[53] Helicopters were not initially intended for use as ambulances, but for rescuing pilots who crash-landed behind enemy lines.[54] However, when the first requests came for patient evacuation, their success was apparent, although not without difficulties. It was a 'learning by doing' process, and technical and medical difficulties were solved through improvisation along the way.[55] The introduction of a helicopter ambulance service enabled battle casualties to be evacuated from battalion first aid to a surgical hospital for surgical procedures. Some of the nurses could not remember having seen a helicopter before arriving in Korea,[56] but they soon learned to distinguish the different sounds made by small Bells carrying only two casualties, big Sikorskys with multiple casualties, and ambulances. Each distinct sound marked a different degree of urgency.

Establishing nursing practice at NORMASH

The centre of a MASH is the operating theatre. A MASH cannot be operable without personnel trained for working in the operation theatre.[57] All other facilities are there to support the operation theatre. Most of the nurses were recruited from civilian hospitals and had not had courses in war surgery or any military experience – they only had their education as nurses and practice and training as theatre nurses upon which to rely. Nevertheless, they constituted the core of a military surgical hospital serving in a bloody war and operating as close as 15 km from the combat zone. The operating theatre nurse was part of an operating team that conducted sophisticated war surgery with a high rate of survival:

> The surgery at a field hospital is characterised by the fact that the hospital is the first place in the evacuation chain where battle casualties are taken care of by a fully trained surgical team. It has surgeons, anaesthetists, operating theatre nurses and orderlies, etc. and, with regard to both quality and quantity, first-class equipment.[58] (Quotation translated by JTL)

> Also our splendid registered nurses fitted into this [MASH] with their thorough education and special education.[59] (Quotation translated by JTL)

> I hope that I, through this, have been able to give you a picture of what modern military medicine is and what it can do, the many special departments and specially educated personnel near the combat zone, the breadth of medical science and the severe wounds a soldier can survive, as well as the low mortality and high rate of healing.[60] (Quotation translated by JTL)

Nursing at NORMASH developed in a different way compared to the other MASHs. The shortage of nurses in the US Army led to use of operating room technicians (ORT) in assisting surgeons with instrumentation, freeing registered nurses to educate and supervise

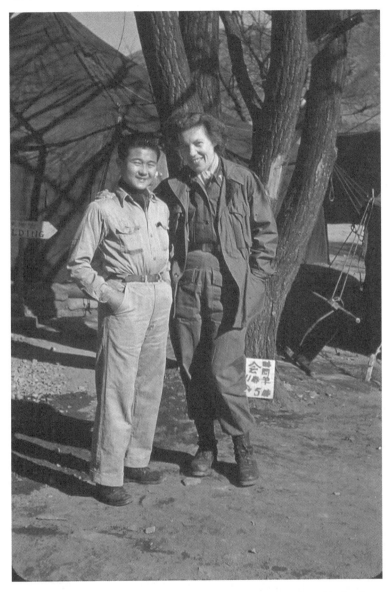

11.4 Kari Roll Klepstad and Chul-Ho (Archie) Lee, reproduced by kind permission of Kari Roll Klepstad auxiliary staff members in addition to nursing surgical patients.[61] Both theatre nurses and registered nurses at NORMASH were obligated by contract to take part in the training of orderlies. Tasks that were the nurses' responsibility but need not necessarily be done by nurses in Norwegian hospitals were often taken care of by soldiers and by 'the boys' under the registered nurse's supervision. 'The boys', as the Korean boys – some of whom were orphans and refugees – were known, were used throughout the whole period by NORMASH. Their tasks were mainly supportive, such as filling up with supplies, cleaning and maintaining surgical instruments, and did not include specialist nurses' work. Training others to do these supportive tasks was already an established practice in Norway. You did not need to be a fully trained nurse but it was the nurses' responsibility, and nurses therefore gave instructions:

> I was in Korea after the armistice. It was amazing to see what the boys could do. I was alone on night duty in post op. I could never have done it all by myself. The boys had learned a little English and translated for us when we had Korean patients. They had learned the names of the different instruments and could prepare packets after lists made by the theatre nurses.[62]

> In my time it was a boy who cleaned surgical instruments. He was careful and often came to show us a surgical instrument and ask if it was well cleaned.[63]

Olav Sandvik was a third-year veterinary student. During his service as a guard soldier at NORMASH he was reassigned to the operation theatre. His training had already included courses on surgery on animals, and he had learned about aseptic procedures under circumstances that were not ideal. All this he found useful working in the operation theatre, a working place of high prestige among his fellow soldiers. Theatre nurses, and also deacons, taught them how to perform practical tasks:

> It was mainly maintaining and autoclaving of surgical instruments, dressings, gowns etc., and it was cleaning after long operations where a lot of equipment and dressings could be left in a mess and even on the dirt floor.[64] (Quotation translated by JTL)

Specialist nurses such as theatre nurses were contracted to work as ward nurses when necessary. In practice, nurses also had to fill the role of theatre nurses when required, often during high-intensity periods when all hands were needed. If no theatre nurses were available, or theatre nurses were exhausted and had to sleep, regular nurses assisted physicians.[65] During periods of intense activity in the operation theatre there were no regulated working hours. All the theatre personnel were required to work until they could not do any more; then they went to sleep, and then up again. On average, there were eight operations every day. If a patient had multiple wounds and underwent surgery for abdominal and limb wounds at the same time, it was recorded as one operation. Once there were 173 operations over a period of seventy-three hours.[66] Over time there were several examples of soldiers being given tasks such as holding retractors and forceps for surgeons.[67] Herman Anker was a guard soldier in the first contingent and, like Sandvik, he was reassigned to the operation theatre where he was soon required to assist surgeons with holding retractors during operations, a task he stated he never felt comfortable with:

> An older surgeon asks me to give narcosis, a task I don't feel competent to do. But he promises to help me keep an eye on the patient and explains how I shall check the size of the patient's pupils. So here I am, sitting at the end of the table dripping ether on mask hour after hour.[68] (Quotation translated by JTL)

Holding retractors had never been seen as a nurse's main task. Only if the surgeons needed an extra hand because of the lack of an assistant would a nurse do this. Theatre nurses had their function during operations, assisting surgeons with instruments and haemostasis. During the busiest periods, theatre nurses stood between two tables and assisted two surgeons.[69] According to Årdalsbakke:

> The soldiers who helped us out in the operation theatre said they viewed holding retractors as a dreadful task. After doing it for some time, they got used to it and did a good job. There was no one we could call in. We also had to teach people from the kitchen how to disinfect their hands and dress in scrub and help hold retractors during particularly intensive periods.[70]

There were never enough nurses to undertake more than the primary nursing tasks. However, despite this, orderlies were not used to support surgeons with tasks such as holding retractors for the whole period of the war:

> I was in Korea very late. Everything was very well organised. We heard that orderlies had been used for holding retractors earlier. We never did that. We did it all by ourselves. Except for the washing. It was the boys, as we said, who did the cleaning of the operation theatre. It was very clean. The floor, of course, was only dirt and could not be washed. But it is amazing what can be done if everyone is willing. I mostly saw wounds of arms and legs. But there were other things. I remember a soldier wounded in the head. I was with a neurosurgeon. We didn't think he would survive. But he did. His parents wrote a letter and thanked us.[71]

NORMASH had two anaesthesia machines. With four operating tables in use during rush hours only two teams could use the machines. The other two used ether dripped on a mask. The first contingent did not have an anaesthesiologist at all, but from the arrival of the second contingent they all had anaesthesiologists.[72] Most of the work with the more sophisticated methods of anaesthesia therefore had to be done by theatre nurses who had undergone additional training. Anaesthetising a patient using ether dripped on a mask was not an easy task, and the risk of vomiting and expiration was high. Experienced theatre nurses were aware that a careful and experienced eye was needed.[73] However, it was still considered a task that surgeons could give to a registered nurse if necessary. At NORMASH there were examples of anaesthesia by this method being done by whomever the responsible surgeon could find.

Modern surgery depends on the prevention of infections, but during the Korean War there were many issues that could easily have led to life-threatening infections among the patients and clinical staff. Bernard Paus, surgeon in contingents 1 and 5, wrote:

> The patients have been wounded on infected Korean soil, they have undergone surgery in a tent with a dirt floor, they are lying in a tent with a dirt floor, and they are lying on stretchers with blankets and no sheets. They are tossing and turning, and the dressings are often on other places than the wounds. The Koreans are also good at plucking at their bandages and taking them off – and still, we hardly ever, ever see an infection.[74] (Quotation translated by JTL)

Several questions could be raised in response to that statement. All patients were routinely given shots of anti-tetanus serum, penicillin and streptomycin. Many of the nurses were used to using only sulpha as antimicrobial medicine, even though penicillin had been used in military medicine since the Second World War. This could have meant that they were exceptionally careful with infection control and with regard to reducing the risk for exogenous wound contamination. Moreover, with a median length of stay for inpatients of three to four days it would be a bit too early for wound infection to manifest itself.[75]

To maintain good hygiene at NORMASH, the water supply for a daily consumption of 15,000 litres was ensured with big tank wagons. The water was disinfected with chlorine and was not suitable for drinking, but was adequate for washing and for personal hygiene. Clothes and linen were washed in a US laundry. An improvised washbasin had been set up at the entrance to the operating theatre so that everybody could wash their hands before entering and before surgical procedures. The theatre nurses organised the operating theatre to ensure that every piece of equipment had its own place. This organisation served many purposes; first it meant that everything was easier to store and keep clean when not in use and also easier to find when needed; moreover, it established clean and unclean areas in the operation theatre and surroundings. Bedpans were washed and disinfected outside. The understanding of the need for good hygiene is fundamental in nursing, and for nurses who went on to become theatre nurses, aseptic procedures became a part of daily life. 'I do believe we had good hygiene at NORMASH. This was instilled in us from home.'[76]

> I will not underestimate the use of penicillin and streptomycin, but when working in a tent on a dirt floor, we became more eager to maintain a good standard in our work. I will say we had the same standards as we did at home with regard to hygiene.[77]

The nurses' testimonies, both from the first and from last days of NORMASH, claim that there was a good standard of hygiene. They believed that it was their job to ensure good hygiene in the hospital, and this was also an important part of their education and the inner core in practice in the operating theatres.[78]

Modern warfare is often total war, with weapons that are designed to kill and maim. Both sides used artillery, anti-personnel mines, anti-tank mines and flamethrowers. The UN forces used napalm bombs, and there are some records of bombing of allied soldiers with napalm.[79] Seeing and handling wounds caused by weapons like this made an impression on the soldiers. 'It is hard for me to remember everything that happened in Korea. The reason can be that so much of what happened makes me sad?' (quotation translated by JTL).[80] Burns did not only kill or wound people for life; they also etched a mark in the memory of helpers: 'It is impossible to describe the suffering and pain' (quotation translated by JTL).[81]

Testimonies from soldiers say that as a soldier one could read about traumatic wounds and even rehearse operating procedures, yet one could never be fully prepared for the smell of burned flesh and blood. Work such as holding retractors and forceps could make a man think about his faith and the future, as well as the future of the patient. For example, one soldier stated that the sight of a man having his fingers amputated might make his think: 'What if he played the guitar?' (quotation translated by JTL).[82] Receiving patients in great numbers could harden staff who were not trained for healthcare, although this does not appear to have had an impact on their ability to empathise with the patients.[83] Nurses also reacted to the Korean War, but they were much better prepared for what they might meet. Inga Årdalsbakke had, as a nurse in training, been called back to duty after the friendly bombing of Oslo on 31 December 1944, when seventy-nine Norwegian civilians and twenty-seven Germans were killed. She thought that if she could cope with it in Oslo, she could do so in Korea.[84] Gerd Semb maintained that she had a wealth of war experience:

> I had seen a lot of war before, and I had seen the sufferings of the civilians in Germany when I was with BAOR. But Korea – it was just a ruin with refugees everywhere. I am not sure that I handled it better than the soldiers. My advantage was that I knew what awaited me. It was work. I knew the work, and I had done it before. Except for the Sunday when the helicopters kept on coming. It was a battle near Imjin – casualties kept on coming; I thought it would never stop. That was the only time I felt that there was so little I could do. I washed many of the casualties that were lying there with a towel moistened with hot water. Many came in already dead. We could only lay them side-by-side outside the tent. That was the only time I felt inadequate in Korea.[85]

Nevertheless, the nursing of wounds and the sight and smell could be compared to daily practice. In some ways the running of a MASH bore similarities with running a civilian hospital. The participating theatre nurses and registered nurses were not given any training in war surgery, even though their mission was to run a MASH 15 km from the combat zone. Operations had to be done, the instruments were the same as they were at home, and many of the surgeons and theatre nurses knew each other from home:

> In many ways it was like back home. We did operations and did not find this to be a new thing. We didn't lack anything or experience any new thing as far as I remember. Everything was well organised.[86]

> I was on a trip in Oslo. On the main street, Karl Johan, I met a physician I had worked with. He told me that he was accepted for duty in Korea, and his wife was also going as a nurse. And then he asked me to apply and come with them. I did so.[87]

Conclusion

NORMASH was an active unit for three years, two years before the armistice and one year afterwards. During the fighting the battle casualties were high; however, the death rate at NORMASH before the armistice was as low as 0.6 per cent. For the whole period it was 1.2 per cent pre-evacuation.[88] It is possible that the low mortality rate was in part due to highly trained and experienced nurses. Without military training and war surgery courses, they were able to operate a military surgical hospital as close as 15 km to the combat zone. The high level of education and training of the nurses also made the staff flexible in the perioperative work and enabled them to train orderlies and local population in supporting tasks at the hospital.

Norway never again operated a MASH. NORMASH was sold back to USA in November 1954, when it was disbanded. Typically, as demonstrated by other historians, the nurses' stories were never sought. But the influence the Korean War had on their lives remained with them throughout their lives. Nursing practice was very little remarked upon at the time, and did not find its way, in any detail, into contemporary accounts of the work of NORMASH. However, the oral history data presented here indicate that the four nurses interviewed were confident in their practice and dedicated to their duties as nurses. The praise of medical officers – who wrote of the nurses' impressive skills, knowledge and professionalism – does find its way into the historical record. Yet, without the study recorded here, the voices of nurses themselves would have been silent. This study demonstrates the value of oral history in both revealing the hidden nature of nursing practice and in offering persuasive evidence for the significance of nursing work.

Notes

1 Margot Isaksen, *Opplevelser ved NORMASH* [Experiences at NORMASH] Transcript of interview conducted by Jan-Thore Lockertsen (Greverud, 27 November 2012).

2 Bernhard Paus (ed.), *Rapport fra Det norske feltsykehus i Korea* (Oslo, Forsvarets sanitet, 1955), 67–8.

3 Trygve Lie, *Syv år for freden* (Oslo, Tiden Norsk forlag, 1954), 305–27.

4 G. Anderton, 'The birth of the British Commonwealth Division Korea', *Journal of the Royal Army Medical Corps* 99 (1953), 43–54, 49.

5 L. U. Pedersen, *Norge i Korea. Norsk innsats under Koreakrigen og senere* (Oslo, C. Huitfeldt forlag AS, 1991).

6 S. C. Woodward, 'The AMSUS History of Medicine Assay Award: The story of the mobile army surgical hospital', *Military Medicine* (July 2003), 503–13.

7 B. King, 'The Mobile Army Surgical Hospital (MASH): A military and surgical legacy', *Journal of the National Medical Association* (2005), 648–56.

8 Paus (ed.), *Rapport fra Det norske feltsykehus i Korea*.

9 Woodward, 'The AMSUS History of Medicine Assay Award, 503–13.

10 Paus (ed.), *Rapport fra Det norske feltsykehus i Korea*.

11 C. Semb, 'Fra sanitetstjenesten i Korea', in Pedersen (ed.), *Norge I Korea*.

12 M. T. Sarnecky, 'Army nurses in "the forgotten war"', *American Journal of Nursing* 11 (2001), 45–9.

13 R. Wüller, 'Med norsk feltsykehus til Korea', *Sykepleien – Organ for Norsk sykepleierforbund* 39 (1 March 1952), 126–32.

14 D. L. Hallquist, 'Development in the RN first assistant role during the Korean War', *AORN Journal* 10 (2005).

15 J. K. Fuller, *Surgical Technology – Principles and Practice*, 6th edition (St Louis, Missouri, Elsevier Saunders, 2013), 3.

16 The Boys were young Koreans who worked at NORMASH. Among them were orphans and homeless children and youngsters.

17 Q. Brunk, 'Nursing at war: Catalyst for change', *Annual Review of Nursing Research* (1997), 217–36.

18 D. F. Polit and C. T. Beck, *Nursing Research. Generating and Assessing Evidence for Nursing Practice* (Philadelphia, Wolters Kluwer Health. Lippincott Willimas & Wilkins; 2012).

19 The Norwegian brigade in BAOR is in Norway called 'Tysklandsbrigaden', The Brigade of Germany.

20 Scandinavian Mission was a joint Project by Denmark, Sweden and Norway for educating Korean health workers. The hospital still exists in Seoul.

21 The project has been ethically approved by Norwegian Social Science Data Services, NSD. Nr 25104.

22 N. S. Egelien, 'Dagbok fra Korea', in Leraand Dag (ed.), *INTOPS – norske soldater internasjonale operasjoner* (Oslo, Forsvarsmuseet, 2012).

23 Woodward, 'The AMSUS History of Medicine Assay Award, 503–13.

24 T, Treider, 'Fra Vinterkrigen til Korea', in Haakon Bull-Hansen (ed.), *I krig for fred* (Oslo, Kagge forlag AS, 2008), 41–3.

25 Paus (ed.), *Rapport fra Det norsk feltsykehus i Korea*; B. King and I. Jatoi, 'The Mobile Army Surgical Hospital (MASH): A military and surgical legacy', *Journal of the National Medical Association* (May 2005), 648–56.

26 Paus (ed.), *Rapport fra Det norske feltsykehus i Korea*; O. F.Apel, jr. and P. Apel, *MASH An Army Surgeon in Korea* (Lexington, The University Press of Kentucky, 1998).

27 S. Florelius, *Rapport fra Norges Røde Kors til Utenriksdepartementet om Det norske feltsykehus i Korea* (Oslo, The Norwegian Red Cross, 1952).

28 P. Lexow, *Opplevelser ved NORMASH* [Experiences at NORMASH] e-mail interview Lockertsen, J-Th. (16 March 2013).

29 I. Årdalsbakke, *Opplevelser ved NORMASH* [Experiences at NORMASH]. Transcript of interview conducted by Jan-Thore Lockertsen (Skei, 7 December 2012).

30 C. Malakasian, *The Korean War 1950–1953* (Oxford, Osprey Publishing, 2001).

31 Årdalsbakke, *Opplevelser ved NORMASH* (Skei, 7 December 2012).

32 Wüller, R., 'Med norsk feltsykehus i Korea', *Sykepleien – Organ for Norsk sykepleierforbund* (Oslo, Norsk sykepleierforbund, 1951), 125–32.

33 Nilssen, R. W., *Med Røde kors i Korea* (Stavanger, Misjonsselskapets forlag, 1952).

34 B. Paus, 'Medisinsk liv ved den koreanske krigsskueplass', *Tidsskrift for Den Norsk Lægeforening* 74 (January 1954), 10–15.

35 L. B. Asbjørnsen, *Fjellet med de fallende blomster – Skisser fra Korea* (Oslo, Fabritius & sønner, 1952).

36 K. R. Kleppstad, *Opplevelser ved NORMASH* [Experiences at NORMASH] Transcript of interview conducted by Jan-Thore Lockertsen (Leknes, 30 March 2011).

37   R. Andresen, *Fra norsk sanitets historie: sjefsøster forteller om kvinners innsats i militære Sykepleie* (Oslo, NKS-forlaget, 1986).

38   Paus (ed.), *Rapport fra Det norske feltsykehus i Korea*.

39   H. Henrichsen, 'Med norsk feltsykehus til Korea', *Sykepleien – Organ for norsk sykepleierforbund* (1952), 62–8.

40   Andresen, *Fra norsk sanitets historie*.

41   Semb, Gerd, *Opplevelser ved NORMASH* [Experiences at NORMASH] Transcript of interview conducted by Jan-Thore Lockertsen (Lørenskog, 20 September 2011).

42   R. Wüller, 'Brev fra Korea-søstrene', *Sykepleien – Organ for norsk sykepleierforbund* Oslo, Norsk sykepleierforbund (1951), 204–7.

43   S. Florelius, *Rapport fra Norges Røde Kors til Utenriksdepartementet om Det norske feltsykehus i Korea*.

44   J-Th. Lockertsen, 'Operasjonssykepleie ved Troms og Tromsø sykehus 1895–1974' (Master thesis, Tromsø, University of Tromsø, 2009).

45   K. Melby, *Kall og kamp – Norsk Sykepleierforbunds historie* (Oslo, J. W. Cappelens forlag AS, 1990).

46   A. Jervell (ed.), *Lærebok for sykepleiersker Vol. 1*, 2nd edn (Oslo, Farbritius og sønner, 1951).

47   Jervell (ed.), *Lærebok for sykepleiersker* vol. 1, 236–42.

48   K. E. Stømskag, *Et fag på søyler* (Oslo, Tano Aschehoug, 1999), 93.

49   Jervell (ed.), *Lærebok for sykepleiersker Vol. 2*, 2nd edn (Oslo, Farbritius og sønner, 1951), 213–41; Lockertsen, 'Operasjonssykepleie ved Troms og Tromsø sykehus 1895–1974'.

50   G. Semb, *Opplevelser ved NORMASH* (Lørenskog, 20 September, 2011).

51   G. Semb, *Opplevelser ved NORMASH* (Lørenskog, 20 September, 2011).

52   O. Schie, 'Korea i september', in Pedersen, *Norge i Korea*, 55–8.

53   T. Treider, 'Fra vinterkrigen til Korea', in Bull-Hansen, *I krig for fred*, 41–63.

54   G. Anderton, 'The birth of the British Commonwealth Division Korea', 43–54.

55   R. S. Driscoll, 'U.S. Army medical helicopters in the Korean War', *Military Medicine* (2001).

56   Årdalsbakke, *Opplevelser ved NORMASH* (Skei, 7 December, 2011).

57   Apel and Apel, *MASH An Army Surgeon in Korea*.

58   B. Paus, 'Kirurgiske erfaringer fra Det norske feltsykehuset i Korea', *Nordisk Medicin* 51, 11 (1954), 374–88.

59   C. Semb, 'Fra sanitetstjenesten i Korea', in Pedersen, *Norge i Korea*, 76–82.

60   Paus, 'Medisinsk liv ved den koreanske krigsskueplass', 10–15.

61   Hallquist, 'Development in the RN First Assistant role during the Korean War'.

62   Kleppstad, *Opplevelser ved NORMASH* (Leknes, 30 March 2011).

63   Årdalsbakke, *Opplevelser ved NORMASH* (Lørenskog, 7 December 2012).

64 O. Sandvik, *Skjebnespill - Fra Kvinnherad til vetrinærvesents innside* (Oslo, Norsk vetrinærhistorisk selskap, 2012), 56.
65 Årdalsbakke, *Opplevelser ved NORMASH* (Skei, 7 December 2011).
66 Paus (ed.), *Rapport fra Det norske feltsykehus i Korea.*
67 D. Randby, 'Fra en elektrikers dagbok', in Bakke Finn (ed.). *NORMASH: Korea i våre hjerter* (Oslo, Norwegian Korean War Veterans Association, 2010), 34-6.
68 H. Anker, 'Morgenstillhetens land', in Pedersen, *Norge i Korea*, 64-9.
69 J.-Th. Lockertsen, 'Operasjonssykepleie ved Troms- og Tromsø sykehus 1895-1974' (Master thesis, Tromsø, University of Tromsø, 2009).
70 Årdalsbakke, *Opplevelser ved NORMASH* (Skei, 7 December 2012).
71 M. Isaksen, *Opplevelser ved NORMASH* (Greverud, 27 November, 2012).
72 Paus (ed.). *Rapport fra Det norske feltsykehus i Korea.*
73 Lockertsen, 'Operasjonssykepleie ved Troms- og Tromsø sykehus 1895-1974'.
74 Paus, 'Kirurgiske erfaringer fra Det norske feltsykehus i Korea', 374-88.
75 Paus (ed.) *Rapport fra Det norske feltsykehus i Korea.*
76 G. Semb, *Opplevelser ved NORMASH* (Lørenskog. 20 September 2011).
77 Årdalsbakke, *Opplevelser ved NORMASH* (Skei, 7 December 2011).
78 Lockertsen, 'Operasjonssykepleie ved Troms- og Tromsø sykehus 1895-1974'.
79 A. D. Dahl, *Koreakrigen og dens erfaringer.* The National Archives of Norway RA/RAFA-2017/D/L0068/0012 (Oslo, Krigsskolen, 1966).
80 T.Treider, 'Fra Vinterkrigen til Korea', in Bull-Hansen (ed.), *I krig for fred*, 41-63.
81 P. Øverland, *Koreasoldat 1953* (Trondheim, Forlaget 90936, 2009).
82 Randby, 'Fra en elektrikers dagbok', 34-6.
83 N. S. Egelien, 'Dagbok fra Korea', in Dag Leraand (ed.) *INTOPS - norske soldater internasjonale operasjoner* (Oslo, Forsvarsmuseet, 2012).
84 Årdalsbakke, *Opplevelser ved NORMASH* (Skei, 7 December 2011).
85 G. Semb, *Opplevelser ved NORMASH* (Lørenskog, 20 September 2011).
86 Isaksen, *Opplevelser ved NORMASH* (Greverud, 27 November 2012).
87 Årdalsbakke, *Opplevelser ved NORMASH* (Skei, 7 December 2011).
88 C. Semb, 'Fra sanitetstjenesten i Korea', in Pedersen, *Norge i Korea.*

12

Moving forward: Australian flight nurses in the Korean War

Maxine Dahl

During the Second World War Australia developed an efficient air evacuation system for its battlefield casualties that saw wounded men transported by air and accompanied by trained flight teams. Management of this system was the responsibility of the Royal Australian Air Force (RAAF). The air evacuation system was based on the US air evacuation model from the Second World War in which the registered nurse assumed the role of team leader for the duration of the flight.[1] For RAAF flight nurses, this was an extraordinary innovation as they had long been used to deferring to the decisions of the male medical officer.[2] Initially, separate units were established which specialised in air evacuation, although these were disbanded at the end of the Second World War as the RAAF adapted to a peacetime role. The flight nurses who worked in these units completed medical air evacuation training courses before being sent to work in these specialised units. Any medical air evacuations carried out post-Second World War were conducted initially by those nurses who had been trained during the war and before air evacuation training was recommenced in 1949.

With the end of the Second World War, many of those nurses still serving found themselves posted to Japan to work as members of the British Commonwealth Occupation Force (BCOF) based in Bofu and then Iwakuni, and these nurses conducted some air evacuation flights back to Australia. On 25 June 1950, with the outbreak of the Korean War, and under the terms of the agreement for the participation of the British Commonwealth Forces in the United Nations action in Korea, the US Eighth Army accepted responsibility for the evacuation of casualties. However, in response to requests from the British

Commonwealth Forces Korea (BCFK), the RAAF gradually assumed responsibility for the evacuation of British Commonwealth casualties from Korea to Japan.[3] By the beginning of 1951, all those casualties evacuated from Korea were transported by the RAAF and Royal Air Force (RAF) medical services.

Prior to 1952, patients were brought from the forward mobile army hospitals to Kimpo airfield in Seoul to await air transportation and received little pre-flight care at the airfield. By this stage casualties had already progressed through a formal evacuation system from the front lines to the rear echelons at Seoul. After assessment by the RAAF air evacuation team, those deemed too unstable for movement by air were then returned to the hospitals from which they had come.[4] Often the evaluation was conducted at the airfield in freezing conditions and patients received little preparation or stabilisation for the forward flight.

By November 1952, the airfield situation had improved with the establishment of a RAAF holding ward within the precincts of the British Commonwealth Communications Zone Medical Unit (BCCZMU). This ward became a much needed casualty staging facility.[5] Initially, one nurse was sent to establish the facility and then two nurses were deployed from Iwakuni for two-month periods to cover the management of the holding ward and occasionally undertake air evacuation flights to Japan. Eventually, the majority of flights were conducted by the RAAF nurses based at Iwakuni.

These flight nurses were part of the RAAF Nursing Service, a feminine gendered organisation which was separate but part of the RAAF. The Nursing Service was led and managed by women, and only women were appointed as its officers. Janette Bomford suggests that this separation 'perpetuated gender stereotypes by defining a discrete women's role'.[6] Bomford also suggests that this 'reflected the thinking of the time that a female organisation was thought to be the best (and only) way to organise, protect, and discipline women but it perpetuated the concept of women as auxiliaries who could make a unique contribution as women rather than as equal members'. The nurses also came from traditional middle-class backgrounds which enabled them to adapt to the requirements of the officer status they had on entry.

This chapter focuses on the RAAF flight nurses who conducted medical air evacuations during the Korean War from 1950 to 1953 – this was part of a wider study on RAAF flight nurses in war. There were very limited secondary sources on air evacuation outside of the Australian Defence Department when the study began in 2001. However, further sources include government files in the Australian War Memorial and the National Archives of Australia, and interviews with ex-RAAF flight nurses who served both in Japan and Korea.[7]

The chapter aims to document the development of the RAAF air evacuation system during the Korean War and to examine the role of the RAAF flight nurses as the war progressed. Further exploration of the training, role and working conditions of this group of flight nurses will illustrate the way in which the flight nurse role evolved and was shaped by the concepts of 'being a good nurse', gender and class. The efforts of this small number of nurses to achieve professional credibility under difficult circumstances and why these efforts are not known will be discussed.

Nursing staff needed for air evacuation

At the time of the outbreak of the Korean War, three RAAF nurses worked at Iwakuni as members of No. 77 Squadron Station Sick Quarters, primarily in the operating theatre or performing rostered ward duties. Not all these nurses were trained in the air evacuation of patients.[8] From 20 October 1950, the Australian forces in Japan were placed on a war footing. RAAF medical support became part of No. 91 (Composite) Wing with the main support elements of No. 391 (Base) Squadron at Iwakuni. From 1950 onwards, there were usually six RAAF nurses on strength at Iwakuni of whom three had undertaken specialised air evacuation training to prepare them for flights into Korea.[9]

When new nurses arrived in Japan, they were met by the medical officer and one of the nurses currently posted to Iwakuni; some nurses also remember the chaplain joining the reception party.[10] They were taken to the Wing Sick Quarters (WSQs) to meet the other nurses over afternoon tea before being shown to their quarters. The nurses were accommodated in houses built for Australian families of servicemen deployed to Japan in the period prior to the declaration of the Korean War. This separated the nurses from where the male officers and other ranks, including the medical orderlies, were accommodated. The allocation of tasks saw one nurse perform the duties of the Senior Sister, one nurse working in the Outpatients Section, two nurses on duty in the operating theatre and the others allocated to casualty air evacuation. At this time, only three nurses were air evacuation trained and routinely participated in the flights into Korea.[11]

As the need for air evacuation increased, it quickly became apparent that there were insufficient medical personnel to meet the commitment from within the Wing resources. Early in 1951, the British Air Ministry offered BCOF a number of RAF medical personnel to assist in casualty air evacuation operations. The offer was gratefully accepted by RAAF headquarters in Melbourne.[12] The RAF personnel who subsequently arrived at Iwakuni included three medical officers and 21 male medical orderlies. Surprisingly, this provision of medical personnel was achieved in the absence of any formal agreement between the RAAF and RAF concerning the status or functional control of these personnel.[13] The records show that this informal arrangement was still in place in April 1953, when correspondence reflects efforts to formalise the arrangement. The RAF medical orderlies were air evacuation trained and assisted the RAAF nurses as members of integrated flight teams but who had little contact outside of flying.

In March 1951, RAF medical staff visited Iwakuni to discuss the provision of RAF Hastings aircraft for a Middle East service to Changi in Singapore as part of an established medical air evacuation route for British casualties.[14] RAAF flight nurses occasionally conducted the first part of the air evacuation flights to Changi. At times one of the nurses would also escort patients back to Australia on Qantas aircraft. At the time, Qantas operated a courier service between Australia and Japan using Lancastrian and later DC-4 aircraft.[15]

From January 1951 onwards, the number of casualties who were air evacuated rose, peaking at 717 in November 1951, the highest number to be evacuated in a month using C-47 Dakota aircraft. The documented patient figures for evacuations during the Korean War from January 1951 to December 1953 total 12,762. In fact, this number may have been higher, as no statistical data could be located for 1950.[16] Patient loads were mixed and comprised some litter patients with the remainder walking patients. Initially, many of the patients suffered from severe frostbite as well as battle injuries.[17]

The RAAF soon realised that it needed a holding ward to stage patients near the airfield until they were uplifted. The closest medical unit in Seoul was the BCCZMU staffed by Army medical personnel from the United Kingdom and Canada. Senior Sister Helen Cleary, Jimmy Morrison (a medical officer) and Sister Pat Oliver were sent over to liaise and negotiate with the BCCZMU staff for the RAAF to use part of an old school as a casualty staging facility.[18] This was an unprecedented situation and demonstrated the nurses' significant level of input into the development of air evacuation in Korea from its very outset. The negotiations successfully completed, a small detachment of RAAF nurses and RAF medical orderlies was sent to the facility to care for patients awaiting air evacuation back to Iwakuni.

Once the number of patients assembled in the Casualty Air Evacuation Flight (CAEF) holding ward reached about 25, aircraft were ordered and the patients were moved to the K16 (Kimpo) airfield, usually by around 8.00 a.m.[19] There they were joined by the more seriously ill patients who had been evacuated through American channels to the 121st Evacuation Hospital in Seoul before being loaded onto RAAF Dakota aircraft for the trip to Japan.[20] On arrival at Iwakuni, patients were transferred to the WSQs for one to two hours before being moved either by hospital train or launch under Australian Army care to the British Commonwealth General Hospital in Kure. The RAAF nurses' responsibility ended with the movement of patients from Iwakuni.

The CAEF represented an ad hoc arrangement which depended on other services in the area to provide accommodation, mess facilities, food and transport. A proposal to formally establish an orthodox CAEF with agreement between RAF and RAAF medical services and which would be jointly staffed by both parties was submitted in March 1953.[21] However, with the declaration of the truce on 27 July 1953, the proposal lapsed with the anticipation that the number of casualties needing evacuation would now diminish.

Training for flight nurses

Medical air evacuation training for nurses in the RAAF recommenced with the establishment of the Air Evacuation and Air Sea

Rescue Course at the Aviation Medical Section at RAAF Station Point Cook (near Melbourne) on 26 April 1949.[22] The first course was conducted by Sister Helen Cleary, an experienced Second World War trained flight nurse. The nurse trainees wore their white uniforms, white stockings and veils for most of the course, although this attire proved impractical for the activities required.[23] Trainees on subsequent courses wore a khaki flight nurse uniform.

The second course was conducted from 28 August to 8 September 1950. The course syllabus indicates an emphasis on training for survival in all types of situations including ocean, land, jungle, desert and Arctic survival.[24] Practical training in sea survival was conducted both at the Melbourne City Baths and in Port Phillip Bay at Point Cook. Additional lectures on the principles of air evacuation, patient loading, in-flight care of patients and anoxia (hypoxia) also formed part of the course. Training in the use of a decompression chamber and the operation of a dinghy was conducted at Point Cook. Trainees were also practised in techniques for loading a patient into an aircraft and a short practice flight was conducted in a C-47 Dakota aircraft.

In 1951, Sister Elizabeth Baldwin assumed responsibility for the conduct of these courses. Like her predecessor, she had completed her flight nurse training late in the Second World War and had considerable air evacuation experience.[25] Changes to the syllabus were proposed in April 1951 and were implemented during the next course, No. 4 Medical Evacuation and Air Sea Rescue Course, which ran from 7 to 18 May 1951. The course was conducted twice in 1952 and attended by eight and nine registered nurses respectively, with the name of the course varying slightly in the official documents of the time.[26] The course was then held annually, in 1953 and 1954, and was known as the Casualty Air Evacuation Course, as stipulated by the policy on casualty air evacuation which had finally been promulgated in November 1952.[27] Official files indicate that syllabuses from both the US Air Force and the RAF were consulted prior to changes in the RAAF syllabus for air evacuation. On completion of their course, which was undertaken separately to the doctors and orderlies, the nurses soon found themselves posted to Japan.

The flight nurse role

Unlike the RAAF flight nurses in the Second World War who undertook flight nurse duties only, the flight nurses in Japan and Korea performed other duties, in addition. These nurses occupied three distinct roles: the flight nurse role, the nursing roles within the CAEF in Korea and the nursing role in No. 91 (Composite) WSQs, which included in-transit care of air evacuated patients and routine nursing duties.[28]

Since its inception in the RAAF, the flight nurse role has been clearly defined at a formal level in policies on medical air evacuation and covers a distinct set of responsibilities. Pre-flight responsibilities included the assessment and briefing of patients; supervising the loading and positioning of the patients within the aircraft; and briefing the pilot on any special requirements for patients in flight with regard to altitude, length of flight or temperature control. Providing in-flight care and writing the reports, completing the flight manifest, supervising the unloading of the patients at the destination airfield, and handing over the patients to the next medical/nursing team completed the responsibilities for the flight nurse for that flight. Clearly, all of these points illustrate the level of professional autonomy given to the flight nurses following successful completion of the training course, yet they had to function within the constraints of the policy.

Once patients were handed over, the flight nurses had to check and restock their flight equipment ready for the next flight. There was little opportunity for any follow-up on the patients they evacuated. The routine for the RAAF flight nurse for the day's flight involved an early pick-up by a Japanese driver who would take her to the hospital to meet the duty medical orderly. There she collected the flight equipment, which consisted of a flight pannier, drug box, and food and drink for the flight.[29] The flight pannier, which was locally made in Japan, was very robust and ideally suited to holding nursing supplies. Its utility was such that it continued to be used for aeromedical evacuation for several decades, although its contents varied. Figure 12.1 illustrates the type of flight pannier used in Korea and Japan. The other equipment taken on the aircraft would have included additional blankets, oxygen cylinder, thermos and drinking mugs.

Aircraft routinely took off at around 5.30 a.m. In winter, ice which

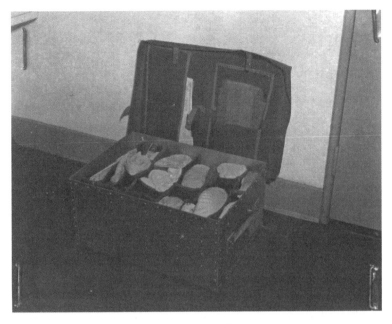

12.1 Flight pannier used during the Korean War

had formed on the wings had to be scraped off by ground crew before departure. The cold affected all the nurses who wore several layers of clothing to keep warm both in the aircraft and on the ground in Japan and Korea. The bitter cold of the winter was one of several stressors associated with the flights noted by nurses interviewed. Others included time spent in holding patterns waiting to land in Korea because fighter aircraft had a higher priority for landing; the number of separate landings before they could finally collect their patients; and the urgency associated with rapidly transporting patients back to Japan for medical treatment. Bad weather often added to the stress of flying, although the nurses had great confidence in the ability of their aircrew.[30]

Once airborne, one of the nurses' first actions was to serve a cup of tea and sandwiches to their patients. Sister Cathie Daniel remembers this as a time when the nurses showed the patients that someone cared, reassuring them with a word and a smile.[31]

In later accounts the nurses often understated the nature of the

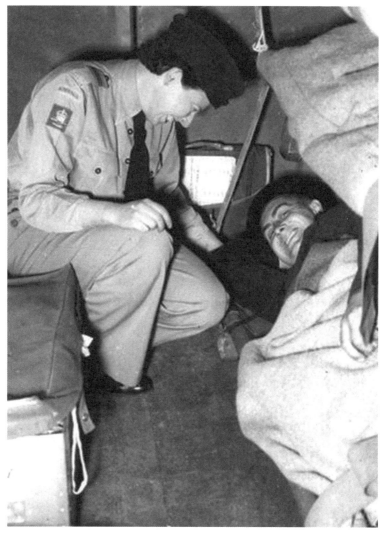

12.2 Sister Cathie Daniel with patient flying from Korea to Iwakuni

injuries of some of their patients, although they did talk about the badly burnt patients, often victims of home-made heaters used in the trenches, and others with amputations, chest wounds and severe blast injuries.[32] Whether this was the nurses' way of not speaking about the terrors of war was not acknowledged by any interviewees. Individual nurses recalled one or two specific cases that warranted their concern and who they were always pleased to land safely and promptly in Iwakuni for further medical attention.

The aircraft usually landed at Iwakuni around 2.00 p.m. and the flight nurse handed over her patients to the waiting staff for transfer by ambulance from the airstrip to the holding ward in the WSQs. The flight nurse then departed to complete paperwork and restock her equipment. The ward was prepared for the arrival of the patients by two other nurses, orderlies and Japanese staff. These nurses took over responsibility for the patients until they were transferred to Army staff for transport to Kure.[33]

Preparing, accepting and looking after the incoming patients from Korea was truly a team effort with all Australian and Japanese staff caring for patients in the holding ward in Iwakuni. Patients usually

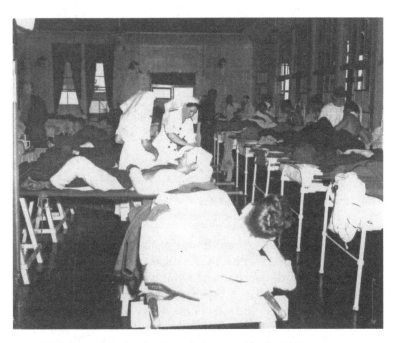

12.3 Recently arrived patients being cared for by RAAF nurses on transfer from Korea to Iwakuni

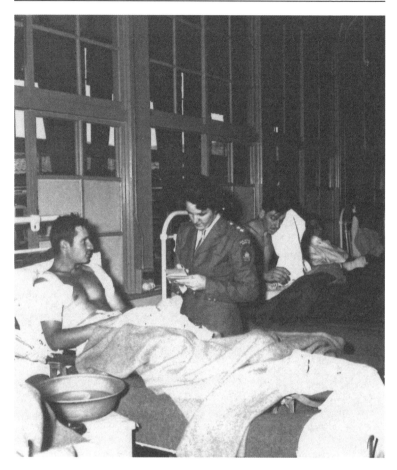

12.4 Sister M. Larsen, Australian Army, reviews patients on arrival from Korea and prior to transfer to Kure

remained in the holding ward from two to five hours before being moved by ambulance to either the ambulance train or a launch for the trip to Kure. Not all patients were fit for travel and all were initially assessed by an Australian Army medical officer and nurse for their suitability for transfer. The roles of the RAAF and army nurses were clearly defined and understood by all staff. Patients deemed unfit for travel would remain in the holding ward for a day or two to be stabilised before proceeding to Kure. After treatment and convalescence, patients were returned to Iwakuni for onward travel either to the UK by RAF Hastings aircraft or to Australia by Qantas Skymaster. These patients had little prospect of being classified fit to return to duty in Korea.

Moving forward into Korea

By June 1952 the improvised CAEF had moved into its quarters at the rear of the BCCZMU. The first RAAF nurse, sent there in October 1952 to establish the CAEF, was Sister Cathie Daniel, who recalls:

> It was an old school and we had the lower floor, it was pretty knocked about, but [we used] the old pot belly stoves to keep warm ... and we had some accommodation upstairs in the building, the ward itself was a big classroom, pretty rough in some places, but it was very much better for holding patients than out on an airstrip.[34]

Initially, Sister Daniel was the only RAAF sister posted to the CAEF for air evacuation duties, although Australian Army nurses and nurses from other British Commonwealth nations also worked at the unit. Sister Nathalie Oldham joined Cathie Daniel in December and remembers that the ward held around thirty patients and that some may have spent one or two days there following surgery before being evacuated.[35] Figure 12.5 illustrates the spartan conditions in the ward and Sister Oldham recalls that it was a luxury to have a sheet or pillowcase, although there were plenty of blankets. Towels were also in short supply and the patients often helped the sisters to wash the used towels. The staff would also use singlets to dry the patients. Eventually the linen supply improved as more equipment was shipped in from Japan.[36]

The nurses' hours were long and they could be very busy depending on the number of patients who came in, the nature of their wounds and the incidence of illness. The sisters saw large numbers of burn patients, particularly during the winter months.[37] Conditions were very difficult for the sisters attached to the CAEF unit in Korea. The weather was much colder than they were used to in Japan and living conditions were cramped and basic. The sisters' quarters were upstairs and were divided into cubicles about six feet wide with just enough space for a stretcher and a trunk. A Korean maid who would

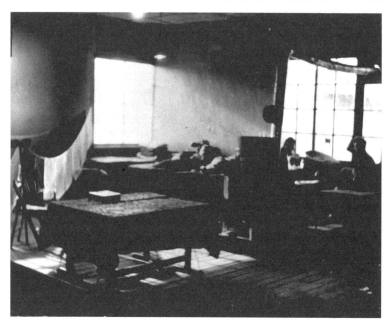

12.5 Casualty Air Evacuation Flight – BCCZMU

look after two or three nurses also did their washing.[38] Personal possessions were kept locked in a trunk as the nurses felt they could not keep an eye on their belongings when so many people were moving in and out of the area. A guard would come up to refill the oil heater several times during the night and would disturb their sleep, but at least they were warm. There was no bathroom in the accommodation block so the nurses used the men's shower block in the compound. Each afternoon at an agreed time a guard would be placed on the men's shower block, which was out in the open, and would stand guard while the nurses showered. In winter, the sisters would trudge back through the snow with all 'the boys' watching them. It was a new experience for nurses such as Cathie Daniel.[39] Despite the fact that the BCCZMU was an operational area, the nurses were unarmed and thus usually accompanied by an armed guard. However, while restricted in some ways, the nurses did manage to take trips forward or to other units such as 77 Squadron or to the US medical facilities.

Given the primitive conditions, long working hours and heavy workload, Cathie Daniel remembers that: 'there wasn't much light heartedness there because you were either waiting for patients to come down from the forward medical facilities, or they were in the holding ward, they were sick, and you were, I would say practically busy the whole time'.[40] Sister Gay Bury recalls her thoughts of being sent to relieve a sick sister in the CAEF in Korea as: 'what a dump this is even dirtier than before, dusty and bedraggled and I have caught the flu again. So that was that anyway we went on as usual.'[41] There was some opportunity for independent decision-making by the nurses responsible for the holding ward care, pre-flight assessment and acceptance of patients for the flight. However, they were not entirely alone and could seek medical help from the staff of the BCCZMU if required. While the nurses retained the right to refuse to take a patient on a flight, there is no evidence that they actually did.[42] The nurses also exercised their own judgement in deciding how patients were loaded into the aircraft. The more serious cases were usually loaded towards the front as this was an area of less turbulence. The nurses also had to assess and monitor the patients' condition during the flight. These roles provided extended practice and the RAAF flight nurses willingly accepted this part of the defined role for flight nurses.

Sometimes one of the nurses from the CAEF would accompany the patients to Iwakuni which would allow her time away from the war zone and precious contact with her nursing colleagues at Iwakuni. At other times, the flight nurse would come over on the aircraft from Iwakuni and return with the patients.

Other flight nurse opportunities

All the RAAF nurses completed air evacuation flights with patients being returned to Australia on Qantas aircraft. The flights back to Australia were long and staged over several days. In the first years of the war, the flight stopped in Manila (Philippines) and Darwin (northern Australia) before the aircraft landed in Sydney. From mid-1952 however, flights flew the alternative route of Iwakuni–Guam–Port Moresby–Sydney which eliminated overnight stops, although the journey still took some 24 hours' flying time.[43] The nurses handed the patients to waiting medical/nursing staff at the airfield for transfer to the 113th Australian General Hospital at Concord (NSW). The flight nurses then returned to Japan on scheduled Qantas flights.

Those flight nurses selected to fly on the RAF Hastings air evacuation flights as far as Changi in Singapore also cherished this as an opportunity for a break from routine. Once in Singapore, they handed their patients to British flight nurses. Each of the RAAF flight nurses conducted at least one such flight. Sister Nathalie Oldham also completed air evacuations with the US 801st Medical Air Evacuation Squadron (MAES) flying out of Tachikawa outside Tokyo. The US flight nurses only performed flight duties and did not work in the hospitals, unlike their RAAF counterparts. Nathalie Oldham also noted other differences: 'They got flying pay. They drove around in convertible cars, and you ate in the Officers Club. They didn't have Mess Halls or anything; a different style of life altogether.'[44]

Flight nurse role as a reflection of social models

Early nursing in Australia incorporated many of the characteristics of the British model of Nightingale nursing and training. This saw nursing shaped by the middle-class female role of Victorian England with women as subservient helpers and 'ladies'.[45] The nurse apprenticeship training which ensued emulated the Nightingale model with long hours, poor remuneration, hard physical work and strict discipline as its hallmarks while working in a subservient role to the doctors. In time, it also came to mean that the ideal nurse was practical, efficient, feminine and altruistic as well mirroring the 'natural' caring and mothering role.[46]

By the 1940s, Australian nurses were invariably female and trained in schools of nursing within the larger teaching public hospitals. Rigid hierarchical structures were also a feature throughout the training period. Helen Gregory notes that even after the Second World War, the rigidness of the nursing hierarchy, long hours of duty, lectures in nurses' own time and shift work remained in place.[47] Yet in the late 1940s a plethora of nursing organisations existed and Russell Smith suggests that 'their functions were overlapping and they were intent on maintaining their own position'.[48] The Australasian Trained Nurses Association, originally set up in New South Wales but subsequently established in the majority of states and together with the Victorian Trained Nurses Association, set the syllabus for hospital-based courses, arranged entrance examinations and approved hospitals as training institutions. Some nurse leaders were trying to improve the education and professional status of nurses.[49] Such struggles occurred in Victoria with establishing the College of Nursing, Australia and in New South Wales with a separate college of nursing being established in 1949. Both colleges had a focus on post-graduate education and improving the nursing profession yet were unable to forgo their own position in favour of a national college for nursing until after the end of the twentieth century.[50]

Heather Harper suggests that two images were prevalent among the nurses who joined the Australian war effort during the Second World War: the 'angel of mercy' and the nurse as 'patriotic heroine'.[51] Harper adds that the visual image of the ministering angel was inseparable from the ideal of tenderness, obedience, dedication, self-sacrifice and a disregard for monetary rewards. Hence, all the qualities of a 'good nurse' in the military were equated with those of a 'good woman' and the images of nursing and Florence Nightingale were intertwined.

Bomford writes that, in the aftermath of the Second World War, the Australian government insisted on the re-establishment of traditional gender roles and that women's work remained undervalued.[52] Nurses comprised one group that appeared unaffected by social changes wrought by female employment during and after the war with some continuing to serve in the military. From 1940, the RAAF Nursing Service was accepted as a separate women's service with its own rules on discipline, accommodation and a lesser rate of pay than male counterparts. Research suggests that the RAAF nurses from this time were women from middle-class backgrounds.[53] The RAAF hierarchy, both male and female, ensured that only the 'right type' of women were recruited and that their behaviour was closely regulated structurally both in their work and living environments. The officer status of the nurses carried with it an expected level of behaviour and leadership in both environments. The character of the 'good nurse' was reinforced and reproduced by the Matron-in-Chief of the RAAF Nursing Service and other nursing leaders who conformed to the prevailing social standards, and by the government and the male military hierarchy.[54] They reinforced these standards through recruitment of nurses of a similar background, the provision of leadership and discipline through a nursing hierarchy and by ensuring that the nurses lived separate and protected lives, suitable for officers and ladies. From the nurses' perspective, the concepts of 'lady' and 'virtue' defined their behaviour and their lives both professionally and socially. The nurses accepted this as 'the way it was'.[55]

The RAAF flight nurse role was modelled on the US model in which registered nurses led the flight team because of the shortage of doctors.[56] The role was detailed in RAAF policies on medical air evacuation and this enabled the nurses to work as part of US or British flight teams when required, one example being when Sister Nathalie Oldham worked with the 801st MAES. The nurses were selected by the nursing hierarchy to undertake the flight nurse training and this depended on a well-reported performance as a RAAF nurse in the formal performance reports and information obtained from the nursing chain of command. The expectation was that the trained flight nurse could be expected to do the 'right thing' under all circumstances.[57] One example was described by Senior Sister Lucy Rule when talking about two air evacuation trips she took into Korea, accompanied by an experienced male nursing orderly,[58] even though she was not trained as flight nurse at that time. She states: 'I would have done more if I'd known that I was allowed. I said to Matron "Why on earth wasn't I trained? Because if an aircraft went down, they would say why wasn't she trained" How would it look if I wasn't trained?'[59] Senior Sister Lucy Rule showed that she was well aware of the responsibilities and boundaries of her role in her position in Japan but wished she could have done more air evacuations while in Japan. This was one example where the nurse stepped outside of the behaviour expected of her.

During the specially designed flight nurse course the nurses were given specific training for their new role and responsibilities. Thus the RAAF flight nurses assumed the lead position and, at times, in consultation with medical staff, took responsibility for decisions concerning the fitness of patients to fly and the nature of in-flight care. The autonomous and extended role of flight nurses was very different to the usual nursing role in settings such as hospitals where the nurse was subservient to the doctor. Flight nurses readily accepted the autonomy and extension of the traditional nursing role during the Korean War. They were prepared to make decisions concerning the fitness of their patients and regarded air evacuation as an exciting new area of nursing.[60] At the same time, flight nurses accepted that they also had nursing roles within the medical facilities in Iwakuni that involved additional duties when they were not flying. These nurses responded eagerly to the opportunity to adapt and expand the traditional nursing role.[61] However, they were also accepting of the more subservient role of the nurse in the traditional hospital setting in Japan.

While readily accepting the responsibilities of the flight nurse role, the nurses were irked by the fact that, unlike the male crew members, they were not entitled to flight pay.[62] In their eyes this amounted to a lack of recognition of their role. While supported at unit level, a submission for flight pay for nurses that went to Treasury in January 1953 was not approved,[63] and they retained their lower pay level for the duration of the Korean War.

The work of these flight nurses was mainly invisible until the 1990s when some of the nurses interviewed began telling their stories. One wonders why the nurses' stories of their work and lives were unheard before this time. For Australians, the Korean War is often referred to as the 'forgotten war' and the nation as a whole was not involved.[64] Joy Damousi in discussing the question of silence in *Living with the Aftermath* suggests that for many veterans silence masked an anguish of the horrors experienced and was often left unarticulated.[65] This could possibly be one reason why nurses did not relate the total picture of their experiences or injuries treated. Sister Mabel Wilson had told her mother that she was going to Japan. She replied: 'Mabel, it is lovely for you to fly there', but Mabel didn't tell her the rest of it. She believed that her mother would have been horrified if she knew she'd been in Korea where people were being killed.[66]

Conclusion

The flight nurse role in Australia was first established in the Second World War, although it was scaled down within the RAAF at war's end. The RAAF recommenced flight nurse training in 1949 and soon newly graduated flight nurses were posted to Iwakuni for duty in Japan as members of BCOF. Australia assumed responsibility for evacuating British Commonwealth casualties from Korea and took on other roles associated with air evacuation. From the period

January 1951 to July 1953, records show that a total of 11,828 patients were evacuated by RAAF nurses. The flight nurse role itself continued to evolve during the war and challenged the parameters of the traditional nursing role.

The development of the CAEF near the airfield in Seoul was an innovation for the Australians and resulted from recognition of the need for improved patient care. Its establishment also saw the RAAF flight nurses move forward into Korea on short-term deployments. Equipment for the air evacuation flights changed according to need, with items such as the flight pannier developed locally and, proving robust and ideally suited to its task, serving on into the future.

The RAAF flight nurse role was established as a female gender role based on the social context of the time, which helped to shape the role and the behaviour of the flight nurses both professionally and socially. This was reinforced by the guidance provided by the RAAF Nursing Service leaders of the time. The social system ensured that the nurse was 'virtuous' and perpetuated the 'good nurse, good woman' concept. However, nurses embraced opportunities to broaden their experience and increase their knowledge within the constraints of the time.[67] Despite these social and structural constraints of being a nurse in the military, flight nurses performed remarkably well, often in stressful and harsh conditions, and worked long hours. Their significant contribution to Australia's casualty evacuation system in the Korean War is still not widely known.

Biographical details of RAAF flight nurses interviewed

Lucy Boland (née Rule)

Sr Lucy Rule N50220 trained at Longreach Hospital and the Brisbane Women's Hospital in Queensland before being appointed to the RAAFNS on 16 March 1942. She was promoted to Senior Sister on 3 January 1947. She was posted to Japan as the Senior Sister on 10 January 1950 and returned to RAAF Station Amberley (near Brisbane) on 7 May 1951. Lucy undertook medical air evacuation training in February 1952. She was awarded an Associate of the Royal Red Cross (ARRC) in 1952 for her work in Japan, Her appointment in the RAAFNS was terminated on 1 October 1952.

Joy Carmody (née Salter)

Sr Joy Salter N504649 was appointed to the RAAFNS on 8 November 1948 and completed the second Air Evacuation and Air Sea Rescue Course after the Second World War. She was posted to Iwakuni, Japan from October 1950 to October 1951 where she undertook operating theatre duties as well as air evacuation duties. She was discharged on 20 June 1952.

Eunice Feil

Sr Eunice Feil N11484 trained at Toowoomba General Hospital and the Brisbane Women's Hospital. She also completed maternal and Child Welfare and Infectious Diseases training prior to being appointed to the RAAFNS on 28 March 1949. She completed the first medical air evacuation course after the Second World War in May 1949 and was posted to Japan from April 1951 to March 1952. She was discharged on 27 March 1953.

Gay Halstead (née Bury)

Sr Gay Bury N35305 trained at Royal Melbourne Hospital and was appointed to the RAAFNS on 5 March 1951. Sr Bury completed Air Evacuation and Air Sea Rescue Course in May 1951. She was posted to Japan on 17 April 1953 and was deployed for a two-month period to Korea returning to Japan on 7 July 1953. She was discharged from the RAAFNS on 13 April 1954.

Elizabeth Marchant (née Baldwin)

Sr Elizabeth Baldwin N500529 trained at the Alfred Hospital (Melbourne) before being appointed to the RAAFNS on 9 April 1944. She completed the No. 3 Medical Air Evacuation (MAETU) Course before being posted to Air Evacuation Station at Garbutt (Townsville) on 11 June 1945 for air evacuation duties. She assisted in evacuating prisoners of war back to Australia in 1945. She was tutor sister for air evacuation training in 1951 and was discharged on 5 November 1951.

Cathie Thompson (née Daniel)

Sr Cathie Daniel N12427 trained at Albury District Hospital and Royal Women's Hospital in Melbourne prior to being appointed to the RAAFNS on 6 November 1950. She was also operating theatre trained. After completing No. 5 Medical Evacuation Course in February 1952, she was posted to Japan on 27 March 1952. She was attached to the CAEF in Korea from late October 1952 until late December 1952. She was discharged from the RAAFNS on 5 November 1954.

Nathalie Wittman (née Oldham)
Sr Nathalie Oldham N35859) trained at Mildura Hospital and the Royal Women's Hospital, Melbourne and had completed an Infectious Diseases Certificate before being appointed to the RAAFNS on 28 March 1949. She completed a medical air evacuation course in February 1952 prior to being posted to Japan. During her time in Japan, Sr Oldham was deployed to work in Korea for two months. She returned to Australia on 6 April 1953 and was discharged on 20 November 1953.

Mabel Wilson
Sr Mabel Wilson trained at the Brisbane General Hospital and the Brisbane Women's Hospital before joining the RAAFNS on 1 March 1950. She completed the Air Evacuation and Air Sea Rescue Course in August 1950 and was posted to Japan on 5 October 1951. She returned on posting to Australia on 12 January 1953 and was discharged on completion of her Short Service Commission on 24 February 1954.

Notes

1 The registered nurses were known as, and were called, 'Sister' during the period of the Korean War.
2 Maxine Dahl, 'Air evacuation in war: The Role of RAAF nurses undertaking air evacuation of casualties between 1943–1953' (unpublished PhD thesis, Queensland University of Technology, Brisbane, 2009), 292.
3 Officer Commanding No. 91 (Composite) Wing, Iwakuni, 'Formation of Air Evacuation Team at K16, "British Commonwealth Casualty Evacuation Flight Proposed Formation – Information"', National Archives of Australia, A12124: 3/8/Air Pt 1, dated 2 April 1953, 1.
4 Interview with Cathie Thompson (nee Daniel), by Maxine Dahl at Wagga Wagga on 13 June 1997. Recording held by RAAF Museum.

5 Gay Halstead, *Story of the RAAF Nursing Service 1940–1990* (Metung, Victoria, Nungurner Press Pty Ltd, 1994), 288.

6 Janette Bomford, *Soldiers of the Queen: Women of the Australian Army* (South Melbourne, Victoria, Oxford University Press, 2001), 10.

7 Details of the ex-RAAF nurses who served in Japan and Korea and who were interviewed are at the end of this chapter.

8 Interview with Lucy Boland (nee Rule) by Maxine Dahl at Brisbane on 12 August 2004. Recording held by interviewee.

9 SMO BCOF, Korea, Monthly Medical Report, June, 1952, National Archives of Australia: Department of Defence; A705, 132/2/866 Part 5, Monthly Reports.

10 Interview with Cathie Thompson (nee Daniel) by Maxine Dahl at Wagga Wagga 1 October 2004. Recording held by interviewee.

11 Telephone interview with J. Carmody (née Salter), by Maxine Dahl on 28 May 2004.

12 'Formation of Air Evacuation Team at K16', National Archives of Australia, A12124: 3/8/Air Pt 1, 1.

13 'Formation of Air Evacuation Team at K16', National Archives of Australia, A12124: 3/8/Air Pt 1, 1.

14 Unit History Records, No. 391 Base Squadron, RAAF Historical Section, OP 0064.

15 Notes from Air Commodore D. Hitchens to Maxine Dahl dated 12 August 2007. Notes held by author.

16 Dahl, 'Air evacuation in war', 246.

17 Department of Veterans' Affairs, *Out in the Cold: Australia's Involvement in the Korean War 1950–53* (Department of Veterans' Affairs, Canberra, 2001), 67.

18 Interview with Cathie Thompson, 13 June 1997.

19 Interview with Nathalie Wittman (nee Oldham), by Maxine Dahl at Canberra on 11 July 1997. Recording held by RAAF Museum.

20 Squadron Leader D. A. S. Morgan, 'Evacuation of Casualties in Korea' (RAAF Museum, handmade book, n.d.).

21 National Archives of Australia, A12124: 3/8/Air Pt 1, dated 2 April 1953, 4.

22 Halstead, *Story of the RAAF Nursing Service 1940–1990*, 381.

23 Interview with Eunice Feil, by Maxine Dahl at Brisbane on 17 February 2005.

24 Medical Training Unit, Syllabus 1950, National Archives of Australia, A705; 208/78/165.

25 Interview with Elizabeth Marchant (née Baldwin), by Maxine Dahl at Melbourne on 25 January 2004. Recording held by interviewee.

26 Department of Defence, RAAF Historical Section, Base Squadron Point Cook, Unit History Sheets 1949–1950, Rolls 168 and 170.

27 Department of Defence, RAAF Historical Section, Air Board Orders Section A – Administrative; A. 154 – Casualty Air Evacuation (132/1/1080, 24

November 1952). This Air Board Order allocates responsibilities for air evacuation during peace and war.

28 Dahl, 'Air evacuation in war', 267.
29 Interview with Eunice Feil, 17 February 2005.
30 Dahl, 'Air evacuation in war', 267.
31 Interview with Cathie Thompson, 13 June 1997.
32 Dahl, 'Air evacuation in war', 227.
33 Interview with Cathie Thompson, 13 June 1997.
34 Interview with Cathie Thompson, 13 June 1997.
35 Interview with Nathalie Wittman, 11 July 1997.
36 Interview with Nathalie Wittman, 11 July 1997.
37 Interview with Nathalie Wittman, 11 July 1997.
38 Interview with Nathalie Wittman, 11 July 1997.
39 Interview with Cathie Thompson, 13 June 1997.
40 Interview with Cathie Thompson, 13 June 1997.
41 Interview with Gay Halstead, by Maxine Dahl at Metung on 4 August 1997.
42 Interview with Eunice Feil, 17 February 2005.
43 Interview with Mabel Wilson, by Maxine Dahl at Brisbane on 13 August 2004. Recording held by interviewee.
44 Interview with Nathalie Wittman, 11 July 1997.
45 Sheryl Delacour, 'The construction of nursing ideology, discourse, and representation', in G. Gray and G. Pratt (eds), *Towards a Discipline of Nursing* (Melbourne, Churchill Livingstone, 1991).
46 Solomon Encel, Norman MacKenzie and Margaret Tebbutt, *Women and Society: An Australian Study* (Melbourne, Cheshire Publishing Pty Ltd, 1974).
47 Helen Gregory, *A Tradition of Care: A History of Nursing at the Royal Brisbane Hospital* (Brisbane, Boolarong Publications, 1988), 94.
48 Russell G. Smith, *In Pursuit of Nursing Excellence: A History of the Royal College of Nursing, Australia 1949–99* (South Melbourne, Victoria, Oxford University Press, 1999), 29.
49 Annette Summers, *Wartime Problems: The South Australian Nurses Registration Board During the Second World War, 1939–1945* (Monograph 2 – Nurses Board of South Australia, Adelaide), 25.
50 Rosalie Pratt and R. Lynette Russell, *A Voice to be Heard: The First Fifty Years of the New South Wales College of Nursing* (Crows Nest, NSW, Allen & Unwin, 2002), 17.
51 Heather Harper, *'Ministering Angels': Australian Nurses and the Nightingale Image during World War II*, Proceedings of the Queensland Nursing History Conference: Queensland Nurses – At War and on the Home Front 1939–1945 (Brisbane, 1995), 20.
52 Bomford, *Soldiers of the Queen*, 7.
53 Dahl, 'Air evacuation in war', 109.

54 Dahl, 'Air evacuation in war', 102.
55 Dahl, 'Air evacuation in war', 288.
56 Dahl, 'Air evacuation in war', 108.
57 Dahl, 'Air evacuation in war', 265.
58 Nursing orderlies were trained second-level nurses who were medical air evacuation trained and possibly with extensive experience in air evacuation.
59 Dahl, 'Air evacuation in war', 219.
60 Interview with Cathie Thompson, 1 October 2004.
61 Dahl, 'Air evacuation in war', 281.
62 Dahl, 'Air evacuation in war', 277.
63 National Archives of Australia, A705, 161/1/2852, Flying pay – RAAF Nursing Service, folio 6A – Royal Australian Air Force Nursing Service – Flying pay dated 8 August 1952 and folio 8A Entitlement to flying pay – RAAF Nursing Service, dated 21 January 1953.
64 Lieutenant-General Sir Thomas Daly KBE, CB, DSO in Foreword to *Korea Remembered*, compiled by Maurice Pears and Fred Kirkland (NSW, Combined Arms training and Development Centre, Georges Height, 1998), iii.
65 Joy Damousi, *Living with the Aftermath: Trauma, Nostalgia and Grief in Post-War Australia* (Cambridge, Cambridge University Press, 2001), 99.
66 Interview with Mabel Wilson, 13 August 2004.
67 Dahl, 'Air evacuation in war', 281.

Select bibliography

Archives

Albert and Shirley Small Library, University of Virginia, Charlottesville, VA, USA

Alderman Library, University of Virginia, Charlottesville, VA, USA

Alfred Hospital Nursing Archives, Sydney, NSW, Australia

Army Medical Museum Archives, Keogh Barracks, Aldershot, UK

Australian War Memorial, Canberra, Australia

British Library, London

Charing Cross Hospital, London

Convent of Mercy, Bermondsey, London

Cornwall Record Office

Department of Defence, Australia

Florence Nightingale Museum

Great Britain, House of Commons, Parliamentary Papers, 1854–55, 1864

Imperial War Museum Archives, London

J. S. Battye Library of West Australian History

Library and Archives Canada

National Archives and Records Administration (NARA), Washington, DC, USA

National Archives of Australia

National Archives of Norway

Plymouth and West Devon Record Office

Red Cross Archives, London

Richmond National Battle Field Park Headquarters, Archives at the Chimborazo Hospital Museum Richmond, VA, USA

State Library of Victoria, Australia

War Department Collection of Confederate Records

Wellcome Archives, London

Oral history interviews

First World War

Curwood, E. I., interview by Vicky Hobbs, 27 October 1975. OH183, J. S. Battye Library of West Australian History, Oral History Programme.

Spanish Civil War

Buckoke, Lillian (née Urmston), interview, Tameside Local Studies Library, Stalybridge, 203.

Craig, Thora (née Silverthorne), interview, Imperial War Museum Sound Archive, London, 13770.

Edney, Patience (née Darton), interview Imperial War Museum Sound Archive, London, 8398.

Edney, Patience (née Darton), interview by Angela Jackson at London on 18 March 1994 and 8 March 1996.

Feiwel, Penny (née Phelps, pen name Fyvel), interview by Angela Jackson at Bournemouth on 22 February 1996.

Green, Nan, interview, Imperial War Museum Sound Archive, London, 13799.

Purser, Joan, interview, Imperial War Museum Sound Archive, London, 13795.

Second World War

Allen, Alice, interviewed by David Justham at Sheffield on 14 July 2008. Began SRN training in London in 1942 (transcript held at UK Centre for the History of Nursing and Midwifery (UKCHNM), University of Manchester).

Bennett, Barbara, interviewed by David Justham at Dyserth on 15 July 2008. Began SRN training in Manchester in 1938 (transcript held at UKCHNM, University of Manchester).

Clark, Carol, interviewed by David Justham at Abergele on 16 July 2008. Began SRN training in Manchester in 1934 (transcript held at UKCHNM, University of Manchester).

Evans, Edith, interviewed by David Justham at Lymm on 18 July 2008. Began SRN training in Manchester in 1936 (transcript held at UKCHNM, University of Manchester).

Farmer, Florence, interviewed by David Justham at Preston on 4 August 2008 at Preston. Began SRN training in Manchester in 1936 (transcript held at UKCHNM, University of Manchester).

Harris, Hilary, interviewed by David Justham at Clitheroe on 6 August 2008. Began SRN training in Manchester in 1934 (transcript held at UKCHNM, University of Manchester).

Jones, Jane, interviewed by David Justham at Preston on 6 August 2008. Began SRN training in Manchester in 1944 (transcript held at UKCHNM, University of Manchester).

King, Kate, interviewed by David Justham at Heswall on 7 August 2008. Began SRN training in Manchester in 1939 (transcript held at UKCHNM, University of Manchester).

Lloyd, Louise, interviewed by David Justham at Grantham on 12 August 2008. Began SRN training in Leicester in 1940 (transcript held at UKCHNM, University of Manchester).

Newton, Nancy, interviewed by David Justham at Sturton by Stow on 19 December 2008 at. Began SRN training in London in the early 1940s (transcript held at UKCHNM, University of Manchester).

Porter, Phyllis, interviewed by David Justham at Nottingham on 24 May 2010. Began SRN training in Nottingham in 1939 (transcript held at UKCHNM, University of Manchester).

Reed, Rita, interviewed by David Justham at Nottingham on 18 May 2010. Began SRN training in Nottingham in 1943 (transcript held at UKCHNM, University of Manchester).

Shaw, Susan, interviewed by David Justham at Nottingham on 18 May 2010. Began SRN training in Nottingham in 1943 (transcript held at UKCHNM, University of Manchester).

Taylor, Thelma, interviewed by David Justham at Nottingham on 24 May 2010. Began SRN training in Nottingham in 1943 (transcript held at UKCHNM, University of Manchester).

Vickers, Violet, interviewed by David Justham at Nottingham on 24 May 2010. Began SRN training in Nottingham in 1947 (Transcript held at UKCHNM, University of Manchester).

Woods, Wendy, interviewed by David Justham at Nottingham on 1 June 2010. Began SRN training in Nottingham in 1950 (transcript held at UKCHNM, University of Manchester).

HX2, interviewed by Graham Thurgood on 25 July 2001. Data extracted 19 July 2010 (transcript held at Huddersfield, University of Huddersfield Archives).

HX5, interviewed by Graham Thurgood on 8 August 2001. Data extracted 19 July 2010 (transcript held at Huddersfield, University of Huddersfield Archives).

HX6, interviewed by Graham Thurgood on 17 August 2001. Data extracted 19 July 2010 (transcript held at Huddersfield, University of Huddersfield Archives).

Korean War

Årdalsbakke, Inga, interviewed by Jan-Thore Lockertsen at Skei on 7 December 2011. Recording held by interviewee.

Boland, Lucy (née Rule), interviewed by Maxine Dahl at Brisbane on 12 August 2004. Recording held by interviewee.

Carmody, Joy (née Salter), interviewed by Maxine Dahl on the telephone on 28 May 2004.

Feil, Eunice, interviewed by Maxine Dahl at Brisbane on 17 February 2005. Recording held by interviewee.

Halstead, Gay (née Bury), interviewed by Maxine Dahl at Metung on 4 August 1997. Recording held by RAAF Museum.

Isaksen, Margot, interviewed by Jan-Thore Lockertsen at Greverud on 27 November 2012. Recording held by interviewee.

Kleppstad, Kari Roll, interviewed by Jan-Thore Lockertsen at Leknes on 31 March 2010. Recording held by interviewee.

Lexow, Peter B., interviewed by Jan-Thore Lockertsen by mail on 3 March 2013. Recording held by interviewer.

Marchant, Elizabeth (née Baldwin), interviewed by Maxine Dahl at Melbourne on 25 January 2004. Recording held by interviewee.

Semb, Gerd, interviewed by Jan-Thore Lockertsen at Lørenskog on 22 October 2011. Recording held by interviewee.

Thompson, Cathie (née Daniel), interviewed by Maxine Dahl at Wagga Wagga on 13 June 1997. Recording held by RAAF Museum.

Thompson, Cathie (née Daniel), interviewed by Maxine Dahl at Wagga Wagga on 1 October 2004. Recording held by interviewee.

Wilson, Mabel, interviewed by Maxine Dahl at Brisbane on 13 August 2004. Recording held by interviewee.

Wittman, Nathalie (née Oldham), interviewed by Maxine Dahl at Canberra on 11 July 1997. Recording held by RAAF Museum.

Primary and secondary sources

Abbott, W. N., 'Sequelae of gas poisoning', *The British Medical Journal* 2 (1938), 597.

Abel-Smith, Brian, *A History of the Nursing Profession* (London, Heinemann, 1964).

Abrahams, Adolphe, 'The later effects of gas poisoning', *The Lancet* 200, 5174 (28 October 1922), 933–4.

Abrams, Lynn, *Oral History Theory* (London, Routledge, 2010).

Adami, J. George, *War Story of the Canadian Army Medical Corps* (London, Colour Ltd and the Roll's House Publishing Co Ltd, for the Canadian War Records Office, 1918).

Anderton, G., 'The birth of the British Commonwealth Division Korea', *Journal of the Royal Army Medical Corps* (London, BMJ Group, January 1953), 43–54.

Andrews, Charles T., *A Dark Awakening: A History of St Lawrence's Hospital, Bodmin* (London, Cox & Wyman, 1978).

Anonymous, 'The nursing of our soldiers', *Nursing Notes: A Practical Journal for Nurses* 23, 147 (1 March 1900), 33.

Anonymous, 'Bloemfontein sister, army nursing notes', *The Nursing Record and Hospital World* 24, 632 (12 May 1900), 376.

Anonymous, 'Army nursing notes', *The Nursing Record and Hospital World* 24, 633 (19 May 1900), 398.

Anonymous, 'Army nursing notes', *The Nursing Record and Hospital World* 24, 635 (2 June 1900), 437.

Anonymous, 'War notes', *Nursing Notes: A Practical Journal for Nurses* 23, 151 (1 July 1900), 91.

Anonymous, 'Army nursing notes', *The Nursing Record and Hospital World* 25, 648 (1 September 1900), 174.

Anonymous, 'The Royal Commission on South African hospitals', *British Medical Journal* (26 January 1901), 234.

Anonymous, 'Dietary of the sick room', *Una* I, 1 (April 1903), 16–20.

Anonymous, 'Detail nursing in case of typhoid fever', No. 2 examination paper answer, *Una* (28 February 1914), 324.

Anonymous, 'Dietetics', *Una* XII, 7 (30 September 1914), 215.

Anonymous [Evelyn Kate Luard], *Diary of a Nursing Sister on the Western Front 1914–1915* (Edinburgh and London, William Blackwood and Sons, 1915)

Anonymous, Column, *The British Journal of Nursing* 54 (1 May 1915), 368.

Anonymous, Column, *The British Journal of Nursing* 54 (8 May 1915), 383.

Anonymous, 'Asphyxiating Gases in War', *The Nursing Times* XI, 523 (8 May 1915), 549.

Anonymous, 'Gas poisoning', *The Nursing Times* XI, 524 (15 May 1915), 585.

Anonymous, Editorial, *The British Journal of Nursing* 54 (15 May 1915), 423.

Anonymous, 'Food value of cheese', *Una* XIII, 10 (30 December 1915), 322.

Anonymous, 'Best answers to medical paper', *Una* (28 February 1917), 377.

Anonymous, 'Savory broths and meat jellies for the sick', *Una* XV, 9 (30 November 1917), 285.

Anonymous, *A War Nurse's Diary: Sketches from a Belgian Field Hospital* (New York, The Macmillan Company, 1918).

Anonymous, Column [Quoting from a letter to the *Australasian Nurses' Journal*] *Nursing Times*, (16 February 1918), 205.

Anonymous, 'Extracts from letters', *Una* XVI, 2 (30 April 1918), 39.

Anonymous, Column, *The British Journal of Nursing* 61 (19 October 1918), 232.

Anonymous, 'Letters: Help for horror camps', *Nursing Mirror* (12 May 1945), 82.

A. N. R., 'Our foreign letter Chieveley, Natal', *The Nursing Record and Hospital World* 24, 637 (16 June 1900), 483.

Andresen, Ruth, *Fra norsk sanitets historie: sjefsøster forteller om kvinners innsats i militær sykepleie* (Oslo, NKS-forlaget, 1986).

Anker, Herman, 'Morgenstillhetens land', Pedersen, Lorentz Ulrik (ed.) *Norge i Korea* (Oslo, C. Huitfeldt forlag AS, 1991).

Apel, Otto F, jr. and Apel, Pat, *MASH An Army Surgeon in Korea* (Lexington, KY, The University Press of Kentucky, 1998).

Asbjørnsen, Lars Bakke, *Fjellet med de fallende blomster – Skisser fra Korea* (Oslo, Fabritius & sønner, 1952).

Ashdown A. Millicent, *A Complete System of Nursing* (London, J. M. Dent & Sons Ltd, 1928).

Ayliffe Graham, A. J. and English, Mary P., *Hospital Infection: From Miasmas to MRSA* (Cambridge, Cambridge University Press, 2003).

Bacot, Ada, *Confederate Nurse*, edited by Jean V. Berlin (Columbia, SC, University of South Carolina Press, 1994).

Baroness de T'Serclaes, *Flanders and Other Fields* (London, George G. Harrap and Co. Ltd, 1964).

Barsoum, Noha and Kleeman, Charles, 'Now and then, the history of parental fluid administration', *The American Journal of Nephrology* 22 (2002), 284–9.

Barwell, M. S. (Nursing Sister), Minutes of Evidence (30.07.1900) *Report of the Royal Commission Appointed to Consider and Report upon the Care and Treatment of the Sick and Wounded during the South Africa Campaign: Presented to both Houses of Parliament by Command of Her Majesty* (London, HMSO, 1901), 82.

Bashford, Alison, *Purity and Pollution: Gender, Embodiment and Victorian Medicine* (Houndmills, Macmillan Press Ltd, 1998).

Bassett, Jan, *Guns and Brooches Australian Army Nursing from the Boer War to the Gulf War* (Melbourne, Oxford University Press, 1997).

Baumgart, Winfried, *The Crimean War 1853–56* (London, Arnold, 1999).

Beardwell, Myrtle, *Aftermath* (Ilfracombe, Arthur H. Stockwell Ltd, *c.*1953).

Bedford Fenwick, Mrs, 'Enteric stalks the British Army', *The Nursing Record and Hospital World* 26, 675 (9 March 1901), 181.

Beer, Fannie A., *Memories: A Record of Personal Experience and Adventure during Four Years of War*, Kindle edn, 23 March 2011 (Philadelphia, J. B. Lippincott, 1888).

Bell, Sir George, *Soldier's Glory* (Tunbridge Wells, Kent, Spellmount, 1991).

Benner, Patricia, *Novice to Expert: Excellence and Power in Clinical Nursing Practice* (Menlo Park, CA, Addison-Wesley, 1984).

Ben-Sefer, Ellen, 'Surviving survival: Nursing care at Bergen-Belsen 1945', *Australian Journal of Advanced Nursing* 26, 3 (2009), 101–10.

Benton, Edward H., 'British surgery in the South African War: The work of Major Frederick Porter', *Medical History* 21, 3 (1977), 275–90.

Berkowitz, Carin, 'The beauty of anatomy: Displays and surgical education in early nineteenth-century London', *Bulletin of the History of Medicine* 85, 2 (2011), 250.

Bevington, Sheila M., *Nursing Life and Discipline: A Study Based on Over Five Hundred Interviews* (London, H. K. Lewis and Co. Ltd, 1943).

Bimko-Rosensaft, Hadassa, 'The children of Belsen', in *Belsen* (no editors acknowledged) (Tel Aviv, Israel, Irgun Sheerit Hapleita Me'haezor Habriti, 1957).

Bisset, Jean, 'Letter from Sister Bisset', *Una* XIII, 11 (29 January 1916), 346.

Black, J. Elliot, Glenny, Elliot T. and McNee, J. W., 'Observations on 685 cases of poisoning by noxious gases used by the enemy. With a note by Colonel Sir Wilmot Herringham', *The British Medical Journal* (31 July 1915), 165–7.

Blanton, Wyndham, *Medicine in Virginia in the Nineteenth Century* (Richmond, VA, Garrett & Massie, Inc., 1933).

Bomford, Janette, *Soldiers of the Queen: Women in the Australian Army* (Oxford University Press, Melbourne, 2001).

Bonham-Carter, Victor (ed.), *Surgeon in the Crimea* (London, Constable, 1968).

Booth, Jeremy, 'A short history of blood pressure measurement', *Proceedings of the Royal Society of Medicine* 70, 11 (November 1997), 793–9.

Bostridge, Mark, *Florence Nightingale: The Making of an Icon* (New York, Farrar, Straus and Giroux, 2008).

Bourke, Joanna, *Dismembering the Male: Men's Bodies, Britain and the Great War* (London, Reaktion Books Ltd, 1999).

Bowden, Jean, *Grey Touched with Scarlet: The War Experiences of the Army Nursing Sisters* (London, Robert Hale Ltd, 1959).

Boylston, Helen Dore, *'Sister': The War Diary of a Nurse* (New York, Ives Washburn, 1927).

Braybon, Gail and Summerfield, Penny, *Out of the Cage: Women's Experiences in Two World Wars* (London and New York, Pandora, 1987).

Brewer, James, *The Confederate Negro: Virginia's Craftsmen and Military Laborers, 1861–1865* (Tuscaloosa, AL, The University of Alabama Press, 1969).

Brittain, Vera, *Testament of Youth* (London, Virago, 1978 [1933]).

Britten, Jessie D., *Practical Notes on Nursing Procedures* (Edinburgh, E. & S. Livingstone Ltd, 1957).

Broadbent, Walter, 'Some results of German gas poisoning', *The British Medical Journal* 2 (14 August 1915), 247.

Brooks, Jane, '"Uninterested in anything except food": The work of nurses feeding the liberated inmates of Bergen-Belsen', *Journal of Clinical Nursing* 21 (2012), 2958–65.

Brown, Kevin, *Fighting Fit: Health, Medicine and War in the Twentieth Century* (Stroud, The History Press, 2008).

Brown, Thomas J., *Dorothea Dix New England Reformer* (Boston, MA, Harvard University Press, 1998).

Bryce, Charles, *England and France Before Sevastopol* (London, John Churchill, 1857).

Burdett-Coutts, William, *The Sick and Wounded in South Africa: What I Saw and Said of Them and of the Army Medical System* (London, Cassell & Co., 1900).

Burdett-Coutts, William, 'Our wars and our wounded', *The Times* 36179 (27 June 1900), 4.

Butler, A. G., *Official History of the Australian Army Medical Services 1914–1918*, vols I–III (Canberra, Australian War Memorial, 1938–43).

Canney, Leigh, 'Typhoid in the Army', *The Times*, no. 36540 (1901), 8.

Canney, Leigh, *Typhoid the Destroyer of Armies and its Abolition Opinions of the Military, Medical and General Press The House of Commons August 17th 1901 The Times* (London, no publisher identified, 1901), E5256, V 9.661.

Cantlie, Neil, *A History of the Army Medical Department*, 2 vols (Edinburgh, Churchill Livingstone, 1974).

Carpenter, Mick, *Working for Health: The History of the Confederation of Health Service Employees* (London, Lawrence & Wishart, 1988).

Celinscak, Mark, 'At war's end: Allied forces at Bergen-Belsen' (unpublished PhD thesis, Toronto, York University, 2012).

Chamberlain, Mrs Richard, 'Condition of base hospitals', *The Nursing Record* 25, 649 (8 September 1900), 189.

Chesnut, Mary, *Mary Chesnut's Civil War*, edited by C. Vann Woodward (New Haven, CT, Yale University Press, 1981).

Cheyne, J., 'Medical Report of the Hardwicke Fever Hospital 1817', in *Dublin Hospital Reports* 1 (1818).

Clampett, Muriel E., *My Dear Mother* (Melbourne, Muriel Clampett, 1992).

Clark-Kennedy, A. E., *The London*, 2 vols (Pitman Medical Publishing, 1962–63).

Clifford, Claudette (ed.), *QE Nurse 1938–1957* (Studley, Brewin Books, 1997).

Clinton, Catherine, *The Plantation Mistress: Woman's World in the Old South* (New York, Pantheon Books, a division of Random House, 1982).

Cohen, Boaz, '"And I was only a child": Children's testimonies, Bergen-Belsen 1945', *Holocaust Studies: A Journal of Culture and History* 12, 1–2 (2006), 153–69.

Collis, W. R. F., 'Belsen camp: A preliminary report', *British Medical Journal* (9 June 1945), 814–16.

Compton, Piers, *Colonel's Lady & Camp Follower* (London, Robert Hale, 1970).

Conan Doyle, Arthur, *The Great Boer War* (London, Smith, Elder & Co., 1900).

Conan Doyle, Arthur, 'The Epidemic of Enteric Fever at Bloemfontein', *British Medical Journal* 2, 2062 (7 July 1900), 49–50.

Coni, Nicholas, *Medicine and Warfare: Spain, 1936–1939* (London, Routledge/ Cañada Blanch Studies on Contemporary Spain, 2008).

Connolly, Maire A. and Heyman, David L., 'Deadly comrades: War and infectious diseases', *The Lancet Supplement* 360 (2002), 23–3.

Cook, G. C., 'Influence of diarrhoeal disease on military and naval campaigns', *Journal of the Royal Society of Medicine* 94 (2001), 95–7.

Cooke, Miriam and Woollacott, Angela (eds), *Gendering War Talk* (Princeton, MA, Princeton University Press, 1993).

Cornell, Judith and Russell, R. Lynette (eds), *Letters from Belsen 1945: An Australian Nurse's Experiences with the Survivors of War, Muriel Knox Doherty* (St Leonards, NSW, Allen & Unwin, 2000).

Coski, John, 'Stroll through the streets or through the collections to meet the women of wartime Richmond', *The Museum of the Confederacy Magazine* (Spring 2010), 18–20.

Cotton, Dorothy, 'A word picture of the Anglo-Russian Hospital, Petrograd', *Canadian Nurse* 22, 9 (1926), 486–8.

Craig, Oscar and Fraser, Alasdair, *Doctors at War* (County Durham, The Memoir Club, 2007).

Craven, Hannah, 'Horror in our time: Images of the concentration camps in the British media, 1945', *Historical Journal of Film, Radio and Television* 21, 3 (2001), 205–53.

Cross, Anthony, 'Forgotten British places in Petrograd/Leningrad', *Europa Orientalis* 5 (2004), part 1, 135–47.

Cullingworth, C. J., *Manual of Nursing Medical and Surgical* (London, Churchill, 1889).

Cumming, Kate, *A Journal of Hospital Life in the Confederate Army of Tennessee: From the Battle of Shiloh to the End of the War* (Louisville, KY, J. P. Morgan and Company, 1866).

Cumming, Kate, *Kate: The Journal of a Confederate Nurse*, ed. Richard Harwell (Baton Rouge, LA, Louisiana State University Press, 1998).

Cunningham, Horace, *Doctors in Gray: The Confederate Medical Service* (Baton Rouge, LA, Louisiana State University Press, 1993 [1958]).

Curtin, Philip D., *Disease and Empire The Health of European Troops in the Conquest of Africa* (Cambridge, Cambridge University Press, 1998).

Dahl, Maxine, 'Aeromedical Evacuation Nurses in the Korean War: Living Through the Experience' (unpublished Master's thesis, Deakin University, Geelong, 1997).

Dahl, Maxine, 'Air evacuation in war: The role of RAAF nurses undertaking air evacuation of casualties between 1943–1953' (unpublished PhD thesis, Queensland University of Technology, Brisbane, 2009).

Damousi, Joy, *Living with the Aftermath: Trauma, Nostalgia and Grief in Post-War Australia* (Cambridge University, 2001).

Darrow, Margaret H., 'French volunteer nursing and the myth of war experience in World War I', *American Historical Review* 101, 1 (February 1996), 80–106.

Das, Santanu, *Touch and Intimacy in First World War Literature* (Cambridge, Cambridge University Press, 2005).

Davies, William A., 'Typhus at Belsen: I. Control of the typhus epidemic', *American Journal of Hygiene* 46, 1 (July 1947), 66–83.

Delacour, Sheryl, 'The construction of nursing ideology, discourse, and representation', in G. Gray and G. Pratt (eds), *Towards a Discipline of Nursing* (Churchill Livingstone, Melbourne, 1991).

Department of Defence (Army), *Korea Remembers: The RAN, ARA and RAAF in the Korean War of 1950–1953* (Combined Arms Training and Development Centre, Georges Heights, NSW, 1998).

Department of Veterans' Affairs, *Out in the Cold: Australia's Involvement in the Korean War 1950-53* (Department of Veterans' Affairs, Canberra, 2001).

Dickens, Charles, *Martin Chuzzlewit*, Oxford World Classics, reprinted with forward notes by Margaret Cardwell (Oxford: Oxford University Press, 2011).

Dingwall, Robert, Rafferty, Anne Marie and Webster, Charles, *An Introduction to the Social History of Nursing* (London, Routledge, 1988).

Donner, Henriette, 'Under the Cross – Why VADs performed the filthiest task in the dirtiest war: Red Cross women volunteers, 1914-1918', *Journal of Social History* 30, 3 (Spring 1997), 687-704.

Dossey, Barbara, *Florence Nightingale: Mystic, Visionary, Healer* (Springhouse, Pennsylvania, Springhouse Corporation, 2000).

Douglas, Mary, *Purity and Danger: An Analysis of Concepts of Pollution and Taboo* (London, Routledge Classics, 2002).

Driscoll, Robert, S, 'US Army medical helicopters in the Korean War', *Military Medicine* (Bethesda, Maryland, April 2001), 290-6.

Driver, Kate, *Experience of a Siege: A Nurse Looks Back on Ladysmith* (South Africa, Ladysmith Historical Society, 1994).

Duncan, Ross, 'Case studies in emigration: Cornwall; Gloucestershire and New South Wales, 1877-1886', *Economic History Review* 16, 2 (1963), 272-89.

Edenhofer, Aurora (née Fernández), 'Unpublished short memoir, Prague', International Brigade Archive, Marx Memorial Library, London, January 1983.

Egelien, Nils, S, 'Dagbok fra Korea', in D. Leraand (ed.), *Intops – norske soldater internasjonale operasjoner* (Oslo, Forsvarmuseet, 2012) 186-90.

Enloe, Cynthia, *Does Khaki Become You? The Militarization of Women's Lives* (Boston, MA, South End Press, 1983).

Enloe, Cynthia, *Maneuvers: The International Politics of Militarizing Women's Lives* (Los Angeles, University of California Press, 2000).

Fause, Åshild, 'Utdanning eller gratisarbeid?', *Et fag i kamp for livet – Sykepleiens historie i Norge* (Bergen, Fagbokforlaget Vigmostad & Bjørke AS, 2002), 225-36.

Faust, Drew, *Mothers of Invention: Women of the Slaveholding South in the American Civil War* (Chapel Hill, NC, The University of North Carolina Press, 1996).

Fetherstonhaugh, R. C., *No. 3 Canadian General Hospital (McGill), 1914-1919* (Montreal, The Gazette Printing Company, 1928).

Fetherstonhaugh, R. C., *McGill University at War, 1914-1918, 1939-1945* (Montreal, McGill University Press, 1947).

Figes, Orlando, *The Crimean War* (New York, Henry Holt, 2010).

Fitzgerald, Gerard, 'Chemical Warfare and Medical Response During World War I', *American Journal of Public Health* 98, 4 (April 2008), 611-25.

Flanagan, Ben and Bloxham, Donald (eds), *Remembering Belsen: Eyewitnesses Record the Liberation* (London, Vallentine Mitchell, 2005).

Foote, Shelby, *The Civil War: A Narrative, Fort Sumter to Perryville* (New York, Vintage Books: A Division of Random House, 1986).

Foote, Shelby, *The Civil War: A Narrative, Fredericksburg to Meridian* (New York, Vintage Books: A Division of Random House, 1986).

Foote, Shelby, *The Civil War: A Narrative, Red River to Appomattox* (New York, Vintage Books: A Division of Random House, 1986).

Fortescue, J. W., *A History of the British Army*, 13 vols (London, Macmillan, 1899–1930).

Fox-Genovese, Elizabeth, *Within the Plantation Household: Black and White Women of the Old South – Gender and American Culture* (Durham, NC, The University of North Carolina Press, 1988).

Fremantle, Francis E., *Impressions of a Doctor in Khaki* (London, John Murray, 1901).

Fyrth, Jim and Alexander, Sally (eds), *Women's Voices from the Spanish Civil War* (London: Lawrence & Wishart, 1991).

Fyvel, Penny, *English Penny* (Ilfracombe, Devon, Arthur H. Stockwell Ltd, 1992).

Gabriel, Richard A. and Metz, Karen S., *A History of Military Medicine Vol. II From the Renaissance through Modern Times* (London, Greenwood Press, 1992).

Gamarnikow, Eva, 'Nurse or woman: Gender and professionalism in reformed nursing 1860–1923', in Pat Holden and Jenny Littlewood (eds), *Anthropology and Nursing* (London, Routledge, 1991).

Gardam, Judith and Charlesworth, Hilary, 'Protection of women in armed conflict', *Human Rights Quarterly* 22 (2000), 148–66.

Goodman, Martin, *Suffer and Survive* (London, Simon & Schuster, 2007).

Grayzel, Susan R., *Women and the First World War* (London, Longman, 2002).

Green, Carol, *Chimborazo: The Confederacy's Largest Hospital* (Knoxville, TN, The University of Tennessee Press, 2004).

Green, Nan, *A Chronicle of Small Beer: The Memoirs of Nan Green* (Nottingham, Trent Editions, 2005).

Gregory, Helen, *A Tradition of Care: A History of Nursing at the Royal Brisbane Hospital* (Brisbane, Boolarong Publications, 1988).

Gowing, Timothy, *A Voice from the Ranks* (Nottingham, privately printed, 1886).

Graves, Robert J., *Clinical Lectures on the Practice of Medicine*, 2nd edn, 2 vols (Dublin, Fannin, 1848).

Guenter, Risse, *Mending Bodies, Saving Souls: A History of Hospitals* (New York, Oxford University Press, 1999).

Gulbransen, Kaare, *Gull og grønne skoger* (Bergen, J. W. Eides forlag, 1956).

Guthrie, G. J., *Commentaries on the Surgery of the War*, 6th edn (London, Henry Renshaw, 1855).

Hagerman, Keppel, *Dearest of Captains: A Biography of Sally Louisa Tompkins* (Richmond, VA, Brandylane Publishers, 1996).

Hall, Richard H., *Women on the Civil War Battlefront* (Lawrence, KA, University Press of Kansas, 2006).

Hallquist, Deborah, L., 'Development in the RN first assistant role during the Korean War', *AORN Journal* 82 (October 2005), 644–7.

Halstead, Gay, *Story of the RAAF Nursing Service 1940–1990* (Nungurner Press Pty Ltd, Metung, Victoria, 1994).

Hardman, Lesley H. and Goodman, Cecily, *The Survivors: The Story of the Belsen Remnant* (London, Vallentine Mitchell, 1958).

Harmer, Michael, *The Forgotten Hospital: An Essay* (West Sussex, England, Springwood Books, 1982).

Harper, Heather, *'Ministering Angels': Australian Nurses and the Nightingale Image during World War II*, Proceedings of the Queensland Nursing History Conference: Queensland Nurses – At War and on the Home Front 1939–1945 (Brisbane, 1995).

Harris, Dora, Manuscript Diary (14.05.1900), 1976–11–17 National Army Museum.

Harris, Kirsty, *More than Bombs and Bandage: Australian Army Nurses at Work in World War I* (Newport NSW, BigSky Publishing, 2011).

Harrison, Brian, *Drink and the Victorians* (Pittsburgh, University of Pittsburgh Press, 1971).

Harrison, Mark, *Medicine and Victory: British Military Medicine in the Second World War* (Oxford, Oxford University Press, 2004).

Hart, Chris, *Behind the Mask: Nurses, Their Unions and Nursing Policy* (London, Baillière Tindall, 1994).

Hawes, Donald, *Who's Who in Dickens* (London, Routledge, 1998).

Hay, Ian, *One Hundred Years of Army Nursing: The Story of the British Army Nursing Services from the Time of Florence Nightingale to the Present Day* (London, Cassell & Company, 1953).

Hayward, T. E., 'A lecture to nurses on typhoid fever', *Nursing Notes A Practical Journal for Nurses* 22, 137 (1 May 1899), 61–3.

Hebblethwaite, A. Stuart, 'The treatment of chlorine gas poisoning by venesection', *The British Medical Journal* 2 (22 July 22), 107–9.

Helmstadter, Carol and Godden, Judith, *Nursing before Nightingale, 1815–1899* (Surrey, Ashgate Publishing Ltd, 2011).

Henrichsen, Hetty, 1952. 'Med norsk feltsykhus til Korea', *Sykepleien – organ for norsk sykepleier forbund* (Oslo, Norsk sykepleierforbund), 62–8.

Herringham, Sir Wilmot P., 'Gas poisoning', *The Lancet* 195, 5034 (21 February 1920), 423–4.

Helmstadter, Carol, 'Early nursing reform in nineteenth-century London: a doctor-driven phenomenon', *Medical History* 46, 3 (2002), 325–50.

Helmstadter, Carol and Godden, Judith, *Nursing Before Nightingale 1815–1899* (Farnham, Surrey, Ashgate, 2011).

Higonnet, Margaret R., 'Not so quiet in no-woman's land', in Miriam Cooke and Angela Woollacott (eds), *Gendering War Talk* (Princeton, Princeton University Press, 1993).

Higonnet, Margaret Randolph, Jenson, Jane, Michel, Sonya and Collins Weitz, Margaret (eds), *Behind the Lines: Gender and the Two World Wars* (New Haven, CT, Yale University Press,1987).

Hill, Douglas (ed.), *Letters from the Crimea* (Dundee, Dundee University Press, 2010).

Hill, Leonard, 'An address on gas poisoning. Read before the Medical Society of London', *British Medical Journal* 2 (4 December 1915), 801–4.

Hitch, Margaret, *Aids to Medicine for Nurses*, 2nd edn (London, Baillière, Tindall and Cox, 1943).

Holcombe, Lee, *Victorian Ladies at Work Middle-Class Working Women in England and Wales 1850–1914* (Devon, David & Charles (Holdings) Ltd, 1973).

Holmes, T., *A System of Surgery*, 4 vols (London, Parker and Son, 1860).

Hoppen, K. Theodore, *The Mid-Victorian Generation 1846–86* (Oxford, Oxford University Press, 1998).

Horder [The Lord] and A. E. Gow, *Bacterial Diseases*, in F. W. Price (ed.), *A Textbook of the Practice of Medicine*, 5th edn (London, Oxford University Press, 1937) 30.

Horwood, Janet G., 'The prevention of gas poisoning', *The British Medical Journal* (24 July 1915), 161.

Houghton, Marjorie, *Aids to Tray and Trolley Setting*, 2nd edn (London, Baillière Tindall and Cox, 1942).

Humphry, Laurence, *A Manual of Nursing Medical and Surgical* (London, Griffin, 1898).

Inder, W. S., *On Active Service with the S.J.A.B., South African War, 1899–1902* (Whitefish, MT, Kessinger Publishing, 2009).

Inglis, K. S., *Hospital and Community: A History of the Royal Melbourne Hospital* (Melbourne, Melbourne University Press, 1958).

Jackson, Angela, *British Women and the Spanish Civil War* (London and New York: Routledge/Cañada Blanch Studies on Contemporary Spain, 2002; revised pb edn, Barcelona: Warren & Pell Publishing/Cañada Blanch Studies on Contemporary Spain, 2009; published in Spanish as *Las mujeres británicas y la Guerra Civil española*, Valencia, Publicacions de la Universitat de València, 2010).

Jackson, Angela, *For us it was Heaven: The Passion, Grief and Fortitude of Patience Darton from the Spanish Civil War to Mao's China* (Brighton: Sussex

Academic Press, 2012; published in Spanish as *Para nosotros era el cielo. Pasión, dolor y fortaleza de Patience Darton de la guerra civil española a la China de Mao*, Barcelona, Ediciones San Juan de Dios, Campus Docent, 2012).

Jones, H. W., Hoerr, N. L. and Osol, A. (eds), *Blakiston's New Gould Medical Dictionary* (London, H. K. Lewis and Co. Ltd, 1951).

Kemp, Edward, *Report of the Ministry: Overseas Military Forces of Canada, 1918* (London, Overseas Military Forces of Canada, 1919).

King, Booker, 'The Mobile Army Surgical Hospital (MASH): A military and surgical legacy', *Journal of the National Medical Association* (2005), 648–56.

Kinglake, A. W., *The Invasion of the Crimea*, 9 vols (Edinburgh, Blackwood, 1891).

Knyvett Gordon, A., 'Notes on practical nursing', *The Nursing Record and Hospital World* 26, 674 (2 March 1901), 165.

Laffin, John, *Digger: The Legend of the Australian Soldier* (Melbourne, Macmillan Australia, revised edn, 1986).

Lasker-Wallfisch, Anita, 'A survivor's memories of liberation', *Holocaust Studies: A Journal of Culture and History* 12, 1–2 (2006), 22–6.

Lataster-Czisch, Petra, 'Patience Edney (née Darton)', in *Eigentlich rede ich nicht gern über mich (Lebenserinnegungen von Frauen aus dem Spanischen Bürgerkrieg 1936–1939)* (Leizpzig and Weimar, Gustav Kiepenheurer Verlag, 1990), 9–105.

Laurence, Eleanor Constance, *A Nurse's Life in War and Peace* (London, Smith, Elder & Co., 1912).

Lawler, Jocalyn, *Behind the Screens: Nursing, Somology, and the Problem of the Body* (Melbourne, Churchill Livingstone, 1991).

Lipscombe, F. M. (Colonel RAMC), 'Medical aspects of Belsen Concentration Camp', *The Lancet* (8 September 1945), 313–15.

Lister, Joseph, 'On the antiseptic principle in the practice of surgery', *The Lancet* 90, 2299 (21 September 1867), 352–6.

Lockertsen, Jan-Thore, 'Operasjonssykepleie ved Troms- og Tromsø sykehus, 1895–1974' (unpublished master's thesis,Tromsø, University of Tromsø, 2009).

Longmore, Surgeon-General T., *Gunshot Injuries* (London, Longmans Green, 1877).

Low-Beer, Daniel, Smallman-Raynor, Matthew and Cliff, Andrew, 'Disease and death in the South African War: Changing disease patterns from soldiers to refugees,' *Social History of Medicine* 17, 2 (2004), 223–45.

Luckes, Eva C. E., *Lectures on Nursing: Lectures on General Nursing, Delivered to the Probationers of the London Hospital Training School for Nurses*, 4th edn (London, Paul, Trench, 1892).

Luckes, Eva C. E., *General Nursing* (London, Taylor & Francis, 1898).

Luddy, Maria (ed.), *The Crimean Journals of the Sisters of Mercy* (Dublin, Four Courts Press, 2004).

Lynch, George, *Impressions of a War Correspondent* (London, Newnes Ltd, MCMIII), Chapter 1, no page number accessed via Project Gutenburg at archive.org/stream/impressionsofawa2166gut/pg21661.txt (22 December 2012).

McBryde, Brenda, *Quiet Heroines: Nurses of the Second World War* (London, Chatto & Windus, 1985).

McBryde, Brenda, *A Nurse's War* (Saffron Walden, Cakebread Publications, 1993).

McCalla, Douglas, 'The economic impact of the Great War', in David Mackenzie (ed.), *Canada and the First World War: Essays in Honour of Robert Craig Brown* (Toronto, University of Toronto Press, 2005).

MacDonald, Lynn, *The Roses of No Man's Land* (Toronto, Penguin Books of Canada, 1993 [1980]).

McDonald, Lynn, *Florence Nightingale: The Nightingale School* (Waterloo, Wilfrid Laurier University Press, 2009).

McDonald, Lynn, *Florence Nightingale: The Crimean War* (Ontario, Canada, Wilfred Laurier University Press, 2010).

McIntyre, Darryl, 'Australian Army Medical Services in Korea', in R. O'Neill (ed.), *Australia in the Korean War 1950–53: Vol. II Combat Operations* (The Australian War Memorial and the Australian Government Publishing Service, Canberra, 1985).

Mackenzie, David, 'Introduction: Myth, memory, and the transformation of Canadian Society', in David Mackenzie (ed.), *Canada and the First World War: Essays in Honour of Robert Craig Brown* (Toronto, University of Toronto Press, 2005).

McLatchey, K. O., 'No. 3 Canadian General Hospital', *Canadian Nurse* 18, 7 (July 1922), 414–18.

Macphail, Andrew, *The Medical Services: Official History of the Canadian Forces in the Great War, 1914–1919* (Ottawa, King's Printer, 1925).

McPherson, James, *Battle Cry of Freedom: The Civil War Era* (New York, Ballantine Book, 1988).

McTavish, Jan R., 'Antipyretic treatment and typhoid fever 1860–1900', *Journal History Medical Allied Science* 42, 4 (1987), 486–506.

Maggs, Christopher J., *The Origins of General Nursing* (London, Croom Helm, 1983).

Malkasian, Carter, *The Korean War 1950–1953* (Oxford, Osprey Publishing, 2001).

Mann, Susan, *Margaret Macdonald: Imperial Daughter* (Montreal, McGill-Queen's University Press, 2005).

Markham, J., *The Lamp was Dimmed: The Story of a Nurse's Training* (London, Robert Hale, 1975).

Marwick, Arthur, *Total War and Social Change* (Basingstoke, Palgrave Macmillan, 1988).

Matheson, Norman M., 'Accidental and surgical wounds', in H. Bailey (ed.), *Pye's Surgical Handicraft: A Manual of Surgical Manipulations, Minor Surgery, and other matters Connected with the Work of House Surgeons and of Surgical Dressers,* 11th edn (Bristol, John Wright and Sons Ltd, 1939).

Maxwell, William, *Lincoln's Fifth Wheel: The Political History of the United States Sanitary Commission* (New York, Longmans, Green & Co., 1956).

Medical Research Council War Wounds Committee and Committee of London Sector Pathologists, *The Prevention of 'Hospital Infection' of Wounds,* MRC War Memorandum No. 6 (London, His Majesty's Stationery Office, 1941).

Meehan, Therese Connell, 'Careful nursing: a model for contemporary nursing practice', *Journal of Advanced Nursing* 44, 1 (2003), 99–107.

Melby, Kari, *Kall og kamp – Norsk Sykepleierforbunds historie* (Oslo, J. W. Cappelens forlag AS, 1991).

Merson, E., 'Nursing in wartime', *International History of Nursing Journal* 3, 4 (1998), 43–6.

Mollison, P. L. (Captain RAMC), 'Observations of cases of starvation at Belsen', *British Medical Journal* (5 January 1946), 4–8.

Moore, Frank, *Women of the War* (Hartford, CT, S. S. Scranton & Co., 1866).

Moorehead, R, 'William Budd and typhoid fever', *Journal of the Royal Society of Medicine* 95 (2002), 561–4.

Mortimer, Barbara, *Sisters: Memories from the Courageous Nurses of World War Two* (London, Hutchinson, 2012).

Murphy, Molly, *Molly Murphy: Suffragette and Socialist* (Salford, Institute of Social Research, University of Salford, 1998).

Nash, Mary, *Defying Male Civilization: Women in the Spanish Civil War* (Denver, Arden Press, 1995).

Neushul, Peter, 'Fighting research: Army participation in the clinical testing and mass production of penicillin during the Second World War', in Roger Cooter, Mark Harrison and Steve Sturdy (eds), *War, Medicine and Modernity* (Stroud, Sutton Publishing 1999).

Nicholson, G. W. L., *Seventy Years of Service: A History of the Royal Canadian Army Medical Corps* (Ottawa, Borealis Press, 1977).

Nicol, Martha, *Ismeer or Smyrna and its British Hospital in 1855* (London, James Madden, 1856).

Nightingale, Florence, *Subsidiary Notes as to the introduction of female nursing into Military Hospitals in Peace and in War. Presented to the Secretary of State for War (Thoughts submitted as to an eventual Nurses' Provident Fund)* (London, Harrison & Sons, 1858).

Nightingale, Florence, *Notes on Hospitals,* 3rd edn (London, Longman, Green, Longman, Roberts, and Green, 1863).

Nightingale, Florence, *Notes on Nursing: What It Is and What It Is Not,* Introductions by Dunbar and Dolan (New York, Dover Publications, Inc., 1969).

Nightingale, Florence, *Notes on Nursing* (London, Churchill Livingstone, 1980[1859]).

Nightingale, Florence, *Notes on the Health of the British Army*, in Lynn McDonald (ed.), *Florence Nightingale: The Crimean War* (Waterloo, ON, Wilfrid Laurier Press, 2010).

Nilssen, Ragnar, W., *Med Røde kors i Korea* (Stavanger, Misjonsselskapets forlag, 1952).

Nochlin, Linda, *Women, Art, and Power and Other Essays* (London, Thames & Hudson Ltd, 1989).

Nolan, Peter, *A History of Mental Health Nursing* (London, Chapman & Hall, 1993).

Norman, Elizabeth, *Women at War: The Story of Fifty Military Nurses Who Served in Vietnam* (Philadelphia, University of Pennsylvania Press, 1991).

Odgers, George, *Remembering Korea: Australians in the War of 1950–1953* (Lansdowne Publishing Pty Ltd, 2000).

Ouditt, Sharon, *Fighting Forces, Writing Women: Identity and Ideology in the First World War* (New York, Routledge, 1994).

Øverland, Per, *Koreasoldat 1953* (Trondheim, forlag 90936, 2009).

Pakenham, Thomas, *The Boer War* (London, Time Warner, 1992).

Palfreeman, Linda, ¡*Salud! British Volunteers in the Republican Medical Service during the Spanish Civil War, 1936–1939* (Brighton, Sussex Academic Press, 2012).

Palmer, Debbie, *Who Cared for the Carers? A History of Nurses' Occupational Health, 1880–1948* (Manchester, Manchester University Press, 2014).

Paus, Bernhard, 'Kirurgiske erfaringer fra Det norske feltsykehuset i Korea', *Nordisk Medicin* 11, 51 (1954), 374–88.

Paus, Bernhard, 'Medisinsk liv ved den koreanske krigsskueplass', *Tidsskrift for Den Norsk Lægeforening* (January, 1954), 10–15.

Paus, Bernhard, *Rapport fra Det norske feltsykehus i Korea* (Oslo, Forsvarets sanitet, 1955).

Pearce, Evelyn, *Medical and Nursing Dictionary*, 6th edn (London, Faber & Faber Ltd, 1933), 574.

Pedersen, Lorentz Ulrik, *Norge i Korea. Norsk innsats under Koreakrigen og senere* (Oslo, C. Huitfeldt forlag AS, 1991).

Pelling, Margaret, 'The meaning of contagion: Reproduction, medicine and metaphor', in Alison Bashford and Claire Hooker (eds), *Contagion: Historical and Cultural Studies* (London, Routledge, 2001), 15–38.

Pember, Phoebe Yates, 'Reminiscences of a southern hospital: By its Matron', *The Cosmopolite* 1, 1 (January 1866).

Pember, Phoebe Yates, *A Southern Woman's Story*, ed. George C. Rable (Columbia, SC, University of South Carolina Press, 2002).

Pennington, Hugh, 'Don't pick your nose', *London Review of Books* 27, 24 (13 December 2005), 29–31.

Pfeiffer, Carl J., *The Art and Practice of Western Medicine in the First Half of the Nineteenth Century* (London, McFarland, 1985).

Pickles, Katie, *Female Imperialism and National Identity: Imperial Order Daughters of the Empire* (Manchester, Manchester University Press, 2002).

Piggott, Juliet, *Queen Alexandra's Royal Army Nursing Corps* (London, Leo Cooper Ltd, 1975).

Powell, Margaret, 'Nurses there work in wards lit by cigarette lighters', *Daily Worker* 7 (January 1938).

Pratt, R., 'Nursing at Lemnos – August–December, 1915', *Reveille* 6, 12 (1 August 1933), 42.

Preston, Paul, *Doves of War: Four Women of Spain* (London, HarperCollins, 2002).

Preston, Paul, 'Two doctors and one cause: Len Crome and Reginald Saxton in the International Brigades', *International Journal of Iberian Studies* 19, 1 (2006), 5–24.

Prime, Peter, *The History of the Medical and Hospital Service of the Anglo-Boer War 1899 to 1902* (Anglo-Boer War Philatelic Society, 1998).

Prochaska, F., *Women and Philanthropy in Nineteenth Century England* (Oxford, Faber, 1980).

Pugh, W. T. Gordon, *Practical Nursing including Hygiene and Dietetics*, 13th edn (Edinburgh, William Blackwood and Sons, 1940).

Quiney, Linda J., 'Assistant angels: Canadian voluntary aid detachment nurses in the Great War', *Canadian Bulletin of Medical History* 15, 1 (1998), 189–206.

Quiney, Linda J., '"Sharing the halo": Social and professional tensions in the work of World War I, Canadian volunteer nurses', *Journal of the Canadian Historical Association* 8 (1998), 105–24.

Rable, George, *Civil Wars: Women and the Crisis of Southern Nationalism* (Urbana, IL, University of Illinois, 1989).

Rafferty, Anne Marie, *The Politics of Nursing Knowledge* (London, Routledge, 1996).

Randby, David, 'Fra en elektrikers dagbok', in Bakke Finn (ed.), *NORMASH: Korea i våre hjerter* (Oslo, Norwegian Korean War Veteran's Association, 2010), 34–6.

Red Cross & St John, *The Official Record of the Humanitarian Services of the War Organisation of the British Red Cross Society and Order of St. John of Jerusalem, 1939–1947* (London, British Red Cross and St John, 1949), 506–8.

Reid, Richard, *Just Wanted to be There: Australian Service Nurses 1899–1999* (Commonwealth Department of Veterans' Affairs, Canberra, 1999).

Reilly, Jo, Cesarani, David, Kushner, Tony and Richmond, Colin (eds) *Belsen in History and Memry* (London, Frank Cass, 1997).

Reverby, Susan, *Ordered to Care: The Dilemma of American Nursing, 1850–1945* (New York and Cambridge, Cambridge University Press, 1987).

Reznick, Jeffrey S, *Healing the Nation: Soldiers and the Culture of Caregiving in Britain during the Great War* (Manchester and New York, Manchester University Press, 2004).

Riddell, Margaret S., *First Year Nursing Manual* 5th edn (London, Faber & Faber Ltd, 1939).

Risse, Guenter B., *Hospital Life in Enlightenment Scotland* (Cambridge, Cambridge University Press, 1986).

Roberts, Hilda and Potter, Petronella, 'Belsen camp', *British Medical Journal* (21 July 1945), 100.

Roberts, M. J. D., *Making English Morals* (Cambridge, Cambridge University Press, 2004).

Rosenberg, Charles, 'The therapeutic revolution', in Morris J. Vogel and Charles E. Rosenberg, *The Therapeutic Revolution* (Philadelphia, University of Pennsylvania Press, 1979).

Rosenberg, Charles E., *The Care of Strangers* (Philadelphia, University of Pennsylvania Press, 1983).

Rosenberg, Charles, *The Care of Strangers: The Rise of America's Hospital System* (New York, Basic Books, Inc., Publishers, 1987).

Rosensaft, Josef, 'Our Belsen', in *Belsen* (no editors acknowledged) (Tel Aviv, Israel, Irgun Sheerit Hapleita Me'haezor Habriti, 1957).

Ryle, John A. and Elliott, S. D., *Septicaemia and Bacteriaemia*, in Humphrey Rolleston (ed.), *The British Encyclopaedia of Medical Practice*, vol. 11 (London, Butterworth and Co., 1939).

Sandvik, Olav, *Skjebnespill – Fra Kvinnherad til vetrinærvesents innside* (Oslo, Norsk Vetrinærhistorisk Selskap, 2012).

Sarnecky, Mary T., *A History of the U.S Army Nurse Corp* (USA, University of Pennsylvania Press, 1999), 36.

Sarnecky, Mary, T, 'Army nurses in "The forgotten war"', *American Journal of Nursing* (November 2001), 45–9.

Saxton, R. S., 'The Madrid Transfusion Institute', *The Lancet* (4 September 1937).

Saxton, R. S., 'Medicine in Republican Spain', *The Lancet* (24 September 1938).

Schie, Ola, 'Korea i september', in L. U. Pedersen (ed.), *Norge i Korea*. (Oslo, C. Huitfeldt forlag AS, 1991; first published in Aftenposten, 20 October, 1951).

Schmitz, Christopher, '"We too were soldiers": The experiences of British nurses in the Anglo-Boer War, 1899–1902', in Gerard J. DeGroot, and Corinna Peniston-Bird (eds), *A Soldier and a Woman: Sexual Integration in the Military* (Essex, Pearson Education Ltd, 2000), 49–65.

Schultz, Bartz, *A Tapestry of Service – The Evolution of Nursing in Australia*, vol. I *Foundation to Federation 1788–1900* (Melbourne, Churchill Livingstone, 1991).

Schultz, Jane, *Women at the Front: Hospital Workers in Civil War America* (Chapel Hill, NC, The University of North Carolina Press, 2004).

Schultz, Jane, 'Nurse as icon: Florence Nightingale's impact on women in the American Civil War', in Simon Lewis and David T. Gleeson, *Civil War – Global Conflict* (Columbia, University of South Carolina Press, 2014).

Schweikardt, Christoph, '"You gained honor for your profession as a brown nurse": The career of a National Socialist Nurse mirrored by her letters home', *Nursing History Review* 12 (2004), 121–38.

Schweikardt, Christoph, 'The National Socialist sisterhood: an instrument of National Socialist health policy', *Nursing Inquiry*, 16, 2 (2009), 103–10.

Scott, Douglas H., *The New People's Physician: A Compendium of Practical Information on Persona Health and Domestic Hygiene*, Vol. 2 (London, Waverley Book Company, undated *c*.1940).

Scott-Ellis, Priscilla, ed. Raymond Carr, *The Chances of Death: A Diary of the Spanish Civil War* (Norwich, Michael Russell, 1995).

Searle, Charlotte, *The History of the Development of Nursing in South Africa 1652–1960: A Socio-historical Survey* (South Africa, Struik, 1965).

Sears, Stephen W., *Gettysburg* (New York, Houghton Mifflin Company, 2004).

Sears, W. Gordon, *Medicine for Nurses* (London, Edward Arnold, 1940).

Sears, W. Gordon, *Medicine for Nurses* (London, Edward Arnold & Co., 1944).

Semb, Carl, 'Fra sanitetstjenesten i Korea', in L. U. Pedersen (ed.), *Norge i Korea.* (Oslo, C. Huitfeldt forlag AS, 1991).

Shephard, Ben, *After Daybreak: The Liberation of Belsen, 1945* (London, Random House, 2006).

Shephard, Ben, 'The medical relief effort at Belsen', *Holocaust Studies: A Journal of Culture and History* 12, 1–2 (2006), 31–50.

Shepherd, John, *The Crimean Doctors*, 2 vols (Liverpool, Liverpool University Press, 1991).

Sington, Derrick, *Belsen Uncovered* (London, Duckworth, 1945).

Sister, Casualty, 'A reformation', *St. Bartholomew's League News* (May 1902).

Sister X, *The Tragedy and Comedy of War Hospitals* (New York, E. P. Dutton, 1906).

Smith, F. B., *Florence Nightingale: Reputation and Power* (Beckenham, Kent, Croom Helm, 1982).

Smith, Russell G., *In Pursuit of Nursing Excellence: A History of the Royal College of Nursing, Australia 1949–1999* (Oxford University Press, South Melbourne, 1999).

Smith, Sarah A., 'Nurse Competence: A Concept Analysis', *International Journal of Nursing Knowledge* 23, 3 (2012), 172–82.

Sondhaus, Laurence, *World War One: The Global Revolution* (Cambridge, Cambridge University Press, 2011).

South, John Flint, *Facts Relating to Hospital Nurses* (London, Richardson Brothers, 1857).

Stanley, Peter, *For Fear of Pain: British Surgery 1790–1850* (New York, Rudopi, 2003).

Select bibliography

Starns, Penny, *March of the Matrons: Military Influence on the Civilian Nursing Profession, 1939–1969* (Peterborough, DSM, 2000).

Starns, Penny, *Nurses at War: Women on the Frontline, 1939–45* (Stroud, Sutton Publishing, 2000).

Steinert, Johannes-Dieter, 'The British teams in Belsen concentration camp: Emergency relief and the perception of survivors', *Holocaust Studies: A Journal of Culture and History* 12, 1–2 (2006), 62–78.

Stewart, A. P., 'Typhoid fever', *British Medical Journal* (15 November 1879), 795.

Stimson, Julia, *Finding Themselves. The Letters of an American Army Chief Nurse at a British Hospital in France* (New York, The Macmillan Company, 1927).

Strømskag, Kjell, E, *Et fag på søyler – Anestesiens historie i Norge* (Oslo, Tano Aschehoug, 1999).

Summers, Anne, *Angels and Citizens: British Women as Military Nurses 1854–1914* (New York, Routledge & Kegan Paul, 1988).

Tate, Trudi, *Modernism, History and the First World War* (Manchester, Manchester University Press, 1998).

Taylor, Eric, *Front-Line Nurse: British Nurses in World War II* (London, Robert Hale, 1997).

Taylor, Eric, *Combat Nurse* (London, Robert Hale, 1999).

Taylor, Eric, *Wartime Nurse: 100 Years from the Crimea to Korea 1854–1954* (London, Robert Hale, 2001).

Taylor, Fanny, *Eastern Hospitals and English Nurses*, 2 vols (London, Hurst & Blackett, 1856).

Terrot, S., *Reminiscences of Scutari Hospitals in Winter 1854–55* (Edinburgh, Andrew Stevenson, 1898).

Thompson, Paul, *The Voice of the Past*, 3rd edn (Oxford, Oxford University Press, 2000).

Toman, Cynthia, '"Ready, aye ready:" Canadian military nurses as an expandable workforce, 1920–2000', in Dianne Dodd, Tina Bates and Nicole Rousseau (eds), *On all Frontiers: Four Centuries of Canadian Nursing* (Ottawa, University of Ottawa Press and Canadian Museum of Civilization, 2005).

Toman, Cynthia, *An Officer and a Lady: Canadian Military Nursing and the Second World War* (Vancouver, University of British Columbia Press, 2007).

Toman, Cynthia, 'Frontlines and frontiers: War as legitimate work for nurses, 1939–1945', *Histoire sociale/Social History* 40, 79 (May 2007), 45–75.

Toman, Cynthia, '"A loyal body of Empire citizens": Military nurses and identity at Lemnos and Salonika, 1915–1917', in Jayne Elliott, Meryn Stuart and Cynthia Toman (eds) *Place and Practice in Canadian Nursing History* (Vancouver, University of British Columbia Press, 2008).

Toman, Cynthia, '"Help us, serve England": First World War military nursing and national identities', *Canadian Bulletin of Medical History* 30, 1 (2013), 156–7.

Tooley, Sarah Southall, *The Life of Florence Nightingale* (New York, Cassell and Company, Ltd, 1914).

Treider, Tor, 'Fra Vinterkrigen til Korea', in H. Bull-Hansen (ed.), *I krig for fred* (Oslo, Kagge forlag AS, 2008), 41–63.

Treves, Frederick, *The Tale of a Field Hospital* (London, Cassell & Co., 1900).

Tyrer, Nicola, *Sisters in Arms: British Army Nurses Tell Their Story* (London, Weidenfield & Nicolson, 2008).

Trueta, Joseph, *Surgeon in War and Peace* (London, Gollancz, 1980).

Valls, Roser (Coordinator), *Infermeres catalanes a la Guerra Civil espanyola* (Barcelona: University of Barcelona, 2008).

Veitch, Zephirina P., *Handbook for Nurses for the Sick* (London, no publisher, 1870).

Waterhouse, Herbert F. W., Harmer, Douglas and. Marshall, Charles J., 'Notes from the Anglo-Russian Hospitals', *British Medical Journal* 2, 2962 (6 October 1917), 441–5.

Watson, J. K., *A Handbook for Nurses* (London, Scientific Press, 1899).

Watson, Janet S. K., 'Khaki girls, VADs, and Tommy's sister: Gender and class in First World War Britain', *The International History Review* 19, 1 (February 1997), 32–50.

Watson, Janet S. K., 'Wars in the wards: The social construction of medical work in First World War Britain', *Journal of British Studies* 41, 4 (October 2002), 484–510.

Watson, Janet S. K., *Fighting Different Wars: Experience, Memory, and the First World War in Britain* (Cambridge, Cambridge University Press, 2007).

Waul, T. N., 'Special report of the committee appointed to examine into quartermaster's, commissary & medical departments, 29 January 1862, US War Department', *War of the Rebellion: A Compilation of the Official Records of the Union and Confederate Armies* (Washington, DC, Government Printing Office, 1880–91).

White, W. Hale, 'The treatment of chlorine gas poisoning by venesection', *The British Medical Journal* 2 (29 July 1916), 159.

Wiener, Martin, *Reconstructing the Criminal* (Cambridge, Cambridge University Press, 1990).

Wilks, Janet, *Carbolic and Leeches* (Ilfracombe, Hyperion Books, 1991).

Williams, Colin, Alexander, Bill and Gorman, John, *Memorials of the Spanish Civil War* (Stroud, Alan Sutton Publishing, 1996).

Williams, Dick (Major) 'The first day in the camp', *Holocaust Studies: A Journal of Culture and History* 12, 1–2 (2006), 27–30.

Wilson, Graham, '"Everything on its belly" – Feeding the first AIF problems and solutions of Australian Army rationing and catering in the First World War (1)', *Sabretache* 41, 3 (1 September 2000), 9–39.

Select bibliography

Wood, Joyce, 'The revolution outside her window: New light shed on the March 1917 Russian Revolution from the papers of VAD nurse Dorothy N. Seymour', *Proceedings of the South Carolina Historical Association* (2005), 71–86.

Woodward, Joan and Mitchell, Glenys, *A Nurse at War: Emily Peter 1858–1927* (New Zealand, Te Waihora Press, 2008).

Woollacott, Angela, *On Her Their Lives Depend: Munitions Workers in the Great War* (California, University of California Press, 1994).

Wootton, David, *Bad Medicine: Doctors Doing Harm Since Hippocrates* (Oxford, Oxford University Press, 2007).

Worboys, Michael, *Spreading Germs: Disease Theories and Medical Practice in Britain, 1865–1900* (Cambridge, Cambridge University Press, 2006).

Wüller, Rønnaug, 'Brev fra Korea-søstrene', *Sykepleien – Organ for norsk sykepleier-forbund* (1951), 204–7.

Wüller, Rønnaug, 'Med norsk feltsykehus til Korea', *Sykepleien – Organ for Norsk Sykepleierforbund* (1952), 126–32.

Young, Margaret (ed.), *We Are Here, Too* (Adelaide, Australian Down Syndrome Association Incorporated, 1991).

Yow, Valerie R., *Recording Oral History: A Practical Guide for Social Scientists* (Thousand Oaks, Sage Publications, 1994).

Zepeda Iturrieta, Juan Roberto and Molino, Jordi Pérez, 'L'Hospital de Sang de Valls', *Quaderns de Vilaniu 51* (Valls: Institut d'Estudis Vallencs, May 2007).

Index